2009 01 21 **and**

reconciliation

D1569798

International Perspectives in Philosophy and Psychiatry

Series editors

Bill (K.W.M.) Fulford
Katherine Morris
John Z Sadler
Giovanni Stanghellini

Volumes in the series:

Mind, Meaning, and Mental Disorder
Bolton and Hill

Nature and Narrative: An Introduction to the New Philosophy of Psychiatry
Fulford, Morris, Sadler, and Stanghellini

The Philosophy of Psychiatry: A Companion
Radden

Disembodied Spirits and Deanimated Bodies: The Psychopathology of Common Sense
Stanghellini

Values and Psychiatric Diagnosis
Sadler

Postpsychiatry
Bracken and Thomas

The Metaphor of Mental Illness
Pickering

The Oxford Textbook of Philosophy and Psychiatry
Fulford, Thornton, and Graham

Dementia: Mind, Meaning, and the Person
Hughes, Louw, and Sabat

Forthcoming volumes in the series:

Reconceiving Schizophrenia
Chung, Fulford, and Graham (ed.)

Body–Subjects and Disordered Minds
Matthews

Empirical Ethics in Psychiatry
Widdershoven et. al

Trauma, truth and reconciliation
Healing damaged relationships

Edited by

Nancy Nyquist Potter
Associate Professor
Department of Philosophy
University of Louisville
USA

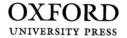

OXFORD
UNIVERSITY PRESS

OXFORD
UNIVERSITY PRESS

Great Clarendon Street, Oxford OX2 6DP

Oxford University Press is a department of the University of Oxford.
It furthers the University's objective of excellence in research, scholarship,
and education by publishing worldwide in

Oxford New York

Auckland Cape Town Dar es Salaam Hong Kong Karachi
Kuala Lumpur Madrid Melbourne Mexico City Nairobi
New Delhi Shanghai Taipei Toronto

With offices in

Argentina Austria Brazil Chile Czech Republic France Greece
Guatemala Hungary Italy Japan Poland Portugal Singapore
South Korea Switzerland Thailand Turkey Ukraine Vietnam

Oxford is a registered trade mark of Oxford University Press
in the UK and in certain other countries

Published in the United States
by Oxford University Press Inc., New York

© Oxford University Press, 2006

The moral rights of the authors have been asserted
Database right Oxford University Press (maker)

First published 2006

British Library Cataloguing in Publication Data

Data available

Library of Congress Cataloging in Publication Data

Trauma, truth, and reconciliation: healing damaged relationships / edited by Nancy Nyquist Potter.
Includes bibliographical references and index.
    ISBN-13: 978–0–19–856943–5 (Paperback)
    ISBN-10: 0–19–856943–2 (Paperback)
    ISBN-13: 978–0–19–856942–8 (Hardback)
    ISBN-10: 0–19–856942–4 (Hardback)
    1. Conflict management. 2. Reconciliation. 3. Forgiveness. 4. Truth commissions. 5. Social
conflict—Psychological aspects. 6. Interpersonal conflict. 7. Psychic trauma. 8. Psychotherapy.
I. Potter, Nancy Nyquist, 1954– . HM1126.T75 2006 303.6'9—dc22 2006014407

Typeset by Newgen Imaging Systems (P) Ltd., Chennai, India
Printed in Great Britain
on acid-free paper by
Biddles Ltd., King's Lynn

ISBN 13: 978–0–19–856942–8 (Hbk.)   ISBN 10: 0–19–856942–4 (Hbk.)
ISBN 13: 978–0–19–856943–5 (Pbk.)   ISBN 10: 0–19–856943–2 (Pbk.)

10 9 8 7 6 5 4 3 2 1

Acknowledgements

I am grateful to members of the Association for the Advancement of Philosophy and Psychiatry, for their enthusiasm in interdisciplinary work and for the forum in which scholars can share research interests; to Linda Muncy, for her organizational abilities for AAPP; and to Kathleen Nagle, who served as my research assistant and has been a delight to work with. Blessings and good will are well-deserved by John Sadler, who is endlessly patient with my endless questions.

Contents

About the contributors

David Brendel, M.D., Ph.D. is Assistant Professor of Psychiatry at Harvard Medical School, Deputy Editor of the Harvard Review of Psychiatry, and Associate Director of the Psychiatry Residency Program at Massachusetts General and McLean Hospitals. He is the author of *Healing Psychiatry: Bridging the Science/Humanism Divide* (MIT Press, 2006).

Gerrit Glas, M.D., Ph.D. is teaching philosophy at the University of Leiden, The Netherlands (special chair in Christian Philosophy). He is also director of a residency training program for psychiatry in Zwolse Poort (Zwolle, NL). He has written extensively on anxiety and anxiety disorders, ethics and professional identity, and other topics in the field of psychiatry and philosophy and psychiatry and religion. He is chairman of both the Section for Psychiatry and Philosophy of the Dutch Association for Psychiatry and of the (Dutch) Foundation for Psychiatry and Religion.

Christa Krüger, M.D. is Associate Professor in the Department of Psychiatry, University of Pretoria, South Africa, and Senior Psychiatrist at Weskoppies Hospital, Pretoria. Her doctoral research was conducted at the University of Warwick, UK. Her research interests include psychosocial, neurophysiological, and religious aspects of dissociation, as well as medical education. Dr Krüger also is currently working toward a master's degree in systematic theology at the University of South Africa.

Sharon Lamb, Ed.D. is Professor of Psychology at Saint Michael's College in Colchester Vermont. She is also a licensed psychologist who practices in Shelburne Vermont. She has written extensively on victimization, publishing *The Trouble with Blame: Victims Perpetrators and Responsibility* with Harvard University Press in 1996 and editing *New Versions of Victims* in 1999 with NYU Press. In 2002 she co-edited with philosopher Jeffrie Murphy the Oxford University Press book, *Before Forgiving*. More recently she has written for therapists on the subject of talking about sex in therapy with children and adolescents. And she has written for the general public on girls' sexual development and the sexualization of girls by the media.

Lewis Mehl-Madrona, M.D., Ph.D. received his M.D. degree from Stanford University and his PhD in clinical psychology from the Psychological Studies Institute of Palo Alto, California. He completed residencies in family medicine and in psychiatry at the University of Vermont College of

Medicine. He is the author of the *Coyote Trilogy*, three books about the contributions that aboriginal culture and philosophy can make to modern medicine and psychology (*Coyote Medicine, Coyote Healing,* and *Coyote Wisdom*). His next book (in preparation) is *Narrative Medicine*. He is currently Associate Professor of Family Medicine (and Psychiatry) at the University of Saskatchewan College of Medicine, in Saskatoon, Canada. His research is on community development using local aboriginal healing knowledge and practices for medical and psychiatric conditions.

Alison Mitchell is a Visiting Scholar at Florida Atlantic University, after spending a post-doc at Warwick University pursuing research in the philosophy of mind, language, and literature. Her doctoral dissertation, *Learning from Literature*, explored the shifts of perspective that take place in our imaginative experience of fictional literature. She is interested in the application of formal philosophical methods and results to practical domains.

Colleen Murphy, Ph.D. is an Assistant Professor of Philosophy at Texas A&M University. Her primary research interest is on the morality of political reconciliation, the process of building healthier political relationships within societies emerging from civil conflict or repressive rule. She has traveled to India, Israel and the Palestinian Territories, Northern Ireland, and South Africa to interview academics, politicians, and human rights workers working for reconciliation.

Christian Perring, Ph.D. is an Associate Professor of Philosophy at Dowling College, New York. He has published in medical ethics and the philosophy of psychiatry. He is editor of *Metapsychology Online Review*.

Nancy Nyquist Potter, Ph.D. is Associate Professor of Philosophy at the University of Louisville. Her publications range from topics such as what role humor plays in defusing conflict, to analyzing the victim empathy portion of a sex offender treatment program in a state prison, to understanding self-injurious behavior. Potter is author of *How Can I be Trusted? A Virtue Theory of Trustworthiness* (Rowman-Littlefield, 2002) and editor of the anthology *Putting Peace into Practice: Evaluating Policy on Local and Global Levels* (Rodopi Press 2004). Her current research project is on Borderline Personality Disorder. She is Vice-president of the Association for the Advancement of Philosophy and Psychiatry and Associate Editor of *Philosophy, Psychiatry, and Psychology*.

Mary C. Rawlinson, Ph.D. is Associate Professor of Philosophy and Comparative Literature at Stony Brook University in New York. She is the co-editor of *The voice of Breast Cancer in Medicine and Bioethics* (Kluwer, 2006), and of *Derrida and Feminism* (Routledge, 1997), as well as the editor of five issues of the *Journal of Medicine and Philosophy*, including *Foucault and the Philosophy of Medicine, The Future of Psychiatry*, and *Feminist Bioethics*. Her publications include articles on Proust, literature and ethics, Hegel, and French feminism. She is currently completing a book on agency that explores detective fiction as a genre of moral philosophy.

Deborah Spitz, M.D. is Associate Professor of Psychiatry at the University of Chicago. She is Past President of the Association for Academic Psychiatry, and has been active on the Scientific Program Committee, the Committee on Women and the Committee on Domestic Violence of the American Psychiatric Association. She is interested in issues of autonomy and self-concept in persons with severe psychiatric disorders, the treatment of refractory affective disorders, and psychiatric education.

Piet Verhagen, M.D. is a psychiatrist and theologian in the Netherlands. He also serves as secretary of the Dutch Foundation for Psychiatry and Religion, and secretary of the World Psychiatric Association (WPA) Section on Religion, Spirituality and Psychiatry.

Peter Zachar, Ph.D. is the chairperson of the psychology department at Auburn University Montgomery. He is a licensed psychologist with scholarly interests in the philosophy of psychiatry and the philosophy of science. He is the author of *Psychological Concepts and Biological Psychiatry: A Philosophical Analysis* (John Benjamins, 2000).

Introduction

Nancy Nyquist Potter

> The psychologists forgive everybody, he [Judge Daniel
> Savage] remembered a colleague saying after one trial,
> because the most important gesture in the modern
> world is to show understanding.
> *Tim Parks*

As gestures go in the modern world, showing forgiveness and understanding
are only one kind, and many of those gestures are private and personal. As
seemingly widespread as the forgiveness turn appears to be in psychotherapy
and politics, it is continually contradicted by declarations of war and revenge.
At the time of this writing, the United States had seen its 2000th American
soldier killed in Iraq, a war inspired by the Al Qaeda bombing of the World
Trade Center on September 11, 2001. No words of forgiveness were urged on
the American people by the Bush Administration at that time; instead, the
pledge of triumph over evil and terrorism shaped American foreign policy
and American military fervor. Forgiveness, it seems, is good for others to do. It
is an open question what psychological toll a passion for justice or oil might
take on people, but one thing is clear: tens of thousands of American and Iraqi
lives have been lost. Forgiveness, reconciliation, and justice are moral terms,
but they have deep psychological implications for the people who embody
those terms. What are those implications, and when should we pursue one
direction rather than another?

This unique collection of essays focuses on intersections between mental
illness and mechanisms for reconciliation and healing from conflict and past
wrongs. Since the trials for human rights violations in Argentina, Brazil, and
Chile in the 1980s, there has been an increase in truth and reconciliation
commissions as a way for people to heal from large-scale wrongdoings that
have lasting damaging psychological effects (Weschler, 1990; Botman and
Peterson, 1990; Nino, 1996). Furthermore, concepts of truth and reconciliation not only have been adopted as means to heal societies that are socially
and politically divided, but they continue to be important concepts in individual psychotherapy (Lamb and Murphy, 2002). Forgiveness therapy, for

example, aims to promote patients' healing from traumatic experiences and the effects of wrongdoing by encouraging those wronged to forgive their wrongdoers and the wrongdoers to seek forgiveness from those they wronged. The assumption in both domains seems to be that sociopolitical and interpersonal suffering and distress caused by trauma, conflict, terror, shame, and displacement can be partly ameliorated by incorporating moral values such as forgiveness, reconciliation, and restorative justice into therapeutic and extra-legal practices such as truth and reconciliation commissions. These assumptions are explored in this anthology, as well as epistemological and metaphysical assumptions that underlie truth commissions, as Alison Mitchell analyzes in this volume.

Restorative justice, forgiveness, and reconciliation have begun, in some domains, to replace more traditional, hard-line approaches to the types of wrongdoing that are especially psychologically damaging. In particular, retributive justice is viewed by many as a morally inferior approach (international relations being the exception.) Peter Zachar, Mary Rawlinson, and Lewis Mehl-Madrona, in this volume, each argue against retributive justice. Yet some people still want to see wrongdoers punished legally and claim to find relief from hatred and rage against their wrongdoers when they see justice meted out. There is even a school of thought that argues that people who commit moral and legal wrongs feel better when punished; the idea is that retributive justice affirms the value of the wrongdoer by treating her as a moral agent worthy of respect and allows the wrongdoer to re-establish self-respect.

Given the increase in violence in our private and public lives, the shift away from revenge and resentment toward more peaceable ways of addressing wrongdoing seems laudable (cf. Fellman, 1998). However, clinical research as to the psychological benefits of these approaches is seriously impoverished, and it is difficult to assess the merits of 'the forgiveness turn' in the absence of rigorous philosophical investigation. This collection begins to correct for this neglect by examining underlying values and assumptions, clinical practices, and research relevant to experiences of trauma and the possibility of healing.

What goes terribly wrong in our lives such that genocide, interventionist wars, legalized racism, and interpersonal violence are ubiquitous and even increasing? One suggestion, advanced by Colleen Murphy, is that these practices are the result of a breakdown of the rule of law. If Murphy is right, then a solution would seem to be found in law as well. But law, too, has its limits, as several of the authors in this book suggest. Laws tell people what is expected of them and what to expect as punishment if they fail to follow the laws of the land, but laws cannot make us into moral beings; laws can punish, but they frequently are a poor substitute for the needs of humans' complex moral psychology. And some of the wrongdoings we inflict on one another do not come under the purview of the law, yet we need ways to address these wrongs in relation to one another if we want to restore ourselves to each other and to avoid inflicting further injury or harm.

Many thinkers locate the value of forgiveness in its healing and restorative capacities—its ability to foster harmony among friends, lovers, kin, and citizens (Shriver, 1995). Truth commissions, like the one in South Africa, are based on this reasoning. The need for harmony is especially salient in nation-states like South Africa whose aim is to become a unified nation after decades of subjugation, divisiveness, and violence. Many local and world leaders believe that not to forgive those who committed human rights violations would allow the history of trauma, deep distrust, anguish, rage, and fear to dominate the political domain in ways that could perpetuate those divisions rather than minimize them, thus undermining the move toward democratization and flourishing. In this volume, authors Piet Verhagen, Gerrit Glas, and Mary Rawlinson argue for the importance of forgiveness and reconciliation, while Sharon Lamb and Deborah Spitz delineate the limits of achieving harmony in an existent world of interlocking oppressions.

Yet it is clear that to be able to forgive is, in general, important to our moral, social, and political lives. Resentment diminishes the quality of our relationships and can fuel violence; overcoming resentment can heal and restore. Having a disposition to hold on to resentments, embitterments, vengeance, and rage is part of the orientation that fuels wars, domestic violence, familial vendettas, and other acts of violence.

Forgiveness is also good in that resentment can be an uncomfortable feeling—whether it is 'naturally' so or because we have been taught that it is undesirable—and so forgiveness is often the preferred response to moral injury. Not only can forgiveness heal divisions; it also means that the victims of wrongdoing no longer have to endure that uncomfortable state. Holding on to hatred, rage, guilt, or shame can exacerbate mental illness or psychological distress (Gilligan, 1996). Being forgiving, then, would seem to cultivate healthier relations both interpersonally and within oneself.

Perpetrators, of course, also benefit from forgiveness. What the wrongdoer wishes, and what a wronged party can grant in the expression of forgiveness, is an affirmation that the wrongdoer did indeed commit these acts but that she is more than the sum total of her wrong acts (cf. Landman, 2002). To grant forgiveness is to say that the wrongdoer is forgivable—that she transcends her acts and her past and is not identical with them. As Afrikaner Constand Viljoen says, 'We must be allowed to make for ourselves an honorable role in the new dispensation. The Afrikaner feels disempowered, unsafe, his language is threatened, his educational structures are in pieces—in short, the Afrikaner feels flooded by the majority and he has nowhere to turn.' (Krog, 2000, p. 166).

This point emphasizes an important counterpart to healing as a victim/ survivor of trauma, and that is the possibility of healing as the wrongdoer. Even in such grotesque circumstances as coming face-to-face with Eugene de Kock, a notorious professional killer during apartheid South Africa, one clinical psychologist argues in favor of finding the human being behind the evildoer's actions and coming to forgive him (Gobodo-Madikizela, 2003). Her forgiveness redeems de Kock and restores him to humanity.

But one concern about the current therapeutic push for forgiveness and reconciliation is that the demand for forgiveness often overly burdens the victims of wrongdoing and mistakenly glosses over *other* requirements neces- sary for members of the full community to continue living together in a just society (cf. Potter, 2001). The demand for forgiveness can become a silencing tool in the name of peaceable living that, in turn, can contribute to even more psychological damage. Lamb, in this volume, raises questions about the ways in which women, but not men, are expected to forgive gendered wrongs against them and argues that truth about the violence and betrayal that women experience in their lives is suppressed in the name of forgiveness.

Just as women may be overly burdened by exhortations to forgive and forget, women may be held up as the paradigm of peaceful values compared with the war-making revengeful attitudes of men throughout the millennia. Nel Noddings (1984), for example, advocates a particularly feminine approach to care and love that is uniquely female, and Sara Ruddick (1989) suggests that maternal tasks and thinking lend themselves to more peaceful endeavors in child-raising and beyond. On such accounts, women are better sources for peacefulness than are men. A quick review of history would seem to support such a view.

But a gendered understanding of men-as-aggressive and women-as- peaceable is, I suggest, too simple. Women of all colors who are mothers or caregivers are the more likely perpetrators of child abuse—three-fifths of all cases of child maltreatment are perpetrated by women (US Department of Health and Human Services, 1998). Even though this figure includes neglect, and fathers are almost never charged with neglect, it undermines claims of 'naturally' peaceful and loving women. While Paula Caplan (1990) argues that our society is prone to mother-blaming and that we must understand the cultural context in which mothering occurs (extraordinary demands, low expectations for fathers as parents, the oppression of women in every arena of their lives), she holds views in tension with Alice Miller (1990), who argues that a failure to hold women responsible for their abuse of children does them no favor at all and simply perpetuates violence and a misguided view of women.

Furthermore, as Claudia Card argues, women are encouraged to remain in relationships where the attachments are unhealthy and even dangerous—all in the name of keeping the peace (Card, 1990). Women abuse women. And women are silent when girls and other women are being harmed. Women should not be valorized or romanticized. Processes of socialization, cultural contexts in which mothering occurs, and internalized oppression that results in horizontal violence against those who are similarly situated need to be taken into account when considering questions of exoneration, blame, and responsibility.

Although women and men are roughly equal when it comes to perpetrating child maltreatment, it is clear that women bear the brunt of rape, sexual assault, trafficking in girls and women, and domestic violence. Philosophical literature extensively covers discussions of moral responsibility and blame. But relatively less consideration has been given to the topic of trauma and recovery from a gendered philosophical view. One notable exception is Susan Brison's *Aftermath: Violence and the Remaking of the Self* (2002). Brison was the victim of rape and attempted murder while out for a walk on a sunny afternoon in the French countryside. In her book, Brison describes the process by which she attempted to heal personally and professionally from events that placed her 'outside the human community' (2002, p. ix). She interweaves her anguished voice with the voice of one who understands trauma theory and with the voice of a feminist philosopher who calls into question the assumptions of what a self is and how it is constituted. Yet Brison says of her healing that 'I am not the same person who set off, singing, on that sunny Fourth of July in the French countryside. I left her in a rocky creek bed at the bottom of a ravine. I had to in order to survive' (Brison, 2002, p. 21). *Trauma, Truth and Reconciliation* is unusual in that it does address gendered aspects of trauma and healing and does so from an interdisciplinary perspective.

But gender is not the only axis of power: gender is always inflected by race, and ethnic and class differences stratify social relations along power dimensions, such as economics, access to health care, safety, social status, and education. How do marginalized and oppressed individuals and communities navigate the difficult terrain of interlocking oppressions and the traumas that oppression produces and reproduces? Would 'speaking truth to power' (Marable, 1996) be a route to healing, for African Americans or indigenous peoples of the Americas? Truth-telling directed at the powerful would seem to require an audience of genuine listeners—what I elsewhere have called 'giving uptake' (Potter, 2000). But it's not clear what will motivate those in power to listen to the oppressed, let alone to care about the damage they are doing to others. We need a theory as well as a plan for what the role of government and the law should be. Would citizens who have been betrayed by their government be better off (i.e., psychologically healthier) if the leaders of nation-states, speaking for their nation, apologized or asked forgiveness for gross injustices and inequalities? Would the leaders?

Theories of reparation argue that people of African descent and indigenous peoples of the Americas would, indeed, be better off. As Thomas McCarthy says, 'redressing past wrongs is essential to establishing conditions of justice in a society scarred by the enduring and pervasive effects of those wrongs' (McCarthy, 2004, p. 751, cf. also Posner and Vermeule, 2003). As long as racism and disenfranchisement continue, the call for reparations is likely to be heard at least in some quarters and, just as resoundingly, opposed. Opposition is not surprising in that, as William Bradford (2002/2003) writes, 'More than any other remedy, reparations transforms the material condition of recipients. Moreover, it connotes culpability . . .'. But most advocates of reparation consider governing bodies the ones that should enact reparations and, again, this raises questions about whether or not government and the law are the best pathways to healing and reconciliation.

At any rate, apologies are easy to give. Reparations—or even genuine remorse—are not. And one might ask whether or not it is in the best psychological interests of the tortured prisoners at Abu Ghraib to forgive their torturers in the absence of evidence of genuine remorse. This is not only a moral question because, as John Conroy (2000) argues in *Unspeakable Acts, Ordinary People*, the experience of being tortured can produce psychiatric symptoms. It is an open question whether or not it is either morally or therapeutically desirable for clinicians to encourage such victims to 'forgive their enemies.'

Questions of complicity in wrongdoing also exist: to what degree should collaborators or bystanders be forgiven? Steven H. Miles, a physician whose work on human rights abuses is invaluable, has uncovered connections between military medical personnel and abuse of detainees in Iraq, Afghanistan, and Guantanamo Bay. Miles found that the 'U.S. military medical system failed to protect detainees' human rights, sometimes collaborated with interrogators or abusive guards, and failed to properly report injuries or deaths caused by beatings' (Miles, 2004, p. 725). Are military medical personnel more culpable than the military for these wrongdoings, because they have a special obligation to treat and heal the medically needy? If so, perhaps detainees should withhold forgiveness from those military workers to a greater extent even than their torturers.

One of the most difficult issues in thinking about how to heal from damaged relationships is how to think responsibly about those who have been victims and perpetrators within the same context. Card (2002), in her wonderful analysis of evil in *The Atrocity Paradigm*, argues that the worst sort of moral damage one can do to another is to corrupt his or her moral standing by making him or her complicit in evil. Rawlinson, in her eloquent essay on Hegel's plea for forgiveness (this volume), also asks how people who have been both victim and perpetrator can live with the knowledge of what they have done and why they have done it. Her answer, following Hegel, is to seek forgiveness through confession. While Card is reluctant to exonerate people whose evildoings are in the 'gray zone,' she too seems inclined to advocate that we forgive those victims who become complicit in inflicting on others the evils that have been wrought on them.

Reconciliation and responsibility are complementary moral concepts, by which I mean that taking responsibility for one's wrongdoings paves the way for reconciliation with those wronged and, at the same time, the desire for reconciliation prompts one to take responsibility for one's actions. Both concepts invoke the inseparability of self-other relations: we cannot either be reconciled or take responsibility if we do not perceive and understand the other as a subject in his or her own right as well as value ourselves as having full moral worth despite what we might have done or failed to do to others. So when we consider questions of accountability for psychological harms, we need to think both individually and sociopolitically about who comprises these groups in various contexts. Trauma can occur in nation-states among large bodies of citizens as well as in families. Authors David Brendel, Christa Krüger, and Colleen Murphy each examine intersections between societal and interpersonal attempts to heal conflict, drawing analogies and noting differences between truth and reconciliation commissions and interpersonal therapy.

Other pressing questions will also be raised and answers sought in this anthology. What is the relationship of truth-telling to psychological well-being? Is there a necessary relationship between truth-telling and reconciliation? Christian Perring and Mehl-Madrona think not; Lamb argues that when truth gets lost, forgiveness is unwise and healing unlikely. What social conditions might prevent victims from being able to heal even when truths are spoken? Deborah Spitz takes up this question by situating the patient in therapy within the larger social context where the oppression of women hinders complete healing and reconciliation. Spitz, Perring, Lamb, and Mehl-Madrona all examine the effects of various forms of oppression both on the production of trauma and in the difficulties of healing in the face of such oppression. How does the value of forgiveness in interpersonal life compare with its value in clinical practice and in political life? The chapters in this anthology work through these and other questions in a variety of ways and provide for readers a complex and stimulating body of reasoning and evaluations by which to formulate their own answers.

The first four chapters examine potential analogies between truth and reconciliation commissions and psychotherapy. In Chapter 1, David H. Brendel carefully sets out similarities and differences between truth and reconciliation commissions and psychotherapy, particularly as they apply to victims of trauma. He argues that both individual and community healing require a dialectic that is dynamic and interactive but that a strict analogy between individual and community healing does not hold. By drawing on clinical experience that involves a conflict between a patient and himself, he makes vivid the dialectical process he envisions.

Christa Krüger, the author of Chapter 2, argues that the South African Truth and Reconciliation Commission (TRC) and many models of interpersonal conflict resolution rely on the idea of a continuous relationship. Drawing on the South African concept of *ubuntu*, she shows how dependent the aims of the TRC were on such continuity. Kruger's objective, instead, is to propose ways in which couples embroiled in conflict can heal when communication has broken down.

Chapter 3 frames both TRCs and psychotherapy as means to manage rage. The author, Peter Zachar, first offers an analysis of rage and argues that rage is a call for justice. He then examines prevailing Western moral theories and theories of justice with respect to forgiveness and securing justice following wrongdoing. The second half of this chapter argues against an overly optimist view of the success of TRCs and psychotherapy. Reconciliation, on his view, is a compromise between the satisfactions of rage and retributive justice, on the one hand, and naïve forgiveness, on the other hand. In Chapter 4, Colleen Murphy sets out the philosophical underpinnings of the rule of law, including the role that mutual expectations play in sustaining a society and the role that the breakdown of the rule of law plays in societal conflict. She then compares that analysis with people who have experienced interpersonal trauma, arguing that patients with post-traumatic stress disorder (PTSD) similarly have undergone a breakdown of expectations. She suggests ways in which this analysis of the effects of a breakdown in expectations can inform both political relationships and psychological research when it comes to healing from traumatic events.

Chapters 5 and 6 expose some of the assumptions embedded in the relationship between truth-telling and reconciliation. Chapter 5, written by Alison Mitchell, challenges a naïve view that truth-telling can bring about the desired aims of TRCs and argues that realist assumptions of TRCs make it unlikely that they can be successful. She proposes an alternative approach toward truth and reconciliation that takes into account the importance of achieving some degree of moral agreement about the significance of past events. In Chapter 6, Deborah Spitz distinguishes between truth-telling and reconciliation: truth-telling is a laudable goal in psychotherapy, but it does not necessarily lead to reconciliation. Spitz identifies three levels of reconciliation: intrapsychic, relational, and social—the latter having to do with a patient reconciling with the social context in which violations occurred. Presenting a case study of a patient with whom she worked, Spitz argues that, while reconciliation with the first two levels is a project that patient and therapist can do together, reconciliation with the social context is a task in which therapist efficacy is limited. Thus, truth-telling in the therapeutic context cannot expect fully to bring about complete reconciliation for the patient.

The next three chapters advocate the place of forgiveness in our lives. Chapter 7 situates questions about forgiveness in the context of former enemies needing to live together after civil wars and wrongdoers having to live with those they have wronged. The way to make that possible, Rawlinson argues, is for people to learn to forgive. Drawing upon Hegel's *Phenomenology of Spirit*, she offers an extended argument on the merits of forgiveness. Hegel explains how dogmatism arises and how it is related to terrorism; dogmatism is the result of one-sidedness, where natural consciousness valorizes itself. Using Hegel's concepts of hard-heartedness and hard-headedness, Rawlinson shows that a Hegelian conception of consciousness and conscience are not a product of the individual but of our embeddedness in sociality. Guilt and wrongdoing are part of our narrative and, so, we need to give and be given forgiveness. That is, forgiveness arises out of the human condition, as Hegel understands it and as Rawlinson persuasively argues. Gerrit Glas, in Chapter 8, similarly writes in a phenomenological vein, setting out a way to understand the dynamics of evil. He characterizes evil as nontransparent and discusses three intersecting dynamics of evil: speechlessness, splitting and denial, and shame. Forgiveness, he suggests, is a way to overcome the dynamics of evil. He ends by contrasting a Nietzschean view of forgiveness with a Christian one. Chapter 9 also defends forgiveness, but the author, Piet Verhagen, provides a theory of forgiveness that is grounded in our relatedness. After examining prejudices against forgiveness, and questions of evidence-based and value-based approaches to it, he sets out models of forgiveness drawn from psychology and psychiatry. While each model makes contributions to an understanding of forgiveness, none adequately captures what is most fundamental about our humanness, and that is our relatedness. Forgiveness is most appropriate, Verhagen argues, when we are committed to a healthy and personal relationship and view forgiveness as a way to honor and sustain that relationship.

The last three chapters examine effects of ongoing oppression on truth-telling, forgiveness, and reconciliation. Sharon Lamb, in Chapter 10, argues that many current psychotherapies appear more concerned to push clients to be forgiving than either to speak the truth or hold people accountable for wrongdoings. Her primary focus is the ways in which forgiveness therapies affect women. To that end, she examines two domains within psychotherapies that require that women, more than men, forgive others' wrongdoings: when women are victims of rape and sexual abuse, and where women's spouses or long-time partners have been unfaithful. The consistent theme of her chapter is the importance of paying attention to differences in gender when considering the application of truth-telling and forgiveness in their lives. Christian Perring, in Chapter 11, focuses his attention on relations between truth, narrative, and oppression. He argues for the use of narrative as story-telling as a way of resisting dominant constructions of the self as members of oppressed groups. Perring argues that, as the trauma and damage done to members of oppressed groups are not only psychological but discursive and political, the healing to be done must also be discursive and political. He uses as an example the ways that transsexual people have sought liberation from debilitating and demoralizing views of difference and then turns to the role narratives can play in creating alternative identities for those with mental illnesses.

The final chapter surveys the deep and pervasive damage done to aboriginal peoples with the invasion of Europeans to North America and the persistent oppression exacted on First Nations people to this day. The author, Lewis Mehl-Madrona, argues that American and European insistence on colonialist values, including Christianity and colonialist law, are abidingly antithetical to traditional ways. Thus, Western models for trauma, truth, reconciliation, and forgiveness cannot be assumed to apply to aboriginal peoples. Mehl-Madrona sets out ways of healing that First Nations people engage in that are responsive to their status as oppressed colonized groups—and ways that are truer to their own pasts and values.

The chapters in this anthology are mostly optimistic about the possibility of healing both from being wronged and from the wrongs we do others; authors variously emphasize truth-telling, dialogue, listening, story-telling, and forgiveness. But those activities aren't always possible. In *Holocaust Testimonies: The Ruins of Memory*, Lawrence Langer (1991) explores the voices of those who 'survived' the camps of Nazi Germany as they were recorded in interviews. Langer notes the persistent gap between what the speaker says and what the listener wants to hear: the listener, coming from a different world than those testifying, longs for a vocabulary of redemption, salvation, heroism, and evidence of 'the indomitable human spirit.' But, if we were to listen carefully—and without imposing our wishful ethical dimensions upon the speakers—holocaust testimonies would reveal, instead, the *absence* of such vocabulary. 'Most of their stories nurture not ethical insight but confusion, doubt, and moral uncertainty,' Langer writes (p. 37). Langer quotes a surviving victim of Auschwitz as saying:

> I am not like you. You have one vision of life and I have two. I—you know—I lived on two planets. After all I was—it seems to me that Hitler chopped off part of the universe and created annihilation zones and torture and slaughter areas. You know, it's like the planet was chopped up into a normal [part]—so-called normal: our lives are not really normal—and this other planet, and we were herded onto that planet from this one, and herded back again, [while] having nothing—virtually nothing in common with the inhabitants of this planet. And we had to relearn how to live again. Literally how to hold a fork, how to wash with soap, how to brush your teeth and... and we have these... these double lives. We can't cancel out. It just won't go away. People will deny it. I mean, probably a greater number will deny it—these memories—than not. But I will tell you, it's terrible... I talk to you and I am not only here, but I see Mengele [she lived in a barrack from which he chose women, including her sister, for his experiments] and I see the crematorium and I see all of that. And it's too much; it's very hard to get old with such—so ungracefully, because that has anything but grace, those memories, you know. It's very hard.
>
> Langer (1991, pp. 53–4)

I add this passage at the end of the Introduction because I believe it is important to respect the intransigence of some traumatic experiences and memories. Sometimes people only continue to live on. Our task, then, is to create a future in which no one ever has to face that as the only option.

Conclusions

This anthology thus takes up the subject of how to heal from psychological suffering caused by wrongdoing and oppression at varying levels within society. While the topics covered do not intersect with all forms of mental illnesses, they may nevertheless have implications for mental illnesses. The after-effects of traumatic experiences on psychological health and well-being seem most relevant to questions about the healing power of forgiveness and reconciliation, but trauma is a stressor that can set off mental illness in someone predisposed towards it, as in schizophrenia or personality disorders, so the domain of inquiry should not prematurely be closed off. Further research might broaden the topic of this book to examine these issues in the context of other mental illnesses. For example, does a role exist for forgiveness for a patient with schizophrenia? How is truth-telling complicated when someone is bipolar and cannot seem to distinguish truth and reality when in a manic phase? Does the trauma of imprisonment spark mental illness, and what would constitute healing for the imprisoned person?

The aim of this anthology has been to unpack some of the assumptions concerning the role of moral values in sociopolitical and interpersonal realms of suffering. Contributors focused primarily on truth-telling, story-telling, the rule of law, forgiveness, reconciliation, and restorative justice. If we are to learn to live together after we wrong one another, to restore ourselves to each other and to prevent further harm, we will likely need to appeal to moral values and frameworks; other moral concepts and values than the ones discussed here should also be examined for their potential to heal and reconcile. Guilt and shame, for example, although discussed by authors within their chapters, are not the central focus of any one chapter. Interdisciplinary and cross-cultural work on these and other concepts needs to be done as well.

Finally, this book offers conceptual and philosophical analyses of some salient issues in philosophy of psychiatry. It does not, itself, offer clinical research or its own empirical findings.

Therefore, *Trauma, Truth, and Reconciliation: Healing Damaged Relationships* needs its arguments tested and extended. It is hoped that readers will join in the expansion of knowledge and understanding in this field.

References

Botman H, Peterson R, and Robin M (eds) (1990). *To Remember and to Heal: Theological and Psychological Reflections on Truth and Reconciliation*. Cape Town: Human & Rousseau Publishers.

Bradford W (2002/2003). With a very great blame on our hearts: Reparations, reconciliation, and an American Indian plea for peace with justice. *Am Indian Law Review* 27(1).

Brison S (2002). *Aftermath: Violence and the Remaking of a Self*. Princeton, NJ: Princeton University Press.

Caplan P (1990). *Don't Blame Mother: Mending the Mother-Daughter Relationship*. New York: Harper and Row Publishers.

Card C (1990). Gender and moral luck. In: *Identity, Character, Morality: Essays in Moral Psychology* (ed. O Flanagan and A Rorty). Cambridge, MA: MIT Press.

Card C (2002). *The Atrocity Paradigm: A Theory of Evil*. Oxford: Oxford University Press.

Conroy J (2000). *Unspeakable Acts, Ordinary People: The Dynamics of Torture*. New York: Alfred A. Knopf.

Fellman G (1998). *Rambo and the Dalai Lama: The Compulsion to Win and its Threat to Human Survival*. New York: State University of New York Press.

Gilligan J (1996). *Violence: Reflections on a National Epidemic*. New York: Vintage Books.

Gobodo-Madikizela P (2003). *A Human Being Died that Night: A South African Story of Forgiveness.* Boston, MA: Houghton Mifflin.

Krog A (2000). *The Country of My Skull: Guilt, Sorrow, and the Limits of Forgiveness in the New South Africa.* New York: Three Rivers Press.

Lamb S and Murphy J (eds) (2002). *Before Forgiving: Cautionary Views of Forgiveness in Psychotherapy.* New York: Oxford University Press.

Landman J (2002). Earning forgiveness: the story of a perpetrator, Katherine Ann Power. In: *Before Forgiving: Cautionary Views of Forgiveness in Psychotherapy* (eds. S Lamb and J Murphy), pp. 232–64. Oxford: Oxford University Press.

Langer L (1991). *Holocaust Testimonies: The Ruins of Memory.* New Haven: Yale University Press.

Marable M (1996). *Speaking Truth to Power: Essays on Race, Resistance, and Radicalism.* Boulder, CO: Westview Press.

McCarthy T (2004). Coming to terms with our past, Part II: On the morality and politics of reparations for slavery. *Political Theory*, **32**(6): 750–72.

Miles SH (2004). Abu Ghraib: Its legacy for military medicine. *Lancet*, **364**: 725–9.

Miller A (1990). *Banished Knowledge: Facing Childhood Injuries* (trans. L Vennewitz). New York: Anchor Books.

Nino CS (1996). *Radical Evil on Trial.* New Haven: Yale University Press.

Noddings N (1984). *Caring: A Feminine Approach to Ethics and Moral Education.* Berkeley, CA: University of California Press.

Parks T (2003). *Judge Savage*, p. 232. New York: Arcade Publishing.

Posner E and Vermeule A (2003). Reparations for slavery and other historical injustices. *The Columbia Law Review*, **103**: 689.

Potter N (2000). Giving uptake. *Social Theory and Practice: An International and Interdisciplinary Journal of Social Philosophy*, **26**(3): 479–508.

Potter N (2001). Is refusing to forgive a vice? In: *Feminists Doing Ethics* (eds P DesAutels and J Waugh), pp. 135–50. New York and Oxford: Rowman-Littlefield Press.

Ruddick S (1989). *Maternal Thinking: Toward a Politics of Peace.* Boston, MA: Beacon Press.

Shriver D (1995). *An Ethic for Enemies: Forgiveness in Politics.* New York: Oxford University Press.

US Department of Health and Human Services (1998). *Child Maltreatment: Reports from the States to the National Child Abuse and Neglect Data System.* Administration for Children and Families; Administration on Children, Youth and Families; Children's Bureau.

Weschler L (1990). *A Miracle, a Universe: Settling Accounts with Torturers.* Chicago, IL: University of Chicago Press.

Chapter 1

Psychotherapy and the truth and reconciliation commission: the dialectic of individual and collective healing

David H. Brendel

1.1 Introduction

What is the relationship between processes of individual healing and collective healing in the wake of profound psychological trauma and unspeakable suffering? Can we attempt to understand the individual victim or perpetrator of a traumatic experience without thinking about the broader community in which he or she lives? Conversely, can we consider the needs of a traumatized community without paying careful attention to the specific experiences and needs of the individuals who comprise it? How mental health clinicians frame these questions and attempt to answer them have important implications for how we understand and try to help victims, perpetrators, and the communities in which they live. Not surprisingly, these questions do not lend themselves to an easy formulation or straightforward answer because of the complex features of particular individuals' lives, their varying levels of resilience and vulnerability to trauma, and the historical, political, and cultural particularities of the societies in which they live. We should be cautious not to generalize about the complex relationship between individual and collective responses to emotionally traumatic experiences. Questions about the nature of this relationship ought to be addressed by paying heed to local conditions, specific circumstances, and practical considerations around the traumatic events and their consequences.

Consideration of people's responses to emotional trauma in particular individual and collective settings can help us to approach this complex set of issues. Two processes designed to address specific forms of emotional trauma—individual psychotherapy for survivors of emotional trauma, and the Truth and Reconciliation Commission (TRC) process that occurred in the 1990s following the dismantling of the apartheid system in South Africa—illustrate that individual and collective healing cannot be understood as entirely distinct. On the contrary, the two processes suggest that individual and collective healing appear to stand in a 'dialectical' relationship to one another. Dialectical reasoning, which can be traced to the early nineteenth century work of German philosopher G.W.F. Hegel, entails serious consideration of both sides of a conceptual dichotomy, recognition of the relevance of both sides, and active efforts to articulate the relation between them. A dialectical approach to individual and community-wide responses to trauma is a dynamic, interactive process, with considerations on both sides of the dialectic constantly informing, shaping, and responding to one another. This chapter presents the argument that the healing of emotional wounds and damaged human relationships following traumatic events depends on appropriate attention being paid to both sides of the individual/community dialectic, regardless of whether an individual or a whole society has been victimized, whether one person or a whole political group has been the perpetrator, and whether the attempts at emotional healing focus on one person participating in a private process (such as psychotherapy) or many people engaging in a public process (such as the South African TRC).

Conceptualizing individual and collective healing in a dialectical relationship to one another empowers mental health clinicians (such as psychiatrists, psychologists, and social workers) and others whose role is to facilitate the post-traumatic healing of individuals and their communities (such as political leaders and public policy makers) to respond flexibly and pragmatically to the needs and concerns of the people whom they aim to help. As soon as we consider what may be healing in individual psychotherapy, we are quickly led to the question of how this therapeutic process can be generalized to benefit many people throughout society—but we are also cautioned against applying the principles of individual therapy too literally to what a society as a whole may require to move beyond the evils of a political system such as apartheid. Similarly, as we consider what underlies a viable truth and reconciliation process like the TRC in South Africa, we can reasonably ask what lessons it might hold for psychotherapy of trauma victims, just as long as we remain mindful of the caveat that the goal of psychotherapy is to heal the individual irrespective of what a sociopolitical system may need to heal itself as a whole. Dialectical reasoning, which aims to integrate both individual and collective models of emotional trauma and healing, enables the clinician to capitalize on the strengths and minimize the shortcomings of both approaches.

1.2 **The individual healing process**

In many contemporary societies, people seek to heal the wounds of emotional trauma in psychotherapy, a process that by its very nature focuses primarily on individual healing. How can an adult come to develop trust for another person within an intimate relationship after having been repeatedly molested by an important childhood figure such as a parent, a sibling, another family member, a family friend, a neighbor, a babysitter, a teacher, or a member of the clergy? How can an individual overcome self-hatred, a self-defeating personality style, and major depression after having internalized a powerfully negative sense of self as a result of unremitting verbal and emotional abuse by someone whom they have depended on and respected? How can an individual who has been victimized by racism, sexism, or some other form of discrimination preserve self-esteem and function successfully in a hostile social environment? The skilled and empathic psychotherapist aims to offer such patients a safe and supportive place in which to share their troubling memories and emotions and to talk openly about their painful experiences. The process, in many cases, can help the patient to develop insight into the origins of day-to-day suffering and to regain confidence that another person can be empathic, respectful, and trustworthy. The resolution of post-traumatic symptoms such as intrusive memories, flashbacks, nightmares, anxiety, and hypervigilance often occurs with psychotherapy and, in some cases, the judicious use of psychotropic medication. The development of a more robust sense of self and satisfying interpersonal relationships may take longer, but many patients find that psychotherapy helps them to achieve these goals as well. The path to the healing of emotional trauma in long-term psychotherapy is deeply personal, individualized, and complex.

Regardless of what any particular person might find helpful in a psychotherapy relationship, the process can be deemed a success if the patient begins to overcome the emotional fallout from past traumatic experiences. The focus here is on what is best for the individual person, regardless of what might be best for other individuals in similar situations or what might be in the best interest of the patient's family or community. As such, the therapist avoids placing the patient on a procrustean bed of what would be helpful to victims of trauma as a general rule or to others in the social environment. In addition, when working with an individual patient, the therapist focuses on providing that patient with optimal care, even if that means excluding other equally deserving patients from his or her practice. The psychotherapist functions as an individual patient advocate who attends to the needs and interests of other people in the patient's world only insofar as it is helpful and desirable to the patient. Exceptions to this general rule occur only in certain extreme cases, such as in the unusual scenario where a psychotherapist may be legally obligated to warn a third party that the patient is threatening to harm him or her imminently (Applebaum, 1985). For the most part, psychotherapists focus their attention on the emotional life of the individual patients they treat, and set aside considerations about what similar patients or other people in the patient's life might find helpful or desirable.

For example, in a family system that has suffered a great deal of trauma, different individuals may have various competing interests and agendas. In such families, some individuals may want to avoid acknowledgement or discussion of past traumas in order to maintain a civil equilibrium in the present, while other individuals in the family may find it helpful to express strong negative feelings openly. Based on what they have endured in childhood, some traumatized people seem to experience and express too little rage for their own good. Instead of directing their anger where it belongs—at those who have abused or victimized them—they turn their anger inward and thereby come to feel guilty, ashamed, depressed, and self-critical. If only they could mobilize these troubling feelings and direct them in a safe and appropriate manner back out into the world, they might find relief from the negative thoughts and feelings that swirl within them. Psychotherapists often aim to facilitate this process of mobilizing and redirecting negative affect so that it is less inwardly directed and pathogenic. In deciding whether and how to pursue such therapy, should the therapist only consider the personal needs and wishes of the patient, or should the therapist also take the needs and wishes of other members of the family (and the family system as a whole) into account? The following clinical case illustrates the complexities of such situations and the need to achieve appropriate balance between the primary focus on the individual and consideration of the interpersonal situation.

A patient of mine in his forties (whose identity has been disguised) had been consistently but unpredictably beaten by his father throughout childhood, but he had no apparent anger toward his father and instead focused on feelings of pity for him and feelings of sadness about his father's death when my patient was a teenager. In his adult life, the patient was extremely self-defeating, unable to motivate himself to find a job (despite his remarkable abilities and sound education), and extremely inhibited in relationships with women. Had he repressed rage toward his father and did his inability to tolerate and talk about that rage cause him to turn it against himself and thereby shut down multiple aspects of his emotional, social, and work life? Ongoing, long-term psychotherapy suggested that he was more proactive and less self-inhibiting when he articulated and explored the negative feelings that he harbored toward his father. Mobilizing the anger toward his father was not what the rest of his family desired; but as it tended to promote his own healing and flourishing, I cautiously supported him in expressing his anger about his father's past behavior in a manner that avoided unnecessary damage to present relationships with family members who were still alive, including his elderly mother. This process mainly involved his openly expressing anger in sessions with me and exhibiting restraint whenever the issue arose in discussions with his mother, as we agreed that expressing anger too harshly toward her would disrupt family life and cause her undue suffering. Even in psychotherapy with a primary focus on individual healing, it may be important to consider the social surround and implications of the individual therapy process for others.

1.3 **The collective healing process**

Unlike psychotherapy, which focuses principally on the individual patient, the process of collective healing of traumatic experiences is oriented primarily toward the needs and interests of the entire community. Countless communities around the world have struggled to heal themselves in the wake of traumas they endured through the twentieth century. How has the community of Japanese-Americans dealt with the history of their internment in the United States during the Second World War? How have Native American groups in the United States come to terms with the profound mistreatment and displacement they endured? How have African-Americans grappled with their history of being enslaved? How has the Armenian community around the world responded as a collectivity to the genocidal war against them in the early twentieth century? How has the Jewish community healed itself in the wake of the Holocaust? What about traumatized peoples of Cambodia, Rwanda, the former Yugoslavia, Tibet, and so many other nations and communities around the world? There is no well-defined recipe for what traumatized groups must do in order to heal themselves, because people respond to trauma in a wide variety of ways that are significantly influenced by the cultures in which they live. Important aspects of collective healing may include sharing stories, ventilating feelings, and finding creative ways to represent the trauma in art. In some cases, the victimized community does not have the opportunity to confront those who abused them, either because of the passage of time or the death of the perpetrators. This is true of many traumatized Native American communities in the United States, which have developed creative processes of healing their trauma (Lyon, 1998) without the presence or involvement of the perpetrators of that trauma.

In other cases, the community of victims and perpetrators has an opportunity to confront one another and engage in an interchange that may involve sharing stories, expressing feelings, apologizing, and forgiving. An example of the latter is the TRC in South Africa, which serves as a useful index example of the process of community healing. Whereas individual psychotherapy is a fundamentally personal process, the TRC process in South Africa was fundamentally political insofar as it aimed to achieve certain societal goals. Emphasizing the principles of collective healing, the African National Congress (ANC) wrote in their *Statement to the Truth and Reconciliation Commission* (available at www.doj.gov.za/trc/submit/anctruth.htm) that the TRC process ought to 'draw the necessary lessons and examples from a wide variety of individual experiences, without it being necessary that everyone appears before the Commission.' While the ANC encouraged many individuals to share their painful stories publicly, it realized that the TRC could not proceed endlessly if it were to achieve 'the broader national goal which relates to the building of a democratic, peaceful, and non-racial South Africa' (www.doj.gov.za/trc/submit/anctruth.htm). They understood that the goal of collective healing in South Africa grew out of political and practical exigencies and could not simply be the process of individual, long-term psychotherapy writ large. At the same time, the ANC realized that an exclusive focus on community healing would be inadequate. The ANC wrote that the primary sociopolitical goal of the TRC was 'achievement of national reconciliation,' but that an important element in achieving this goal would be 'personal catharsis' for individuals who had suffered under apartheid. South Africa's TRC website (www.doj.gov.za/trc/reparations/policy/htm) noted that the collective process 'restores dignity' to individual victims and would help them 'to take control of their own lives.'

Notwithstanding the recognition of the role of the individual in the TRC, the process was primarily sociopolitical and community-oriented, with less attention paid to its effects on individuals. A primary focus on collective healing can be problematic, however, because some trauma victims find that describing (and thereby reliving) their experiences actually may worsen their suffering, that forgiving perpetrators may not promote healing, and that suppression of anger toward perpetrators may be counter-therapeutic and lead to depression and self-criticism. In an article titled 'The Cultural Construction of Healing in the Truth and Reconciliation Commission: Implications for Mental Health Practice,' South African psychologists Leslie Swartz and Gerard Drennan (2000) argued for these points and presented clinical material to support them. They questioned the assumption implicit in the South African TRC process that collective healing would in fact help to heal particular individuals who had suffered under the apartheid system. Their arguments point out some of the limitations on taking a strictly communitarian approach to healing trauma and damaged interpersonal relationships. For example, the community-wide injunction to forgive South African perpetrators for racially driven crimes is morally and psychologically problematic, as it may be understandable and healthy for some individual victims to feel angry and unforgiving about how they suffered under the apartheid system.

Swartz and Drennan worried that the TRC's promotion of 'healing by decree' and 'absolution' of perpetrators might get in the way of some individuals' being able to explore a wide range of feelings (such as anger, rage, resentment, and hatred) by way of the psychotherapeutic process of 'working through, a process which is private and time-consuming' (Swartz and Drennan, 2000, p. 212). They described the case of a woman who had been involved in humanitarian work in South Africa in the 1980s and later was suffering with feelings of humiliation and confusion around her husband having an affair with another woman. The husband had had a history of being physically violent toward the patient in years past. Her psychotherapy focused on how to endure these humiliations and whether or not to leave the marriage, but the TRC process seemed to obstruct her personal healing. 'A major sticking point in her treatment,' Swartz and Drennan wrote, 'was her insistence that she should be able to reconcile and forgive as this was what was being called for nationally. She found it extremely difficult to accept her own anger and her sense of betrayal' (p. 212). Her inability to tolerate her anger and act on it to protect her personal interests seemed to have been exacerbated by the culture of the TRC process, which may have prematurely advocated forgiveness for undeserving perpetrators and unnecessarily increased the emotional turmoil of trauma victims who could neither forgive nor adequately express their rage.

Another case presented by Swartz and Drennan (2000) addressed the problems that may emerge when an individual is encouraged to reawaken a deeply buried psychic trauma. The patient was a South African man who for many years harbored a nagging suspicion that his son's death had come at the hands of the apartheid government. He had attempted to deal with the pain of losing his son by sealing it off emotionally and trying to forget about his suspicions of state violence. Years later, he had a chance encounter with somebody from the TRC, who encouraged the man to submit a statement about his son's death and thereby prompt an investigation into its cause. After reluctantly deciding to pursue this course of action, he waited many months for a response and then received what appeared to be a form letter, carefully and sympathetically worded, stating that there was insufficient evidence to investigate the case.

The man then came to psychotherapy 'feeling bewildered and angry at the extent of his emotional reaction to this letter, and full of regret at having been persuaded not to let sleeping dogs lie' (p. 212). This kind of reaction to exploring a suppressed or sealed off traumatic memory is not uncommon in psychotherapy: some trauma victims respond more favorably to therapy that focuses on relationships and life challenges in the here-and-now rather than to interventions that re-expose the patient to suppressed traumatic memories. The collective healing interests of processes like the TRC and the individual healing goals of psychotherapy may conflict in some situations. Is there a way to work through this dilemma on both the individual and collective level so as to promote the healing of traumatic wounds and the avoidance of doing further harm along the way?

1.4 **The dialectic of individual and collective healing**

Individual and community-wide healing from emotional trauma are not mutually exclusive processes. While in some situations the primary focus is on the former (as in individual psychotherapy) and in other situations it is on the latter (as in the TRC), mental health clinicians ought to consider seriously both individual and collective factors when determining the appropriate approach to helping traumatized people and communities to heal themselves. When focusing on the experiences and needs of the traumatized patient in individual psychotherapy, the clinician should consider the role that other people in the patient's world will play in the therapy or the implications of the therapy for those other people. Conversely, when concentrating on the construction of a fairer and more enlightened social order, a TRC should not overlook the experiences and needs of particular traumatized people or the wide range of consequences for individuals of participating in the national process. A dialec-tical approach to healing emotional trauma—in which individual and collective factors deeply shape and influence one another—can help mental health clinicians to balance all of these disparate concerns.

At a TRC or other such community-wide venue for healing trauma, it is critical to attend carefully to the needs and the welfare of individual participants even though the principal aim of the process is to heal the community as a whole. This major concern was highlighted by Swartz and Drennan's case of the father who was persuaded by someone involved in the South African TRC to request an investigation into the death of his son, which led to the father's feeling overwhelmed and re-traumatized—and wishing he had 'let sleeping dogs lie.' It may have been prudent for those running the South African TRC to encourage participation of only those victimized individuals for whom describing and experientially reliving their trauma would have been helpful, or at least would have been unlikely to do significant harm. How might a future TRC ensure the participation of such individuals and, at the same time, glean important evidence from others without requiring that they present their narratives in a manner that would cause them to relive their trauma? In addition, in light of the concerns raised by Swartz and Drennan's case of the South African woman with trouble tolerating her well-justified rage toward her abusive and unfaithful husband because of the national climate of forgiveness, how can people in a society engaged in a collective process such as the TRC avoid the potential risks and pitfalls of applying community-wide principles (such as total forgiveness of perpetrators) to the healing of their individual lives?

Clearly, there is no easy, boilerplate solution to these vexing questions. Perhaps it would help to employ individual psychotherapists to screen for those TRC participants who would be unlikely to suffer serious adverse reactions to presenting their narratives. To ensure fairness, such psychotherapists should be provided at no cost to potential TRC participants, as screening traumatized individuals ultimately would serve the purpose of promoting community-wide healing and reconciliation. The screening therapists, of course, should offer advice rather than make binding decisions; a traumatized individual may wish to present his or her story to the TRC despite running the risk of experiencing further pain and suffering in the process. Dialectical reasoning here leads to an approach that integrates individual and collective concerns. Screening individuals for participation in the TRC, and informing them of the psychological risks of participating, would help to protect individuals and, at the same time, promote a process that is mainly sociopolitical in its aims. In addition, government and other policy-making institutions could assume the responsibility of providing widespread education that conveys the message that the collective ideals of amnesty and forgiveness do not necessarily apply to deeply personal struggles of individuals in their day-to-day lives. Educational programs or advertising campaigns promulgating this message may not have assuaged all of the guilt of Swartz and Drennan's patient with the abusive husband, but in her individual psychotherapy it might have reinforced the critical message that it is understandable and healthy to feel enraged and unforgiving when one has been emotionally abused by a spouse for so long. This case also points out the problematic nature of the South African TRC's focus on unquestioning forgiveness of perpetrators of apartheid crimes: if it is not healthy for certain individual victims of apartheid to renounce their rage, then perhaps the TRC's absolute norm of forgiveness was too strict.

The individual/community dialectic applies as much to psychotherapy of patients with trauma histories as it does to devastated societies trying to heal themselves through processes such as the TRC. The therapist listens empathically to the patient's account of the trauma and helps the patient to understand its repercussions and manifestations in his or her current life. At the same time, the therapist retains curiosity about what happened to the patient, as any narrative telling of a life story is shaped by psychological defenses as well as cultural and interpersonal factors. Is the patient presenting the traumatic memory in a somewhat exaggerated fashion, depicting himself or herself as a helpless victim in order to avoid acknowledging his or her own aggression or jealousy toward the identified perpetrator? Or, on the other hand, is the patient downplaying the trauma because of guilt that he or she provoked the perpetrator to engage in the beating or the molestation? In psychotherapy, it is often difficult for the clinician to know exactly what happened to the patient, as the description of the traumatic events comes by way of the patient's own report. At times, a family member may confirm what occurred, but the family member's memories also may be distorted. Patient and clinician in psychotherapy often need to grapple with deep uncertainties about the line between narrative truth and historical truth, which underlies an ongoing controversy in contemporary psychotherapy (Person and Klar, 1994). The psychotherapist works dialectically by empathizing with the patient's reported experience while also considering the perspectives of other people and the overall socio-cultural context in which both the trauma and the subsequent therapeutic interaction take place.

These points were highlighted in my psychotherapy work with a man (whose identity has been disguised) with a drug-addicted mother who used to take money he earned as a newspaper delivery boy during childhood and gamble it away at the horse track. Even when sober, she never apologized to my patient for this behavior and never returned his hard-earned money. In adulthood, he severely mistreated his wife, who had a debilitating physical and mental illness. In a case of 'identification with the aggressor' (in which the trauma victim assumes the role of the perpetrator), my patient often left his ill wife at home for long stretches of time so that he could spend the day gambling at a casino. He came to therapy with intense anger toward his mother, but he minimized the problems of how he and his wife related. If I had unquestioningly accepted his description of his childhood experiences and his marital situation, I would not have challenged him to consider whether he was harming his wife in much the same way that he reported he had been harmed by his mother in childhood. By looking at his interpersonal world and heeding our cultural sensitivity to abusive relationships, I was in a position to confront him about the problems of how he was treating his wife. As he came to realize that he was acting in the same selfish manner that he recalled his mother acting during his school years, he felt guilty and ashamed but also motivated to change. A dialectical approach in psychotherapy, which acknowledged his personal suffering but balanced it with attention to his wife's suffering and sensitivity to the insidious nature of abusive marital relationships, helped him to understand better the complexities of his relationship with his mother and to heal his marriage by achieving a better balance between his wife's needs and his own. He felt increasingly satisfied with his life as he began to gamble less, plan a vacation with his wife, and return to work so that he was adding to their savings account rather than depleting it.

Another aspect of the individual/community dialectic as applied to psychotherapy concerns the need at times to expose the private, one-to-one process of therapy to public scrutiny. With the permission of one of my patients, I published an account of our work together in a professional journal in which I disguised his identity and, for didactic purposes, provided an exaggerated account of his somewhat formal demeanor (Brendel *et al.*, 2002). After the article was published, I gave him a copy of it with the caveat that I had overemphasized some aspects of his case but played down others in order to make certain points. Despite this warning, he felt hurt and enraged by the portrayal, such as my use of the terms 'stilted' and 'pedantic' to describe his interpersonal style. He noted that I had protected his privacy by disguising personal details about him, but he felt shamed and criticized by me in much the same way that he often had felt shamed and criticized by his parents and schoolmates throughout his unhappy childhood. Over the ensuing months, he confronted me with his anger in our sessions and also worked it through by seeking a consultation with another clinician. I apologized for how I had hurt him and wondered aloud whether the shame I felt about hurting him helped me to better empathize with the shame that he had experienced all his life. Offering an apology, which plays so many functions in troubled relationships (Lazare, 2004), was an important first step toward repairing our damaged patient/therapist relationship.

But still feeling guilty and bewildered about how I could have upset my patient so badly, I presented the situation to a medical school ethics consortium and published an account of the specific course of events and the ethical issues they highlighted, with the patient's identity still disguised (Brendel, 2003). This follow-up article was published side-by-side with an essay written under a pseudonym by my patient on what he had experienced in reading my case report (Carter, 2003), as well as commentaries by clinicians with an interest in the ethics of writing about patients (Halpern, 2003; Howe, 2003; Joffe,

2003; Mitchell and Truog, 2003). The follow-up publications provided an opportunity for me to reflect on my preconceptions and missteps, and for my patient to gain a voice about his experience in an article in the medical literature. The multifaceted response to this traumatic experience helped us to move beyond it and gave us tools for how a perpetrator and a victim might usefully work through an interpersonal trauma. In fact, the response looked like a small-scale version of a TRC, in which the victim airs grievances and expresses hurt feelings, the perpetrator listens and apologizes, and others observe, support, and comment upon the entire process as it unfolds. The trauma that my patient had experienced as a child and in psychotherapy with me clearly had not been erased but had been therapeutically transformed by way of dialogue and apology in a public setting.

This process, which empowered us to continue our therapeutic work together during the ensuing year, depended on a medical school ethics consortium. The existence of this consortium was a godsend for my patient and me, because on our own we might not have been able to turn a profoundly painful experience for both of us into an occasion for insight, empathy, mutual respect, and healing. In the future, rather than relying on the good fortune that a local medical school or other institution could provide a setting for this TRC-like exchange to take place, psychotherapists and the institutions with which they affiliate (such as psychoanalytic institutes) may want to create such venues for themselves, so that there is a consistent forum for discrete but public discussion of certain private matters that can arise in individual psychotherapy. Like the South African TRC, this venue would not function as a source of moral judgment, discipline, or punishment, but instead would provide a safe and future-oriented place for patients and therapists to engage in a process of dialogue, apology, and forgiveness. Such a venue would embody the principles of dialectical reasoning at its best, with mental health clinicians doing all that they can to promote the healing of emotional trauma and damaged relationships by paying equally careful attention to traumatized individuals, perpetrators, and the complex communities in which they live.

References

African National Congress, Statement to the Truth and Reconciliation Commission, August 1996. Accessed from www.doj.gov.za/trc/submit/anctruth.htm.

Applebaum PS (1985). Tarasoff and the clinician: problems in fulfilling the duty to protect. *American Journal of Psychiatry*, **142**: 425–29.

Brendel DH (2003). Complications to consent. *Journal of Clinical Ethics*, **14**: 90–4.

Brendel DH, Bodkin JA, Hauptman B, and Ornstein A (2002). 'I see dead people': Overcoming psychic numbness. *Harvard Review of Psychiatry*, **10**: 166–78.

Carter J (2003). Looking into a distorted mirror. *Journal of Clinical Ethics*, **14**: 95–100.

Halpern J (2003). Beyond wishful thinking: facing the harm that psychotherapists can do by writing about their patients. *Journal of Clinical Ethics*, **14**: 118–36.

Howe EG (2003). Lessons from 'Jay Carter.' *Journal of Clinical Ethics*, **14**: 109–17.

Joffe S (2003). Public dialogue and the boundaries of moral community. *Journal of Clinical Ethics*, **14**: 101–8.

Lazare A (2004). *On Apology*. New York: Oxford University Press.

Lyon WS (1998). *Encyclopedia of Native American Healing*. New York: WW Norton & Company.

Mitchell C and Truog R (2003). Seeking blinded consent. *Journal of Clinical Ethics*, **14**: 88–9.

Person ES and Klar H (1994). Establishing trauma: the difficulty distinguishing between memories and fantasies. *Journal of the American Psychoanalytic Association*, **42**: 1055–81.

Swartz L and Drennan G (2000). The cultural construction of healing in the Truth and Reconciliation Commission: Implications for mental health practice. *Ethnicity & Health*, **5**: 205–13.

Chapter 2

Spiral of growth: a social psychiatric perspective on conflict resolution, reconciliation, and relationship development

Christa Krüger

The worldwide wave of political truth commissions in the last 20 years has generated widespread interest in possible ways of managing conflict and reconciliation in political contexts (Meiring, 1999; Susin and Aquino, 2003). Most of these truth commissions have relied on business principles of conflict management, sometimes also on judicial principles, and have been effective to varying degrees.

The South African Truth and Reconciliation Commission (TRC) (1996–98) is generally accepted as having been successful and effective. It relied heavily on religious principles and on the South African *ubuntu* culture. Ubuntu (the Xhosa version of the term) is an African concept, a social perspective/philosophy, that includes the meanings of collective personhood, harmony in the community, a culture of communalism, shared fellowship, and cooperation for the common good (Masina, 2000). In the 10 years since democracy there has been ongoing reconciliatory work in South Africa, *inter alia*, in the political and religious spheres. Several conferences have been held locally, where issues such as reconciliation have been discussed at length (Du Toit, 1998; Van Der Walt and Naudé, 1996; Van Vugt and Cloete, 2000). For example, Cornel Du Toit led a conference held by the Research Institute for Theology and Religion (RITR) at the University of South Africa in March 1998 (Du Toit, 1998). The pamphlet by Van der Walt and Naudé refers to a conference on Christianity and Democracy in South Africa, July 10–12, 1996 (Van der Walt and Naudé, 1996). The volume by Van Vugt and Cloete (2000) resulted from a conference at the University of the Western Cape in January 1999 on race and reconciliation in South Africa. This conference sought to create a multicultural, scholarly dialogue on the history, theology, philosophy, and politics of race and reconciliation in South Africa.

The question arises whether the successful politico-religious approach of the South African TRC to intergroup conflict could also be applied to resolve interpersonal conflict (conflict between two people), as encountered in our professional context in a state psychiatric hospital and a university department of psychiatry, where the resolution of various types of conflict forms a part of our core work. No formal distinction will be made between conflict in mental health and conflict in mental illness, as the former may be a frequent antecedent to the latter, and since a categorical distinction between the former and the latter is a debatable issue.

However, it will be shown in the course of this chapter that not only the TRC approach but also other existing strategies for interpersonal conflict resolution and reconciliation, such as couples psychotherapy and negotiation theory, rely on a continuous relationship between two willing parties. All these approaches are likely to fail in 'dead-end' situations of interpersonal conflict where the relationship and meaningful communication have broken down. These approaches appear to be inadequate for situations where either or both of the parties do not contribute constructively to the relationship.

The aim is to explore a perspective on interpersonal conflict resolution and reconciliation that does not rely on a continuous relationship between two willing parties. It should be possible to apply such a perspective unilaterally where the relationship has broken down. In these cases the perspective should contribute to re-establishing a relationship between the conflicting parties. The perspective should emphasize relationship development despite conflict. Moreover, this perspective should ideally foster moral development in both parties and in the relationship.

The above question, problems, and aims are approached here from a social psychiatric perspective in which social and sociological concepts are applied in the context of interpersonal conflict. Although the currently fashionable understanding of social psychiatry revolves around social factors that influence mental disorders and their rehabilitation, as well as the organization and delivery of mental health policy and care (Sartorius, 1988; Sartorius et al., 2002), the approach followed here can probably be categorized as social psychiatric, as it explores the interface between psychiatry/psychology, social/political science, and religion/theology in which the concepts of conflict and reconciliation are embedded. This approach follows the general example set by the field of social psychology (Sears et al., 1988; Meyers, 1993, 1994; Higgins and Kruglanski, 1996; Aronson et al., 1999; Kenrick et al., 1999; Smith and Mackie, 2000; Delamater, 2003; Fiske, 2004), by combining and integrating ideas from different theoretical traditions. The approach here is not eclectic, but integrative, with a view to contributing to an interdisciplinary dialogue that might ideally yield emancipatory strategies for application in both interpersonal and intergroup situations of conflict.

One of my assumptions is that, without denying the qualitative difference between the two levels, political conflict may be approached as a larger-scale expression of interpersonal conflict as is found, for example, in couples conflict. The players in political conflict are people, the same people who may experience conflict in their personal contexts. Although political conflict may occur on a more abstract level than, for example, couples conflict, the groups in political conflict often know a lot about each other, and might share time and space (as they have done in South Africa). Such a context for political conflict might even be regarded as a kind of intimate context. A related assumption is that effective conflict resolution principles should ideally apply on all levels—international/global conflict, business disputes, domestic tensions, and inner personal struggles (Heitler, 1990)—and contribute to the emancipation and empowerment of powerless or oppressed groups of people, as part of a transformative agenda.

These assumptions are supported by contributions from the fields of social psychology, clinical psychology, narrative therapy/counseling, and international conflict analysis and resolution. In the edited volume by Lawler and Markovsky (1993) on the social psychology of groups, two of the chapters show how small group processes activate social networks or politically active generations, and how microsociological and macrosociological phenomena are interconnected (Braungart and Braungart, 1993; Fine and Stoecker, 1993). Moreover, intergroup conflict has been explained on the basis of individuals' cognitive categorization of who is in and who is out (Rusbult and Van Lange, 1996; Stainton Rogers, 2003). The mutual influence between culture and individual psychology has also been examined by Markus et al. (1996). They illustrate how psychological processes vary with socio-cultural context by referring to the example of Japanese culture that is highly relational, resulting in intense attunement to interpersonal conflict and hence prevention of conflict by anticipatory management. In the field of clinical psychology, Sue Van Zyl (1999) points toward a psychoanalytically informed treatment of the sequelae of trauma on a social level, and Marc Ross (1995) offers a psychocultural interpretation theory, i.e., a socially rooted psychoanalytic theory. John Neal et al. (1999) describe a postmodern narrative approach in which the therapist helps clients to separate from the problem story through the process of externalization, and to notice that the problem is not about personal deficiency, but, rather, is an effect of cultural discourse (and in the context of couples therapy, an effect of the operation of cultural discourse through gender). The dominant cultural perspective on problems is said to leave people with little room to make sense of problems other than as reflecting some defect in them and their relationships. Thus the authors demonstrate a connection between interpersonal and intergroup conflict. The next phase in the therapy is then re-authoring and reconnection to preferred identities and histories by 'co-constructing a coherent narrative truth about them' (Neal *et al*.1999, p. 389). In the field of international conflict analysis and resolution, Hicks (2001) applies the principle of identity development to interactions between two people or between groups of people. In contrast, it should be noted that Worthington (2001), a psychologist who also applied concepts of couples and individual psychotherapy to societal and international relations, concluded that one could not generalize from individuals to couples to groups.

Given the two above assumptions, the potential applicability of the inter-personal perspective that is developed here, in contexts of intergroup conflict on a larger scale, e.g., a political scale, should eventually be examined thor-oughly. However, an exploration of such applicability in contexts of inter-group conflict falls outside of the scope of this chapter. This chapter will only concern the potential value of the perspective in an interpersonal context.

A search of the literature relevant to the interpersonal focus of this chapter showed that the fields of politics and religion have yielded numerous publica-tions in the last 10 years, which contribute new thought concerning conflict and reconciliation, as well as truth and forgiveness between groups of people. A similar search in the field of clinical psychology, on intra-individual and interpersonal conflict, couples conflict and psychotherapy yielded less than the search on political conflict and reconciliation, and not much on potential links and applications between these fields. Moreover, a search in social psy-chology did not reveal many relevant recent developments. A search in the field of systemic therapy, in anticipation that potential links between inter-group conflict and interpersonal conflict might draw on systems theory, was also disappointing. Contributions from the latter field have concerned mainly therapy for couples and families, extending to cultural issues in the context of such therapy rather than to intergroup conflict.

The four elements of my hypothesis represent an integration of contribu-tions from various fields/approaches in a proposed perspective on conflict resolution, reconciliation, and relationship development:

- A contribution from game theory means the proposed perspective may be applied unilaterally where the relationship has broken down, to encourage repeated choices for cooperation in successive rounds of interaction.
- A contribution from systemic thinking means the proposed perspective may help to re-establish and sustain an improved relationship between the

conflicting parties, through reintroduction, focusing on the style rather than the content of the conflict, and narrative reconstruction of their identities.

- A developmental view of relationships may situate conflict in the larger context of human development, may relativize the role of conflict in relationships, and may foster optimism about gradual reconciliation despite conflict.

- A contribution from moral philosophy means the proposed perspective may foster moral development in both parties and the relationship, through re-establishing relatedness.

Given the potential scope of this chapter, I shall not venture into great detail about the relevant background in all the relevant fields, but focus only on some details in some fields of study. Accordingly, in a political sense, the focus will be limited to the South African TRC. Although some of the concepts in this chapter, e.g., reconciliation, apply to many of the world's religions, the focus will be restricted to their relevance in Christianity, the latter being the professed faith of about 87% of the South African population, according to the 1996 South African national census (Chapman and Spong, 2003). Furthermore, even though the concept of truth featured prominently in the South African TRC, a detailed philosophical or theological discussion of truth falls outside of the scope of this chapter. Suffice it to point out that in the field of religion, the truth tends to be regarded in absolute terms (Biggar, 2001). A notable exception was Dietrich Bonhoeffer (1949/1966) who emphasized the contextual nature of truth. In interpersonal conflict the truth may often be elusive and the different parties may have divergent views on what the truth is. Even so, I think that interpersonal conflict can be resolved or at least relationships can be improved without getting caught up in what the 'truth' of the matter is. Similarly, forgiveness has been a topic of concern in theology, moral philosophy, political ethics, psychology, and feminism [see especially Nigel Biggar's review of the literature on forgiveness in the twentieth century (2001), as well as the chapter by Pamela Sue Anderson in the same volume (2001)]. For Ron and Pat Potter-Efron (1995), forgiveness is an intrapsychic, unilateral, voluntary act that helps the individual overcome his/her own anger—a gift of relief to oneself, a choice, an act of free will—with no relational implications such as that the perpetrator should change or return to the relationship. Although many authors accommodate both forgiveness and reconciliation as parts of a single process, some say forgiveness precedes reconciliation (Staub and Pearlman, 2001), while others claim the opposite, that reconciliation precedes forgiveness (Worthington, 2001).

The two concepts that remain within the focus of this chapter are conflict and reconciliation. I shall take conflict to refer broadly to disagreement between two parties, a bilateral problem, which may or may not be accompanied by anger or abuse. Although I recognize the positive impetus for growth that conflict may provide in various situations, including in relationships between individuals and groups of people, the focus here is on situations where conflict has led to relationships being 'messed up'. Reconciliation will be taken to refer to re-engagement in relationship as far as the two parties are able to do so—not in the same relationship as before, but aiming towards an improved, morally more accountable relationship. I tend to regard reconciliation as a process rather than as an outcome. The focus will be on interpersonal reconciliation between the conflicting parties, rather than on the religious (divine) reconciliation between a perpetrator and God, or between a perpetrator and a caring church community, which has been regarded as a fundamental symbol of the Christian tradition (Livingston, 2002). Note that in the context of the TRC, reconciliation followed the broad outline of confessing sin, asking for forgiveness and mercy, and making amends, thus suggesting that reconciliation overlapped with forgiveness, yet also implied justice, responsibility, and restitution (Meiring, 1999, 2000). This TRC definition seems to have derived from the concept of reconciliation as used by the National Initiative for Reconciliation (NIR) (Nürnberger and Tooke, 1988), a predecessor of the TRC, which was launched in September 1985 in South Africa at a conference of 400 church leaders from many denominations. The NIR defined reconciliation as the agreement between two parties in a conflict to forgive and accept each other. Their concept of reconciliation was based on Christian reconciliation where God reconciled people to himself in Christ, and Christ restored people to the fellowship with God and with each other. Notwithstanding this strong theological focus, Tooke, in the same volume (Tooke, 1988), warned that the South African issues should not be spiritualized endlessly, but that reconciliation was primarily to be understood in socio-economic–political terms. The ideas of making amends and restitution have a parallel in the field of psychology, where, e.g., Staub and Pearlman (2001) and Worthington (2001) argue that reconciliation includes a restoration of trust in a relationship.

2.1 The Truth and Reconciliation Commission of South Africa

The TRC that consisted of 17 commissioners and 11 committee members operated for $2^{1}/_{2}$ years beginning February 1996 (Meiring, 1999). For example,

Piet Meiring, a theologian from the Dutch Reformed Church, served on the Reparation and Rehabilitation Committee of the TRC, and represented the Afrikaans Churches of South Africa (Meiring, 1999). The TRC aimed to promote national unity and reconciliation in a spirit of understanding that transcends the conflicts and divisions of the past, *inter alia*, by establishing as complete a picture as possible of human rights violations since March 1, 1960 and the context of such violations, by finding victims and restoring their human and civil dignity, by facilitating the granting of amnesty to perpetrators, by providing support and counseling to victims, perpetrators and their families, and by making recommendations to prevent future human rights violations (Meiring, 1999, 2000).

It should be noted that the TRC represented only one of several approaches followed in South Africa towards reconciliation. Other approaches included, e.g., pursuing the superordinate goal of creating a single rainbow nation, changing racist perceptions through public education in the media, and implementing increased contact between different cultural groups through desegregation and affirmative action. These other approaches to intergroup conflict resolution were based more on social identity theory and negotiation theory (Meyers, 1993; Stainton Rogers, 2003) than on theological or ubuntu principles.

The TRC held, *inter alia*, human rights violations hearings, where the victims, who came from all cultural groups, seemed to derive great benefit from being heard in public and from sharing past traumas that had haunted them for decades in some instances. Amnesty hearings were also held, where perpetrators (again of all cultural groups) were granted amnesty if they made full disclosure of all relevant facts and if the violations had been made in the context of political motives, orders by seniors, or military battle. A demonstration of remorse or expression of regret was not required, as it was thought that such would encourage dishonesty. The TRC did not look for what a court would require (proof beyond reasonable doubt), but rather demanded that the evidence be 'reasonably true, on a balance of probability' (Tutu, 1998). Thus, the TRC helped the nation to come to terms with its past not by amnesia or trials, but by amnesty and storytelling (Tutu, 1998).

Led by Archbishop Desmond Tutu, the work of the TRC was based on theological principles. It seems as if the government, through the TRC, moved from crime to sin (Connor, 1998) in order to gain hope that the South African problems would be remediable and that a fresh start could be made. Chapman and Spong (2003) point out that there was a predominance of conventional Christian participation in the work of the TRC. This may seem appropriate, as the apartheid policy had benefited hugely from theological justifications made by Christian church leaders at the time, and on the other hand, Christian church leaders were among those dedicated to fighting the apartheid policy. However, as Chapman and Spong illustrate through their series of interviews with leaders from the African indigenous churches, the Jewish faith, the Muslim faith, and other religious traditions, the process of reconciliation in South Africa also benefited greatly from multifaith inputs. Hence, conventional Christian leaders cannot claim ownership of the TRC's work.

Desmond Tutu emphasizes some of the theological truths that underpinned the work of the TRC, namely, the concepts of original sin (there is sin in all humans), the grace of God, and a nonjudgmental attitude (Meiring, 1999). However, he did not refer in Meiring's book to his own ubuntu theology that, to my mind, was a more important guiding force in the TRC's work than were the more generic theological truths mentioned in Meiring (1999).

Tutu's ubuntu theology, as studied by Michael Battle for his doctoral degree (1995) and published later in book form (Battle, 1997), is based on a Trinitarian image of God, i.e., the correct relation of Persons, and as such remains conventional and orthodox. What seems to be unique is the way that Tutu narrates Christian orthodoxy in a context of conflicting racial identities, which may be inspired by his Anglican ecclesiology (way of thinking about the church) and his African concept of community (ubuntu), according to which, loosely interpreted here, the image of God is found in human interdependence. This ubuntu theology aims to liberate oppressed people, *inter alia*, by emphasizing that all humans, including African people, are created in God's image. Ubuntu is called 'the environment of vulnerability, i.e., a set of relationships in which persons are able to recognize that their humanity is bound up in the other's humanity' (Battle, 1995). Ubuntu is also considered the quality of interaction in which one's own humanness depends upon its recognition in the other. Moreover, each individual's humanity is ideally expressed in relationship with others, and in turn, individuality is truly expressed. Battle calls Tutu's theology significant because one cannot distinguish his theory from his praxis. In the context of the TRC, Tutu's theology seems to have enhanced ubuntu, which made possible the confession and forgiveness of sin by perpetrators and victims respectively, within the safety of a mutually empathic relationship. Owing to space constraints, Tutu's ubuntu theology will not be described in further detail here. Neither will the criticisms leveled against Tutu's theology by Itumeleng J. Mosala and James Cone, as representatives of African theology and black (African American) theology respectively as discussed by Battle (1995, 1997), be discussed here.

There were some problems in the work of the TRC, such as that some parties did not want to participate in the process. For example, the TRC put three questions to all South African faith communities: To what extent had the faith community suffered or benefited from apartheid? What had the faith community done to support or oppose apartheid? What kind of expertise can the faith community contribute in the future to foster reconciliation and restitution? The response by the Synod of the Reformed Church of South Africa (RCSA), the teaching school or seminary for ministers in the smallest, most conservative (even fundamentalist), and most male-dominated of the three Afrikaans churches, was to refuse to make a submission to the TRC. Instead, a delegation of two members prepared a submission to the TRC in their personal capacities (Van der Walt and Naudé, 1996; Van der Walt and Venter, 1998). In their submission this delegation endorsed the same sequence of events that theoretically constituted reconciliation as defined by the TRC. However, it seems to me as if the delegation tended to defend themselves (hardly the spirit of reconciliation), and insisted on spiritualizing the gospel rather than engaging in socio-political dialogue like many of the other churches in South Africa had done. Moreover, it seems as if the elusiveness and relativity of the 'truth' was a convenient loophole for not naming specific human rights violations as was advocated by the TRC.

An unwillingness to confess turned out to be problematic in some instances. For example, the then leader of a right-wing political movement, Eugene Terre'blanche, declared that he would confess only to God and to no man. In another famous example, Ms Winnie Madikizela-Mandela spent many hours at the TRC vehemently denying numerous allegations brought against her, and then eventually, after being encouraged to do so, she acknowledged that some things had gone wrong and said that she was sorry, but it was not clear exactly what it was that she was sorry about (Meiring, 1999). In contrast, the necessity and reasons for confession were examined at the conference held by the Research Institute for Theology and Religion (RITR) at the University of South Africa in March 1998, led by Cornel W du Toit (1998). Prior to the conference, in July 1997, the RITR had sent an open letter of confession to 12 000 ministers and church leaders, had a 5% signed and returned rate, and had submitted the letter to the TRC. Although many of the church leaders had expressed hostility towards the TRC, by March 1998, 34 submissions had been made to the TRC by churches and religious bodies. Du Toit concluded that the offer of forgiveness and amnesty by the TRC had played a large role in the amount of truth that was confessed. He maintains that no forgiveness is possible without confession, and that the TRC made it possible for perpetrator and victim to face each other with confession and pardon.

Let us now consider the question raised at the beginning of this chapter, whether the approach adopted by the TRC with respect to intergroup conflict could also be applied to resolve interpersonal conflict.

It seems to me that within the ubuntu base of the TRC, the interpersonal and intergroup contexts overlapped, and the psychological construct of empathy that was experienced between individuals at the TRC became paradigmatic of intergroup empathy. The daily proceedings of the TRC seem to have relied on the empathy that was felt between individual perpetrators and victims, and by the audience at large, as the horrors of the human rights violations were shared. I think it became less important who was technically guilty of what, in the face of the shared human suffering. Although the TRC did not explicitly promote a role for empathy in the process of reconciliation, later work by Worthington, who was aware of the activities of the TRC as well as of the ubuntu culture in South Africa, did incorporate empathy (especially empathy for the transgressor) in a six-part model of reconciliation that he called 'FREE' ('Forgiveness and Reconciliation through Experiencing Empathy') (Worthington, 2001).

The narrative approach taken in the TRC's work represents another potential link between the interpersonal and intergroup contexts. Referring to the political process, Connor (1998) writes that reconciliation begins by a sharing of stories in a context of supportive understanding. The different stories then become a single story of common pain. Of course this would be the ideal outcome. In reality, the parties' stories might be so opposing that a gradual weaving together of those stories might appear unattainable at the outset. Or, for example, pride, rather than remorse, might drive amnesty-seekers' stories, complicating and possibly jeopardizing progress towards a single political story of common pain. If one considers the interpersonal context on the other hand, the value of a narrative therapeutic approach has been emphasized by Glick *et al.* (2000) and many others. More locally, for example, Christina Landman (1996a, b, 1998, 1999, 2000, 2001) uses a narrative approach for healing in the contexts of theology and religious counseling. She focuses, *inter alia*, on making audible the unheard stories of women, in a way that is comparable with that of the TRC that made audible the untold stories of political suffering.

I think the primary strength of the TRC probably lay in its ubuntu base, i.e., the ubuntu theology, as well as the ubuntu culture as lived by most South African people. In a context of ubuntu, relationships are preserved almost at all costs. The potential impact of such an ubuntu base has been recognized by Richard Bell (2002), who considers ubuntu and the South African truth and reconciliation process as substrates for African moral philosophy, which has implications for universal human issues such as restorative justice, communitarian civic order, and compassion-based morality. Secondarily, the approach of the TRC gained strength from its reliance on empathy and shared narrative.

Additionally, possibly, the success of the TRC also lay in the softening of polarities to find common middle ground and the softening of theological dualisms such as sin versus righteousness, or truth versus falsehood. As Masina also points out, ubuntu at the philosophical level seeks to find a balance between self and other, the destructive and the creative, good and bad; it moves away from dualisms in working toward mutually beneficial solutions (Masina, 2000). A further strength of the TRC might have been its facilitation of moral development in the different parties (this will be discussed later in this chapter).

However, if it was not for the given ubuntu culture and the strong religious adherence of the large majority of South Africans, I think the TRC might have failed in its aim of promoting national unity and reconciliation. Thinking more generally, not specifically of the South African context, I have reservations about the potential applicability of the TRC approach in other situations of political conflict, especially, for example, in Western contexts that might value individualism highly. Similarly, in the interpersonal context, I suspect that the value of the TRC approach (confessing sin, asking for forgiveness and mercy, and making amends) would be limited in situations where the conflicting parties do not value each other's humanity, or where the relationship and meaningful communication have broken down.

If the TRC approach might not work in situations of bad interpersonal conflict, would existing psychotherapeutic or other political approaches fare better? It seems odd, as will be shown below, that most psychotherapeutic approaches to couples conflict resolution, as well as the negotiation approach to solving political conflict, are based on the unrealistic assumption that conflicting parties would necessarily cooperate in the interests of reconciliation.

2.2 Psychotherapeutic approaches to conflict resolution require continuing relationships

Notwithstanding the immense benefit that many people derive from various types of psychotherapy, there are limitations to the value of psychotherapeutic approaches. Specifically in the context of couples therapy, where conflict resolution is often an issue, it seems that most approaches depend on a continuing relationship between two willing parties, or at least on some degree of cooperation between the conflicting parties. Moreover, these psychotherapeutic approaches are usually only said to be appropriate for relationship problems where the conflict has not been very severe, and are not considered appropriate where there has been partner abuse. However, the reality in many cases is that the conflict between the parties is quite severe and that the relationship between the parties has indeed deteriorated to the extent that one might describe it as having broken down. The parties might have very negative attitudes toward each other and might not value each other's humanity. In other words, the relationship might not resemble ubuntu. In these instances, I think the value of psychotherapeutic approaches is limited.

For example, James Donovan's psychodynamic-psychoanalytic approach to couples group therapy is one example of a psychotherapeutic approach that relies on a continuing relationship between two willing parties (Donovan, 1999). Each member of each of the couples gets turns to have his or her hidden feelings and defensive solutions probed and interpreted in the group situation. Donovan applies Malan's triangle of conflict (wish/hidden feeling/self-care—anxiety/self-blame—defensive solution/self-protection) to his own 'triangle of focus' (fight—family of origin—character conflicts) (1999). The fight is seen as a comment on the couple's relationship and as an interlocking defensive solution to each partner's family-of-origin and character conflicts. In group therapy, with each member of each couple, the defensive solutions are interpreted first, then the anxieties responsible for these solutions are probed, and finally the hidden feelings beneath are uncovered. The key is gaining insight and 'affective breakthrough'. Clearly such a procedure can only work if both members of each couple are motivated to benefit from the therapy.

In the cognitive-behavioral field, Weeks and co-workers give guidelines to 'fair fighting' as a method to resolve conflict, where they want partners to start by trying to understand the functions of each other's anger (Weeks and Treat, 1992; Weeks and Hof, 1995). For example, if one partner fears intimacy, anger might serve to regulate the distance between the partners. If one partner wishes for closeness, yet fears rejection or abandonment, anger might serve the function of testing the commitment of the other partner. If one partner fears being controlled and is unwilling to negotiate, anger might serve the function of asserting power and control. Moreover, the anger might be expressed directly or indirectly. Weeks and Hof list eight ways in which anger between partners can be expressed indirectly: collusion, passive aggression, moral one-upmanship, intellectualization, being nonrewarding and creating doubt, and being the 'helpless aggressor', 'sickness tyrant', or 'Red Cross nurse aggressor' (1995). In the latter three ways weakness is used as a vehicle for expression of anger. The next phase in 'fair fighting' then includes the learning of problem-solving techniques. This method relies on good communication skills and negotiation between the partners. Importantly, Weeks and Hof (1995) offer their conflict utilization model only for situations of 'low-level conflict' where anger and conflict are not instrumental or purposeful, and have not reached the level of abuse.

Similarly, the primarily cognitive-behavioral approach by Glick and colleagues (2000) considers couples in which active violence has been present, as not suitable candidates for couples work unless the therapist believes that the couple could hold to a no-violence contract. This guideline is based on the negative effect that violence has on the couple's honesty in therapy. For example, a wife who is afraid of being hit is anticipated not to be honest in therapy. The same restriction applies to Kim Halford's (2001) brief self-regulatory couples therapy. All these cognitive-behavioral approaches to couples therapy are only suitable where the members of a couple are on nonabusive speaking terms.

If we consider the psychotherapies that are informed by object relations, Susan Johnson bases her emotionally focused perspective of marital distress and adult intimacy on, *inter alia*, the attachment theory of Bowlby (Johnson, 1999). Marital distress is understood in terms of separation distress and an insecure bond between the partners. Anger, fear, and sadness are said to arise when an attachment figure is perceived as inaccessible or unresponsive. The resultant loss of connection is addressed in therapy by helping the couple to find the 'soft' emotions beneath the angry recriminations and to share empathic experience. In her words, 'placing distressed responses in an attachment context allows spouses to see and relate to their partner's pain'. Another example from object relations comes from Judith Siegel (1992), who links ego psychology and systems theory, and demonstrates how the object relations of each spouse affect the boundaries and defenses of the marital couple. According to this approach, the partners' internalized representations and introjects influence their subjective experience of relationships. Struggles from the family of origin are perpetuated in the dynamics of marriage. When unconscious conflicts from the representational world are re-enacted in the marital relationship, projective identification is said to occur interpersonally. Such projective identification makes an individual prone to deny the present reality or truth (Siegel, 1992). The idea is then to examine the representational worlds of both partners, and for the couple to develop insight into this—again, something that could only happen in a continuous relationship.

In a different vein, structural family therapy with couples deals 'not just with the dynamics of interaction between partners, but also with the boundaries around and between them' (Nichols and Minuchin, 1999). This kind of therapy relies on enactment in the therapy, to demonstrate the couple's interaction. Like the other therapies above, it relies on ongoing relationships and assumes that even conflictual relationships endure.

The few examples above do not represent an attempt to do justice to the vast field of psychotherapy, but merely serve to illustrate the point in a few instances that these forms of couples psychotherapy cannot be effective where relationships have broken down and couples are not willing to cooperate in therapy. At best, I think the value of these approaches is limited to situations where there is indeed some degree of cooperation. Critics of psychotherapeutic approaches might refer also to problems other than a reliance on a continuing relationship. Other problems might include, for example, that those psychotherapeutic approaches that are based on what might be considered patriarchal Freudian theory, might maintain the patriarchal system in couples to the detriment of the women partners. Or, for example, some psychotherapeutic approaches might, by their 'inward' emphasis, amount to 'blaming the victim' in cases where more assertive partners cannot understand why the less assertive partners might have a problem with the assertive ones' behavior.

2.3 Negotiation theory also depends on cooperation between conflicting parties

An attempt to apply principles from the business world in a psychotherapeutic context has not solved the above problem in the traditional psychotherapies. In her book on individual, couples and family therapy, Heitler uses negotiation theory, as contributed by the field of social psychology, and later by schools of law, business, and international relations, as a cornerstone for the development of her conflict resolution ideas in the context of psychotherapy (Heitler, 1990). Negotiation theory contributes the following elements to successful conflict resolution: clarification of issues, improvement of mutual understanding, reduction of hostile attitudes, assistance by a third party as a mediator, separation of broad issues into manageable subunits, identification of common superordinate goals, establishment of mechanisms for resolving future conflicts, and an awareness of the problems in an organization. A full understanding of oneself and one's opponent is taken to be the key to optimizing one's gain. Whereas mediators or negotiators help to resolve conflicts in the realms of government, law and business, counselors or therapists are said to do the same in the realms of personal and family distress (Heitler, 1990).

Heitler distinguishes positional bargaining from interest-based bargaining. In positional bargaining the parties initially have opposing positions, where their demands cannot be reconciled. Both parties eventually compromise towards common middle ground (as in haggling). This process appears rather two-dimensional. In interest-based bargaining, the assumption is that although the parties' positions may be opposed, their underlying interests may be shared or at least compatible. This allows for alternative solutions, other than the initial opposing demands or a compromise between them, which might still satisfy the interests of both parties. She then outlines three phases in her suggested route from conflict to resolution in psychotherapy: expressing the parties' initial positions, exploring the underlying concerns, and selecting mutually satisfying solutions (that are responsive to all the significant underlying concerns).

There are, however, drawbacks to using negotiation theory in psychotherapy. There are many steps in the process, and numerous potential substeps, which would require note keeping in order not to get lost in the details or to lose sight of some details. Owing to this heavy agenda, the process of negotiation seems to be quite time-intensive. Like other psychotherapies, it still relies on mutual cooperation between the conflicting parties, as well as the presence initially of a mediator (or therapist). The process cannot be effective if the two parties are not on speaking terms. Furthermore, the emphasis on the concrete issues about which there is conflict may detract from the deeper meanings and emotions that may underlie the conflict and may obscure problematic interactional styles (see below, Section 2.6—A developmental view of relationships may relativize the role of conflict in relationships); hence, the negotiation theoretical approach seems superficial. Moreover, the deeper issues might contribute to the process of negotiation being sabotaged. Also, the power gradients that often exist between conflicting parties may make negotiation difficult, even with the help of a mediator. Note that even in international politics recently, a number of instances of negotiation with mediation have not been very successful, e.g., the South African delegates' attempts to mediate in the Northern Ireland situation, and some of the more recent South African mediation attempts in the Ivory Coast situation. It may be possible that the failure of negotiation with mediation in these instances had something to do with deeper issues that were not being accommodated by the negotiation paradigm, or with power issues.

It seems, then, that for situations where a relationship has deteriorated beyond the possibility of cooperation, we would need to turn to contributions from other fields for a fresh perspective.

2.4 Game theory may offer a useful unilateral approach to conflict resolution where the relationship has broken down

Heitler's (1990) other application in the psychotherapeutic context of an idea that originated in a foreign field is more promising. She draws on mathematical game theory, from which cooperative versus competitive strategies for resolving conflicts have been developed. Briefly summarized from her book, Luce and Raiffa developed 'The Prisoner's Dilemma', a game theory paradigm, in

1957. According to this hypothetical problem, two prisoners facing long jail terms are given the options of confessing against the other ('defecting') or refusing to do so ('cooperating'). In short, prisoner A will be freed if he confesses against B, leaving B to serve the full sentence, but only if B did not confess against A (and vice versa). If A and B both confess against each other, both will serve the full sentence. If neither A nor B confesses against the other, both will serve lesser sentences. In the game of repeated choices, based on this dilemma, players A and B may not communicate about the option each will choose (defection or cooperation) in any given round of play. The game consists of a set number of rounds of play. Points are accrued so that in any one round, being freed translates to earning, e.g., 5 points, serving the full sentence translates to earning no points, and serving a lesser sentence translates to earning, e.g., 3 points. Axelrod, in 1984, investigated the benefits of choosing cooperation versus choosing self-interest at the expense of the other player in a game of Prisoner's Dilemma, by inviting game theorists to submit computer programs for playing this game. The winning program that offered the most effective strategy for earning points over multiple rounds of play, was Rapoport's 'Tit for Tat'. 'Tit for Tat' begins with a cooperative move (starting 'nice') and thereafter proceeds by returning cooperative for cooperative moves (kindness for kindness) and selfish moves for selfish moves (meanness for meanness), depending on what the other player chose. This proved to be the most robust, successful long-term strategy over a wide range of opponents' game plans.

Heitler (1990) then applies the above to real-life interpersonal relationships, in the form of general guidelines: although acting selfishly may maximize gain in brief encounters, solutions that optimize what both parties receive yield higher gains in ongoing relationships. Niceness pays and selfishness costs. Moreover, whereas excessive pessimism is expensive, optimism or basic trust (the expectation that the other will cooperate) yields higher gains. She also illustrates how 'forgiveness' can be built in (doing more than one nice move despite a selfish response by the opponent), which enhances the effectiveness of the 'Tit for Tat' approach.

The above contribution from game theory offers a potential way to approach conflict in interpersonal relationships, which maximizes mutual benefits by handling conflict cooperatively. Moreover, game theory is particularly useful in the context of this paper, as it depends neither on communication between the partners (which may often have broken down), nor on the presence of a third party as a mediator, as is often employed in couples therapy and in the resolution of political conflicts. Instead, either party can apply the approach unilaterally. Game theory also supports the developmental view of relationships that I shall discuss below.

However, there are potential pitfalls in this game theoretical approach. For example, one of the parties might play deviously, e.g., by deliberately acting selfishly in order to stall potential cooperation, regardless of the resultant loss of benefit to themselves. Furthermore, in situations of heterosexual couples conflict, one might anticipate that stereotyped gender role expectations might influence the moves that each partner makes. For example, a stereotyped expectation that 'women should be subordinate to men' might encourage a woman to err on the side of being too cooperative, and her partner to err on the side of being too selfish in their playing. This might jeopardize a good outcome, i.e., an outcome where conflict is minimized and cooperation is maximized.

Notwithstanding the potential utility of the available model of the Prisoner's Dilemma, Ellis, a South African applied mathematician and Quaker, points out a need for additional models from game theory, which might be more suitable to the issue of forgiveness (Ellis, 2001).

For now, let us keep in mind the above contribution from game theory, while we turn to systemic thinking next.

2.5 Systemic thinking may help to re-establish and sustain an improved relationship over time

Systems theory has mainly been applied to situations of family therapy, where the world is seen in relational, reciprocal terms, and where the concern is as much about the process as the content of a given relationship (Becvar and Becvar, 1988). Dorothy and Raphael Becvar (1988) contrast the Lockean approach of individual psychotherapy, where attention is invested in individuals and individual problems, and in why things happen, with the Kantian approach of systemic family therapy, where attention is turned towards relationship and relationship issues, and towards what is happening rather than why.

One of the strong points of therapies based on systemic theory is the stance of neutrality/curiosity that is encouraged by these approaches (Selvini et al., 1980; Aponte, 1985; Campbell and Draper, 1985; Boscolo et al., 1987; Cecchin, 1987), according to which the therapist models an attitude of respect, nondiscrimination, and acceptance of each system member's perspective as valid. Another strong point is the so-called circular thinking (Selvini et al., 1980; Aponte, 1985; Campbell and Draper, 1985; Boscolo et al., 1987; Cecchin, 1987), according to which interactional patterns are identified and potentially altered to improve relationships. One might have anticipated that these strong points would contribute toward the leveling out of power gradients among a system's members and a reduction in the frequency and intensity with which some members might violate the rights of other members. In other words, one might have anticipated that wrongs might not necessarily always be followed by more wrongs (as dictated by the old idea that every action has a reaction), if systemic thinking is applied in therapy.

On the other hand, in a very different context, the religious discourse of 'sin—confession—forgiveness' has traditionally been the discourse where wrongs were not necessarily followed by more wrongs. Instead, through the grace of God, wrongs could be undone, forgiven, and reversed. Whereas this religious discourse is quite linear, the question arises whether the more circular systemic thinking might also have something to offer with a view to conflict resolution and reconciliation in instances where the relationship has broken down as a result of human rights violations, and with a view to moral development of the parties.

However, the problem seems to be that systemic therapy as used for family problems (Campbell and Draper, 1985; Becvar and Becvar, 1988; Boscolo et al., 1987), does not focus on conflict resolution and reconciliation in the same way as is done in theology, psychology, or politics. It is as if the discourse of truth, forgiveness, and reconciliation is foreign to systemic thinking. Although the terms 'marital conflict' and 'tension' are used in systemic therapy, no reference is made, e.g., in Becvar and Becvar (1988) to 'forgiveness', 'reconciliation', 'anger', 'aggression', 'violence', or 'abuse'. Systemic therapists tend not to assign blame, or call abuse, abuse. This might be due to the neutrality advocated by systemic approaches, their descriptive stance, and their permissiveness. In such a context of neutrality, the most value-laden or 'worst' descriptor that a systemic therapist might assign to a family is probably 'conflictual', possibly 'dysfunctional'. Instead of forgiveness or reconciliation, systemic therapists might talk of 'accommodation' or 'negotiation' as keys to the successful navigation of life as a family (Becvar and Becvar, 1988).

Notwithstanding the value of several aspects of systemic therapeutic thinking, it runs the risk of dismissing a phenomenon such as interpersonal abuse, as a part of a functional system. In this regard, George Steinfeld (1997), an experienced couples therapist, points out that systemic, interactional neutrality is not therapeutic in cases of family violence: 'Therapeutic neutrality in these cases are acts of omission (thereby subtly reinforcing the *status quo*) and, as a result, contributes to the maintenance of the problem.' Thus systemic therapy might gloss over human rights violations without having anything to offer to the victims. This point is also acknowledged by Claire Worrell Haslam and Phyllis Erdman (2003) when they refer to some feminist researchers who dispute the appropriateness of applying a systems approach to conceptualizing couples violence, as the systemic approach relieves the perpetrator of responsibility for the violence. However, Worrell Haslam and Erdman still find it useful to link systems and attachment theories to provide a conceptual framework for marital violence.

Despite this problem, systemic thinking can be useful for the purpose of the perspective explored in this paper, in the following ways: it supports reintroduction of parties to each other, and it also supports narrative reconstruction of identity in both parties. Additionally, it contributes towards the developmental perspective on relationships that is discussed in the next section.

2.5.1 Systemic thinking supports reintroduction of parties to each other

The sharing of stories in the context of the TRC makes sense from a systemic perspective, where such sharing reintroduces the parties to each other. The parties then get to know and understand each other in a spirit of neutral curiosity. Thus the parties establish and sustain a (new) relationship (Connor, 1998; Long and Brecke, 2003), as if on a new playing field. Such mutual introduction and understanding would then foster mutual empathy, which in turn might redress the balance of power and control between conflicting parties. Of course the previously powerful party might have a vested interest in maintaining the *status quo* and might therefore not participate empathically in the process. Perhaps such an approach of reintroduction might only be useful in instances where the party that wielded the power also happens to possess a sense of moral responsibility.

Although this idea of re-getting to know each other seems to be particularly systemic, it has also been advocated in nonsystemic couples–psychotherapeutic contexts. For example, Margaret Waller and Michael Spiegler (1997) work with the assumptions that an intimate relationship requires a sense of freedom to be one's uncensored self in the presence of the loved one, that intimacy involves extensive self-disclosure, and that intimate partners cannot conceal essential parts of themselves without jeopardizing the relationship. Although they focus on cross-cultural differences, they offer their model of accepting differences, managing maladaptive reactions to differences, and co-constructing 'a common couple culture' as applying to all types of differences between partners. 'Truth' often emphasizes 'difference' (and might seem to preclude reconciliation), but the acceptance of those differences (on a new playing field) and the construction of a new 'truth' might actually help the relationship problem. In another example of a nonsystemic context, namely, a social psychology context, or more specifically a social constructionist context, Holmes and Murray (1996) advocate the creation of a new truth in the process of interacting, in situations of couples conflict.

2.5.2 Systemic thinking supports narrative reconstruction of identity

The above systemic reintroduction of conflicting parties to each other may contribute to a narrative reconstruction of identity in both parties, as suggested by a number of authors. For example, Long and Brecke (2003), who studied 11 case studies of civil war and eight of international conflict, refer to the redefinition of the identities of former belligerents. The strategy of changing social identity to facilitate conflict resolution is also advocated by Smith and Mackie (2000, pp. 503–48). For the purpose of this chapter, the focus will be on the work of Hicks (2001), an expert in international conflict analysis and resolution, as contained in the edited volume by Helmick and Petersen (2001) that followed a symposium held at Harvard University in 1999. The volume includes contributions from the fields of theology, ethics, Christian ethics, social psychology, clinical psychology, political psychology, political science, strategic and international studies, public law and security, public policy and administration, diplomatic service, social science, human rights law, and applied mathematics.

Hicks' assumptions about identity include the idea that identity has two aspects—a core identity and a socially constructed identity. She states that the process of identity development requires social interaction in the context of relationship. Moreover, she considers identity development as a life-long process—or in other words, identity is in constant evolution if one is open to learning (Hicks, 2001).

She claims that when one's learning mechanisms are overloaded, one's beliefs about oneself and others freeze as a stabilizing mechanism, and one's beliefs become rigid and resistant to change in the interests of self-protection. Conflict may cause one's learning mechanisms to become overloaded. When the nature of interaction between two people or groups becomes threatening (as in conflict), the process of identity formation may shut down, along with other learning mechanisms. The threat thus also applies on an existential level to the participants' identity. The normal flow of identity development is interrupted and the parties' identities do not develop further, as both parties may be unable to learn from information they receive from the other party. Instead, both parties' beliefs about themselves and the other remain static and become rigid, and both may be certain that they are right. This might in turn lead to reduced interaction and a further diminished chance of incorporating disconfirming information from the other (i.e., information that would challenge each party's beliefs about themselves and the other).

The problem with identity in inter-ethnic conflict seems to be that an acknowledgement of the identity of the other is perceived as an act of self-destruction. This happens because a recognition of the experiences of the other brings into question one's own interpretation of history, the conflict, and of the responsibility one holds for the past, present, and future shared realities. Conflict acts as a threat to the parties' identities, and more broadly, a threat to the way we maintain our inner sense of coherence and stability.

Hicks points out that current political conflict resolution and reconciliation processes have not addressed the issue of identity. She advocates the reconstruction of identity through narrative as a critical component to the process of reconciliation. Hicks refers to Kelman's description of 'negotiating identity', where both sides engage in a reciprocal examination of their identities. Each party would narrate their version of the conflict story and both parties would examine the implications of these narrated versions for their respective identities (in other words, what the stories say about the parties). Such negotiation with a view to reconciliation is likely to be more fruitful if the individuals have progressed from an egocentric stance (embedded in one's own perspective, unable to tolerate ambivalence) to a more sociocentric stance (capable of tolerating multiple perspectives, able to accept uncertainty and ambivalence) (Hicks, 2001). The parties should open themselves up to new information about the other and oneself. For example, the group that she calls the 'high power group' or 'dominators' have to accept those aspects of their identity that were capable of traumatizing the other, while still protecting their human dignity. On the other hand, the 'low power group' or 'dominated' have to let go of the moral advantage that has been the source of their power for the duration of the conflict. The moral advantage of the victims arises from the fact that they are not the ones who are or were guilty of perpetrating the wrongdoing, e.g., violence or abuse. (cf. Claudia Card's reference to the moral power of victims of oppression; Card, 1999). Notwithstanding the moral advantage of those who are victims of oppression, the victims are at risk of moral compromise in ambiguous moral 'gray zones', and at risk of complicity, under stress, in perpetrating oppression on others (Card, 1999).

Hicks' reconciliation depends on the restoration of human dignity to both groups, and a reconstruction of both sides' narratives so that a 'mutually tolerable interpretation of the past' is achieved, paving the way for a shared future in the context of a relationship that permits both groups' identities to develop and flourish. For example, whereas party A might previously have regarded party B as terrorists who undermine democracy, party B's interpretation might have been that party A were completely disinterested in party B's attempts to have their (party B's) needs met in a reciprocal relationship. A 'mutually tolerable interpretation of the past' might, for example, be that the previous power imbalance between the two parties had oppressive consequences that were intolerable to party B. Thus the new joint narrative may be more than just an appreciation of the other's story, but may involve corrections, new interpretations, and sometimes integrations. The process of storytelling itself seems to reveal each party's story in new ways, so that neither of the parties keeps on telling the same old story with their same interpretations. Rather, they discover themselves and the other through creating a new story that is more accurate and acceptable to both parties and that accounts for both parties' previous experiences.

Although this narrative-based, systemically sensitive approach appears very valuable on the whole, there seems to be a risk, in cases of protracted conflict and associated long periods of interrupted identity development, especially as is found, e.g., in ideological contexts such as paternalism or patriarchy where roles and identities are socially entrenched, that the parties might not be able to engage without fear in a process of negotiating and reconstructing their identities. For example, an abused woman might be too afraid of further abuse to tell her side of the story in the context of couples therapy, based on previous experiences of suffering abuse whenever she dared to differ from her abuser or whenever she did not comply with the abuser's demands.

Similarly, on a more concrete level, the ideological context of apartheid in South Africa would have jeopardized the chances of mutual reconstructing of identities by keeping groups of people physically separated from each other. In such instances of relationship breakdown, it might be fruitful for either party to revert initially to a unilateral approach to the relationship (for example, the game theoretically informed developmental approach discussed below) until an atmosphere of cooperation can be re-established.

Another problem would arise if, in the process of reintroduction or identity reconstruction, one party gets to know the other party as seemingly incapable of engaging meaningfully in the relationship. Here, too, the first party might consider reverting to a unilateral, more behavioral, less abstract, game theoretically based approach.

2.6 A developmental view of relationships may relativize the role of conflict in relationships

If one combines aspects of game theory, as discussed by Heitler (1990), and a systemic view of conflict in relationships, with a developmental view of relationships, the role of conflict is relativized. In such a perspective, each instance of conflict represents merely another 'speech act' or 'relationship act' in an ongoing relationship, or a single 'round' in the ongoing game of the relationship. The conflictual relationship act can be considered as the undesirable outcome of a specific round of interaction in the relationship. A regular pattern of interaction where a conflictual relationship act tends to be the usual outcome would indicate 'stuckness' and a failure of the relationship to continue its desired natural development and growth.

Rather than harping on a single instance of conflict that needs to be resolved, the game theoretical contribution to the suggested perspective would encourage the making of repeated choices for cooperation over time in successive rounds of play. Each instance of conflict represents a single round in a longer game. The round is played, and then that instance of conflict is 'dropped', forgotten, or at least relativized as one enters the next round in the game. An instance of conflict might also be regarded as a dead-end in the developmental road of the relationship, where there are no more options for development. In such a scenario, the thing to do would be to go back along the road to find an alternative route (for the next round in the development of the relationship). Such a view might relieve the urgency for dramatic intervention at a specific instance of conflict in an ongoing relational problem.

The systemic contribution to the above perspective informs a potential approach to bring about change in situations of repetitive conflict. The approach would be to focus away from the content, i.e., the specific topic of the conflict, and rather to look at the process, i.e., the way or style of interacting. The parties would gradually become reintroduced to each other's patterns of interaction, and this might facilitate reconstruction of both their identities. The aim would be to facilitate a shift in the system's pattern of interaction in successive rounds, so that a conflictual relationship act is not always the outcome of interaction. Such a shift in the system's way of interacting might well entail that the interactions more frequently end up being 'cooperative' rather than 'selfish', in the game theoretical sense.

The above developmental view of relationships as informed by aspects of game theory and systemic thinking is compatible with more traditional psychotherapeutic approaches. For example, Sheila Sharpe (2000) augments object relations approaches to couples therapy by adding a multifaceted view of relationship development. She presents an object relations based, developmental formulation of how love relationships consist of multiple patterns of relating that develop in parallel over time in an interrelated fashion. She identifies seven universal, central relationship patterns, including patterns of connection (nurturing, merging, and idealizing) and patterns of separateness (devaluing, controlling, competing for superiority, and competing in love triangles). These patterns are said to reflect everyone's relational needs. The patterns have their origins in the individuals' early relationship development. An optimal outcome is a balance between a mutual relationship and individual growth. However, when one of these patterns dominates or rigidifies, the relationship cannot grow and becomes stagnant or destructive. Therapy would focus on understanding the couple's patterns as reflecting each partner's wishes for and fears of intimacy and self-development.

It might seem that if one applies game theory and systemic thinking to a developmental view of relationships, one might have a practical solution for situations of conflict where the relationship has largely broken down and, e.g., couples therapy using Sharpe's method (2000) is not possible, or where a couple is not on speaking terms to allow, e.g., the weaving in of their respective narratives into the fabric of a new relationship. In the above developmental approach, no cooperation between the partners would be required at the outset. One of the parties might start the game of developing the relationship in the direction of cooperation. Moreover, the process need not concern hot, conflictual issues initially; the process could be practiced first on lesser, more mundane issues. All that seems to be needed is a little bit of daring on the side of the first player, a small act of optimism, and a single act of 'niceness' to serve as an invitation to the other party to play another round in the game of developing the relationship. Arguably, this approach might also be used by a group of people in situations of political conflict.

Note that the suggested rounds in the game of this relationship would be simple instances of interaction. The focus for change would be on the process (style of interacting) rather than on the content (the topics around which the parties tend to get stuck). Of course the content of conflict is important, as it represents the substrate in which the relationship grows or does not grow, but the content cannot be resolved without mutually suitable interactional skills. The idea would be to aim for repeated choices for cooperation.

However, it could be argued that such an approach might be too naïve to be of help in tough cases of relationship breakdown. For example, in some cases of protracted conflict, a single instance of conflict might endure. The parties might be unable to 'drop' the issue, especially if it is ideologically based and maintained, or socially entrenched. In such cases, the relationship would become stuck and it might be impossible for the relationship to develop beyond that point. This would result in a pernicious and deep division in the relationship. Furthermore, the above approach might fail where either or both of the parties are so psychologically and morally damaged that they are devious, mean, and unwilling to contribute towards an improved relationship. In such cases the prognosis for relationship development would seem poor.

Notwithstanding these problems, one of the potential positive side-effects of the above approach might be the moral development of the second player from playing 'selfishly' to playing 'cooperatively' despite her/himself (see below). The desired outcome would be a situation where conflict is no longer the defining characteristic of the relationship and where both parties are able to engage in further cooperative relationship development, which would ideally include the integration of their respective historical narratives in an improved relationship.

2.7 The suggested perspective on conflict resolution and reconciliation may foster moral development

The question is: What are the implications of the developmental perspective on conflict resolution and reconciliation for the issue of moral development?

Again, the example of the TRC will be considered before focusing on interpersonal conflict. It is not only in perpetrators that moral growth might occur, in cases of conflict where there is indeed a perpetrator, but victims would also be involved in a process of moral development. Although moral development is used here primarily in an individual sense, it might also be useful at another time to consider the implications of reconciliation for moral development in an anthropological sense (Hallpike, 1998/2001). Furthermore, the quality of the relationship as an abstract entity might develop with respect to its moral sophistication. Owing to the potential scope of this section of the chapter, I shall focus only on a few contributions from the field of moral philosophy.

The work of the South African TRC has been recognized to contribute to the moral development of the participants, and this moral development has been considered in religious terms. The South African NIR's (Nürnberger and Tooke, 1988) official theological statement on reconciliation (also referred to earlier in this chapter) seems to hinge on moral development: 'In reconciliation, God's suffering acceptance of people's unacceptability transforms them into what He intends them to be.' This transformation happens, *inter alia*, through redressing wrongs, which may need to take the form of social action for justice. Connor (1998) also supports the idea of moral development in his Roman Catholic interpretation of forgiveness in the South African TRC experience when he refers to regaining dignity and true humanity so as to serve others better. He emphasizes that such reconciliatory development takes time and cannot be rushed. In contexts other than the South African TRC, such moral development has been described as 'the 'opponent' being weaned from error by patience and sympathy' (Da Silva, 2001) and 'a complex dynamic of disciplined watchfulness and patient encouragement' (Livingston, 2002).

Alternatively, for the purpose of evaluating the TRC's contribution to moral development in the light of other moral theories, I shall briefly consider only a few of these theories.

According to Lawrence Kohlberg's theory, moral development is a social process linked to the general physical, psychological, social, and spiritual development of the individual (Kohlberg 1817/1981, 1817/1984). 'Social process' means that an individual develops her or his morality in interaction with others. Kohlberg's model of moral development occurred in a linear way, through three levels, with each level consisting of two stages, for a total of six stages: In Level 1 (Pre-conventional morality), Stage 1 refers to whether behavior should be rewarded or punished, and Stage 2 refers to what can be gained. In Level 2 (Conventional morality), Stage 3 concerns approval, and Stage 4 concerns respect for authority and the best interest of society. In Level 3 (Post-conventional morality), Stage 5 distinguishes between an orderly society and a just society, and Stage 6 refers to a universal system of ethical principles (Kohlberg 1817/1981, 1817/1984). His theory has been said to strive towards objective, hierarchical principles of justice (Gilligan, 1997a,b).

However, Kohlberg's theory is flawed in that it was developed through studying boys, without studying girls, yet presented itself as pertaining to 'human' moral development. Carol Gilligan studied girls, first using Kohlberg's theory, then independently of his theory (Gilligan, 1982/1993, 1995, 1997a,b, 2000; Bernstein and Gilligan, 1990; McLean et al., 1996). She discovered a 'different voice'—a voice of an ethic of care (Gilligan, 1982/1993, 1997a, 2000), according to which moral development occurred through three levels: Level 1 refers to an orientation to individual survival. Then the first transition occurs from selfishness to responsibility. Level 2 refers to goodness as self-sacrifice. This stage is said to engender psychological violence. The second transition occurs from goodness to truth. Level 3 subsumes the injunctions to 'care for others' and to 'care for self' under the moral principle of nonviolence (Gilligan, 1997a). Gilligan's levels have parallels with Kohlberg's levels in that they progress from pre-conventional through conventional to post-conventional. However, whereas Kohlberg described a post-conventional justice and rights-based morality, Gilligan described a post-conventional contextualism (Benhabib, 1997). Gilligan's work suggests that patterns of moral thinking might be gender-related. Whereas a man-way of reasoning about relationships might conjure an image of hierarchy, a woman-way of thinking about relationships might conjure an image of a web (Norlin et al., 2003). Gilligan's work deservedly has had a major impact in the field of moral philosophy

(Gilligan, 1995, 1997a, b, 2000; Moody-Adams, 1991; McLean *et al.*, 1996). It should be noted that critics of Gilligan find her model as stereotyped as Kohlberg's and claim that her model does not allow for diversity in moral discourse (Moody-Adams, 1991).

Other theories of moral development include that of Martin Hoffman (2000), where the focus is on empathy. Furthermore, John Gibbs (2003) integrates Kohlberg's and Hoffman's theories and offers an approach to understanding and treating antisocial youths.

In a different vein, Krebs challenged the notion of linearity when he viewed Kohlberg's model from the perspective of evolutionary biology (2000). According to Krebs, people's real-life moral decisions usually advance their adaptive interests. He also considers game theory research on adaptive strategies of cooperation and concludes that adaptive interests might lead people to uphold systems of cooperation. Krebs (2000) suggests that the evolution of morality parallels the evolution of cooperation. He contrasts selfish individualism with indiscriminate altruism and the 'Tit for Tat' of Axelrod and Rapoport (cf. Heitler, 1990). Hence, Krebs considers Kohlberg's Stage 1 to correspond to selfish individualism and deferring to more powerful people; Kohlberg's Stage 2 corresponds to systems of direct reciprocity where the aim is to maximize individual returns, e.g., gains in trade; Stage 3 corresponds to systems of indirect reciprocity among members of in-groups, based on the reputation of its members; Stage 4 corresponds to complex social systems of indirect reciprocity where reward and punishment are institutionalized. According to Krebs' empirical research, the first three stages usually are affectively based and used in real-life situations, whereas Kohlberg's Stages 5–6 are 'colder', more logical, and seldom used in real-life situations. Even so, he suggests that when Stages 5–6 are implemented, it is done in order to uphold the systems of cooperation from which the person stands to benefit. Krebs does not consider moral development as a linear process; instead, he says, people retain what they learned earlier, so that they acquire a broad range of moral strategies for use in different situations.

If the TRC's work is interpreted superficially according to Kohlberg's theory, then the initial moral inadequacy of the perpetrators of human rights violations might point towards a Kohlbergian developmental level in the very early stages. Appropriately then, the TRC approach that focused on confession and forgiveness in a theological sense might be considered to have represented a moral developmental strategy aimed at orienting perpetrators towards a concern with the approval of God and respect for authority and the best interests of society as served by the rule of law (cf. Kohlberg's Stages 3 and 4—a justice-based approach to moral development).

However, if one takes Krebs (2000) seriously, one can recognize elements of several Kohlbergian stages concurrently in the victims who participated in the TRC. Alongside Stage 2 strategies, e.g., as demonstrated in the armed struggle for democracy, the victims' use of Stage 5 and 6 strategies could be considered to have served their adaptive interests, as changing and improving the society would end the unjust oppression that the victims had suffered.

If the moral developmental contribution of the TRC is evaluated in the light of Gilligan's model, it might be thought of as an example of Level 3 post-conventional contextualism, i.e., care for self (using principles of justice to protect human rights and effect restitution) and care for others (offering forgiveness and amnesty), under a morality of nonviolence (that included the renunciation of the armed struggle for democracy).

Notwithstanding the moral value of the theological underpinnings of the TRC's work and the value of the abovementioned moral theories for understanding the TRC's contribution to moral development, I think the TRC also contributed to moral development via its underlying driving force of ubuntu. The TRC remained true to the ubuntu principle of preserving the relationship between victims and perpetrators. This ubuntu driven preservation of the relationship in the context of the TRC might exemplify the abovementioned web-based way of moral thinking about relationships as opposed to the more hierarchical way of thinking found in societies dominated by men, such as most Western societies and also South Africa. The preservation of the 'pre-Colonial', 'alternative' ubuntu morality right inside a male-dominated society might have had something to do with the surprising success of the TRC project in South Africa, despite the surface inadequacies of the TRC process.

Furthermore, the ubuntu contribution of the TRC might have ensured that the process of (theologically informed) moral development did not run the risk of ending up as a spiritual abstraction, but became translated in many instances into concrete social action for justice in a context of communal empathy. In this case, social (moral) action for justice included things such as regulating measures of restitution for victims of human rights' violations, and on a wider scale, regulating a more equitable distribution of resources, *inter alia*, through reversing the previous forced removal of people from land, where possible.

Let us return now to the above-suggested potential developmental perspective on conflict resolution and reconciliation in the interpersonal context and the question of whether it might foster moral development. Clearly, neither theologically based nor ubuntu based moral development, as happened in the intergroup context of the TRC, could occur in situations of interpersonal conflict where the relationship and meaningful communication have broken down. Furthermore, Kohlberg's (1817/1981, 1817/1984) theory of moral development cannot contribute much to explaining potential moral development in situations of interpersonal conflict with relationship breakdown either. According to his theory, progression from one moral stage to the next happens in a childhood context where there is ongoing (healthy) social interaction, rather than the scenario that is the focus of this chapter (an adult context of interpersonal conflict where the relationship has broken down).

Krebs' point (2000), drawing on game theory research, that people's adaptive interests might lead them to uphold systems of cooperation, and his point that the evolution of morality parallels the evolution of cooperation, might help to explain potential moral development in the suggested developmental perspective on conflict resolution and reconciliation in situations of interpersonal conflict with relationship breakdown. In such cases, if a victim party (e.g., a victim of psychological abuse) were to initiate a cooperative 'relationship act' unilaterally, the perpetrator party would in effect be invited to re-engage in relationship and be called on to react. Game theory and a 'Tit for Tat' approach by the victim party would dictate that even though the perpetrator party might be inclined to react selfishly, she or he would gradually be conditioned to react cooperatively, as this would maximize his or her own gains through repeated rounds of interaction. Thus the perpetrator party would develop in a moral sense from playing 'selfishly' to playing 'cooperatively' despite him- or herself.

In the scenario sketched in the previous paragraph, moral development might also occur in the victim party, possibly along the lines of Gilligan's theory again (Gilligan, 1982/1993, 1995, 1997a, 2000): The victim of psychological abuse might obtain a balance between 'caring for other' (by continually re-inviting the other party to engage in relationship), 'caring for self' (surviving, for example, by pursuing justice in a tit for tat way) and doing so under a principle of nonviolence (by rewarding with cooperation only those interactions from the perpetrator's side that do not, through their own selfishness, demand self-sacrifice from the victim).

Notwithstanding the potential moral development of either of the parties, the concept of moral development might also apply in a spiral kind of way to the conflictual relationship between the parties, in which the quality of the interactional style might gradually improve over time in successive rounds of interaction. Such improvement in interactional style might be thought of as moral growth of the relationship. The desired outcome might be a situation where conflict is no longer the defining characteristic of the relationship and where both parties are able to engage in further cooperative relationship development, which would ideally include the integration of their respective historical narratives in an improved relationship.

Although a more detailed discussion of the potential fostering of moral development by the developmental approach to interpersonal conflict will not be undertaken here, it appears as if, despite starting from a situation of relationship breakdown, this approach might foster moral development in a number of different ways. Perhaps the key is that the suggested approach might provide a potential route for re-establishing relatedness—a relationship that might then serve as the substrate upon which further moral development can occur.

2.8 **Conclusions**

The argument was that the (successful) politico-religious approach of the South African TRC to intergroup conflict cannot be applied directly in the resolution of interpersonal conflict in situations where the relationship has broken down, because the TRC's success hinged, *inter alia*, on its ubuntu base, or its embeddedness in a social context of human interrelatedness. Similarly, most of the existing approaches to couples psychotherapy, as well as negotiation theory, rely on a continuing relationship between two willing parties. Hence, they have limited value in situations of relationship breakdown.

The aim was to explore a perspective on conflict resolution and reconciliation that does not rely on a continuous relationship between two willing parties. This social psychiatric perspective on conflict resolution and reconciliation—developed with reference to existing models in the fields of game theory, negotiation theory, systemic therapeutic thinking, various psychotherapies, Christian theology, and South African culture—appears to have a structure of its own, of which the potential theoretical and practical applications might fruitfully be explored further.

This proposed model might be called a 'spiral of growth' model for conflict resolution, reconciliation, and relationship development. It was suggested that conflict resolution and reconciliation might be facilitated if conflict is conceptualized (and hence contextualized and relativized) as one round in a developing spiral of relationship, after which round the parties are reintroduced to each other and establish an alternative relationship. The idea of each conflictual relationship act representing a round, or a circle, enables the parties to obtain closure and leave that round of conflict behind in their progression along the line of relationship development. The act of applying the model constitutes a willingness to re-engage in a reciprocal relationship, albeit a new version of the relationship, with new rules (including adaptive strategies of cooperation) and 'new' players (reintroduced to each other, and in the process of reconstructing their identities). Furthermore, the act of applying the model also constitutes optimism about the future developmental potential of the relationship, including the potential for moral growth of both parties, as well as the moral development of the relationship as such.

More specifically, the contribution from game theory (the 'Tit for Tat' approach to the 'Prisoner's Dilemma') means the proposed perspective may be applied unilaterally where the relationship has broken down, to encourage repeated choices for cooperation in successive rounds of interaction. The contribution from systemic thinking means this perspective may help to re-establish and sustain an improved relationship between the conflicting parties, through reintroduction, focusing on the style rather than the content of the conflict, and narrative reconstruction of their identities. A developmental view of relationships relativizes the role of conflict and fosters optimism about gradual reconciliation despite conflict. The contribution from moral philosophy (especially the ethic of care for self and others) means this perspective may foster moral development in both parties and the relationship, through re-establishing relatedness.

The model's greatest strength probably lies in its nonreliance on continuous, cooperative relationships between two willing parties. In cases where the relationship between two conflicting parties has broken down, the model might initially be applied unilaterally by one of the parties. Arguably, the effect might be similar whether the party might be an individual or a group of people. An oppressed party might also be able to apply the model to the relationship with the oppressor, in cases where the latter consistently and deliberately damages the relationship. Thus an oppressed party might contribute to their own emancipation and development as well as to the development and growth of the relationship to an improved version. This is not to say that I hold only the oppressed party responsible for developing the relationship. Indeed, oppressors should be held accountable not only for the way that they treat others in their relationships, but also for developing their relationships.

Admittedly, a unilateral application of the model might yield neither immediate, nor longer-term returns in terms of a rewarding relationship. Furthermore, reconciliation might be fraught with problems, even if both parties participate actively in the process. For example, if in the reintroduction process, the parties get to know each other as subscribing to incompatible ideologies or points of view on a certain matter, reconciliation would be jeopardized. Even in situations of cooperative relationship development, reintroduction might bring surprises, and reconstruction of identities is unlikely to overlap completely between the parties.

Although reconciliation is not guaranteed, this 'spiral of growth' model might at least initiate and maintain a series of relationship acts where there might have been none, or establish a better pattern than there might have been before. And if mathematical game theory is sound, then the chances seem good that even such a seemingly meaningless series of relationship acts might develop into a more cooperative pattern, and might improve from a moral point of view. Thus this proposed model might help to fill the gap between protracted conflict (possibly with violence and/or minimal contact between the parties) and successful reconciliation (potentially including confession, forgiveness, and meaningful cooperation).

From a methodological perspective, this model derives strength from its integration of apparently opposing ideas from various fields on a number of levels. It integrates the idea of continuous psychological development with the 'stop–start–stop–start' quality that seems to characterize so many interpersonal relationships. Also, it integrates and cross-fertilizes between the fields of interpersonal relationships and intergroup relationships, illustrating a holistic approach to people in their social contexts. Furthermore, it represents an example of potential conceptual integration between the seemingly irreconcilable fields of psychiatry/psychology and religion/theology.

Notwithstanding the potential problems, it might be worthwhile to develop this model further, especially with respect to the prognosis for reconciliation towards a sustained, mutually enriching relationship, with respect to the possibilities for moral development in both parties and the relationship, and with respect to its potential for empowerment of oppressed parties in both interpersonal and intergroup conflict.

References

Anderson PS (2001). A feminist ethics of forgiveness. In: *Forgiveness and Truth: Explorations in Contemporary Theology* (eds AI McFadyen and M Sarot), pp. 145–55. Edinburgh: T & T Clark.

Aponte HJ (1985). The negotiation of values in therapy. *Family Process*, **24**: 323–38.

Aronson E, Wilson TD, and Akert RM (1999). *Social Psychology*, 3rd edition. New York: Longman Publishing.

Battle MJ (1995). The Ubuntu theology of Desmond Tutu: How Desmond Tutu's theological model of community facilitates reconciliation among races in a system of apartheid (Dissertation for the degree of Doctor of Philosophy in the Department of Religion in the Graduate School of Duke University). Ann Arbor, MI: UMI Dissertation Services.

Battle M (1997). *Reconciliation: The Ubuntu theology of Desmond Tutu*. Cleveland, OH: The Pilgrim Press.

Becvar DS and Becvar RJ (1988). *Family Therapy: A Systemic Integration*. Boston: Allyn and Bacon.

Bell RH (2002). *Understanding African Philosophy: A Cross-Cultural Approach to Classical and Contemporary Issues*. New York: Routledge Publishers.

Benhabib S (1997). The generalized and the concrete other: The Kohlberg-Gilligan controversy and moral theory. In: *Feminist Social Thought: A Reader* (ed. DT Meyers), pp. 736–56. New York: Routledge Publishers.

Bernstein E and Gilligan C (1990). Unfairness and not listening: Converging themes in Emma Willard girls' development. In: *Making Connections: The Relational Worlds of Adolescent Girls at Emma Willard School* (eds C Gilligan, NP Lyons, and TJ Hanmer), pp. 147–61. Cambridge: Harvard University Press.

Biggar N (2001). Forgiveness in the twentieth century: a review of the literature, 1901–2001. In: *Forgiveness and Truth: Explorations in Contemporary Theology* (eds AI McFadyen and M Sarot), pp. 181–217. Edinburgh: T & T Clark.

Bonhoeffer D (1949/1966). *Ethics* (ed. E Bethge) (trans. NH Smith). London: Collins Press.

Boscolo L, Cecchin G, Hoffman L, and Penn P (1987). *Milan Systemic Therapy: Conversations in Theory and Practice.* New York: Basic Books.

Braungart RG and Braungart MM (1993). Generational conflict and intergroup relations as the foundation for political generations. In: *Social Psychology of Groups: A Reader* (eds EJ Lawler and B Markovsky), pp. 253–77. Greenwich, CT: JAI Press.

Campbell D and Draper R (eds) (1985). *Applications of Systemic Family Therapy: The Milan Approach.* London: Grune & Stratton, Harcourt Brace Jovanovich.

Card C (1999). Groping through gray zones. In: *On Feminist Ethics and Politics* (ed. C Card), pp. 3–26. Lawrence, KS: University Press of Kansas.

Cecchin G (1987). Hypothesising, circularity, and neutrality revisited: An invitation to curiosity. *Family Process* 26 (4): 405–413.

Chapman AR and Spong B (eds) (2003). *Religion and Reconciliation in South Africa: Voices of Religious Leaders.* Philadelphia, PA: Templeton Foundation Press.

Connor BF (1998). *The Difficult Traverse from Amnesty to Reconciliation.* Pietermaritzburg, South Africa: Cluster Publications.

Da Silva A (2001). Through nonviolence to truth: Gandhi's vision of reconciliation. In: *Forgiveness and Reconciliation: Religion, Public Policy, and Conflict Transformation* (ed. RG Helmick and RL Petersen), pp. 305–27. Philadelphia, PA: Templeton Foundation Press.

Delamater J (2003). *Handbook of Social Psychology.* New York: Kluwer Academic/Plenum Publishers.

Donovan JM (1999). Short-term couples group psychotherapy: A tale of four fights. In: *Short-term Couple Therapy* (ed. JM Donovan), pp. 43–62. New York: The Guilford Press.

Du Toit CW (ed) (1998). Confession and Reconciliation: A Challenge to the Churches in South Africa (Proceedings of a conference held by the Research Institute for Theology and Religion at the University of South Africa on 23 & 24 March 1998). Pretoria, South Africa: Research Institute for Theology and Religion.

Ellis GFR (2001). Afterword: Exploring the unique role of forgiveness. In: *Forgiveness and Reconciliation: Religion, Public Policy, and Conflict Transformation* (eds RG Helmick and RL Petersen), pp. 395–410. Philadelphia, PA: Templeton Foundation Press.

Fine GA and Stoecker R (1993). Can the circle be unbroken? Small groups and social movements. In: *Social Psychology of Groups: A Reader* (eds EJ Lawler and B Markovsky), pp. 225–52. Greenwich, CT: JAI Press.

Fiske ST (2004). *Social Beings: Core Motives in Social Psychology*. New York: Wiley Publishers.

Gibbs JC (2003). *Moral Development and Reality: Beyond the Theories of Kohlberg and Hoffman*. Thousand Oaks, California: Sage Publications.

Gilligan C (1982/1993). *In a Different Voice: Psychological Theory and Women's Development*. Cambridge: Harvard University Press.

Gilligan C (1995). The centrality of relationship in psychological development: A puzzle, some evidence, and a theory. In: *Identity and Diversity: Gender and the Experience of Education* (eds M Blair, J Holland, with S Sheldon), pp. 194–208. Clevedon, Avon: Multilingual Matters Ltd.

Gilligan C (1997a): In a different voice: Women's conceptions of self and of morality. In: *Feminist Social Thought: A Reader* (ed. DT Meyers), pp. 549–582. New York: Routledge Publishers.

Gilligan C (1997b): Woman's place in man's life cycle. In: *The Second Wave: A Reader in Feminist Theory* (ed. L Nicholson), pp. 198–215. New York: Routledge Publishers.

Gilligan C (2000). Selection from: In a different voice. In: *Ethical Theory: A Concise Anthology* (eds H Geirsson H and MR Holmgren), pp. 273–84. Peterborough, Ontario: Broadview Press.

Glick ID, Berman EM, Clarkin JF, and Rait DS (2000). *Marital and Family Therapy*, 4th edition. Washington, DC: American Psychiatric Press.

Halford WK (2001). *Brief Therapy for Couples: Helping Partners Help Themselves*. New York: The Guilford Press.

Hallpike CR (1998/2001). *Moral Development from the Anthropological Perspective*. UK: Prometheus. 4 January 2005
http://prometheus.org.uk/Publishing/Books/HallpikeOnEMU

Heitler S (1990). *From Conflict to Resolution: Strategies for Diagnosis and Treatment of Distressed Individuals, Couples, and Families*. New York: WW Norton & Company.

Helmick RG and Petersen RL (eds) (2001). *Forgiveness and Reconciliation: Religion, Public Policy, and Conflict Transformation*. Philadelphia, PA: Templeton Foundation Press.

Hicks D (2001). The role of identity construction in promoting reconciliation. In: *Forgiveness and Reconciliation: Religion, Public Policy, and Conflict Transformation* (eds RG Helmick and RL Petersen), pp. 129–49. Philadelphia, PA: Templeton Foundation Press.

Higgins ET and Kruglanski AW (eds) (1996). *Social Psychology: Handbook of Basic Principles*. New York: The Guilford Press.

Hoffman ML (2000). *Empathy and Moral Development: Implications for Caring and Justice*. Cambridge: Cambridge University Press.

Holmes JG and Murray SL (1996). Conflict in close relationships. In: *Social Psychology: Handbook of Basic Principles* (eds ET Higgins and AW Kruglanski), pp. 622–54. New York: The Guilford Press.

Johnson SM (1999). Emotionally focused couple therapy: straight to the heart. In: *Short-term Couple Therapy* (ed. JM Donovan), pp. 13–42. New York: The Guilford Press.

Kenrick DT, Neuberg SL, and Cialdini RB (1999). *Social Psychology: Unraveling the Mystery*. Boston: Allyn & Bacon.

Kohlberg L (1817/1981). *The Philosophy of Moral Development: Moral Stages and the Idea of Justice. Essays on Moral Development,* Vol 1. San Francisco: Harper & Row Publishers.

Kohlberg L (1817/1984). *The Psychology of Moral Development: The Nature and Validity of Moral Stages. Essays on Moral Development,* Vol. 2. San Francisco: Harper & Row Publishers.

Krebs DL (2000). The evolution of moral dispositions in the human species. *Annals of the New York Academy of Sciences,* **907**: 132–48.

Landman C (ed.) (1996a). *Digging Up Our Foremothers: Stories of Women in Africa.* Pretoria, South Africa: Unisa Press, University of South Africa.

Landman C (1996b). *Wat Nou Van Isebel? Verhale van Vroue in die Bybel.* [So What About Jezebel? Stories of Women in the Bible.] Cape Town, South Africa: Human & Rousseau Publishers.

Landman C (1998). *Nagstukke vir Een Maand . . . Oor Vrywees en Vrouwees en Goed Voel Oor Jouself.* [Night Pieces for One Month . . . About Being Free, Being a Woman, and Feeling Good About Yourself.] Cape Town, South Africa: Lux Verbi.

Landman C (1999). *The Piety of South African Women.* Pretoria, South Africa: CB Powell Bible Centre, University of South Africa.

Landman C (2000). *Woorde Wat Heel Maak: Jesus Maak Heel Waar Vroue Seerkry.* [Words That Heal: Jesus Heals Where Women Hurt.] Wellington, South Africa: Lux Verbi.

Landman C (2001). Vryers en Vennote: Bevry jou Verhoudings. [Lovers and Partners: Liberate your Relationships.] Cape Town, South Africa: Struik Christelike Boeke.

Lawler EJ and Markovsky B (eds) (1993). *Social Psychology of Groups: A Reader.* Greenwich, CT: JAI Press.

Livingston DJ (2002). *Healing Violent Men: A Model for Christian Communities.* Minneapolis, MN: Fortress Press.

Long WJ and Brecke P (2003). *War and Reconciliation: Reason and Emotion in Conflict Resolution.* Cambridge, MA: MIT Press.

Markus HR, Kitayama S, and Heiman RJ (1996). Culture and 'basic' psychological principles. In: *Social Psychology: Handbook of Basic Principles* (eds ET Higgins and AW Kruglanski), pp. 857–914. New York: The Guilford Press.

Masina NM (2000). Xhosa practices of Ubuntu for South Africa. In: *Traditional Cures for Modern Conflicts: African Conflict 'Medicine'* (ed. IW Zartman), pp. 169–81. Boulder, CO: Lynne Rienner Publishers.

McLean Taylor J, Gilligan C, and Sullivan AM (1996). Missing voices, changing meanings: Developing a voice-centred, relational method and creating an interpretive community. In: *Feminist Social Psychologies: International Perspectives* (ed. S Wilkinson), pp. 233–57. Buckingham: Open University Press.

Meiring P (1999). *Chronicle of the Truth Commission: A Journey Through the Past and Present—Into the Future of South Africa.* Vanderbijlpark, South Africa: Carpe Diem Books.

Meiring P (2000). Truth and reconciliation: the South African experience. In: *Race and Reconciliation in South Africa: a Multicultural Dialogue in Comparative Perspective* (eds WE Van Vugt and GD Cloete), pp. 187–99. Lanham, MD: Lexington Books.

Meyers DG (1993). *Social Psychology,* 4th edition. New York: McGraw-Hill.

Meyers DG (1994). *Exploring Social Psychology*. New York: McGraw-Hill.

Moody-Adams MM (1991). Gender and the complexity of moral voices. In: *Feminist Ethics* (ed. C Card), pp. 195–212. Lawrence, KS: University Press of Kansas.

Neal JH, Zimmerman JL, and Dickerson VC (1999). Couples, culture, and discourse: a narrative approach. In: *Short-term Couple Therapy* (ed. JM Donovan), pp. 360–400. New York: The Guilford Press.

Nichols MP and Minuchin S (1999). Short-term structural family therapy with couples. In: *Short-term Couple Therapy* (ed. JM Donovan), pp. 124–43. New York: The Guilford Press.

Norlin JM, Chess WA, Dale O, and Smith R (2003). *Human Behavior and the Social Environment: Social Systems Theory*, 4th edition. Boston, MA: Allyn and Bacon.

Nürnberger K and Tooke JV (eds) (1988). T*he Cost of Reconciliation in South Africa*. Cape Town, South Africa: Methodist Publishing House.

Potter-Efron R and Potter-Efron P (1995). *Letting Go of Anger: the 10 Most Common Anger Styles and What to Do About Them*. Oakland, CA: New Harbinger Publications.

Ross MH (1995). Psychocultural interpretation theory and peacemaking in ethnic conflicts. *Political Psychology*, **16**(3): 523–44.

Rusbult CE and Van Lange PAM (1996). Interdependence processes. In: *Social Psychology: Handbook of Basic Principles* (eds ET Higgins and AW Kruglanski), pp. 564–96. New York: The Guilford Press.

Sartorius N (1988). Future directions: a global view. In: *Handbook of Social Psychiatry* (eds AS Henderson and GD Burrows), pp. 341–46. Amsterdam: Elsevier.

Sartorius N, Gaebel W, López-Ibor JJ, and Maj M (2002). *Psychiatry in Society*. New York: John Wiley & Sons. E-book, accessed 26 January 2005.

Sears DO, Peplau A, Freedman JL, and Taylor SE (1988). *Social Psychology*, 6th edition. Englewood Cliffs, NJ: Prentice-Hall International.

Selvini MP, Boscolo L, Cecchin G, and Prata G (1980). Hypothesising—circularity—neutrality: three guidelines for the conductor of the session. *Family Process*, **19**: 3–12.

Sharpe SA (2000). *The Ways We Love: a Developmental Approach to Treating Couples*. New York: The Guilford Press.

Siegel JP (1992). *Repairing Intimacy: an Object Relations Approach to Couples Therapy*. Northvale, New Jersey: Jason Aronson.

Smith ER and Mackie DM (eds) (2000). *Social Psychology*, 2nd edition. Philadelphia, PA: Psychology Press.

Stainton Rogers W (2003). *Social Psychology: Experimental and Critical Approaches*. Maidenhead, Philadelphia, PA: Open University Press.

Staub E and Pearlman LA (2001). Healing, reconciliation, and forgiving after genocide and other collective violence. In: *Forgiveness and Reconciliation: Religion, Public Policy, and Conflict Transformation* (eds RG Helmick and RL Petersen), pp. 205–27. Philadelphia, PA: Templeton Foundation Press.

Steinfeld GJ (1997). The cycle of violence: an integrative clinical approach. In: *When One Partner is Willing and the Other is Not* (ed. BJ Brothers), pp. 49–81. New York: The Haworth Press.

Susin LC and Aquino MP (eds) (2003). *Reconciliation in a World of Conflicts*. London: SCM Press.

Tooke JV (1988). Fourteen theses on justice and reconciliation. In: *The Cost of Reconciliation in South Africa* (eds K Nürnberger and JV Tooke), pp. 126–30. Cape Town, South Africa: Methodist Publishing House.

Tutu D (1998). The truth and reconciliation commission: preamble. In: *Confession and Reconciliation: A Challenge to the Churches in South Africa* (Proceedings of a conference held by the Research Institute for Theology and Religion at the University of South Africa on 23 and 24 March 1998) (ed. CW Du Toit), pp. 3–6. Pretoria, South Africa: Research Institute for Theology and Religion.

Van der Walt BJ and Naudé CFB (1996). Christianity and democracy in South Africa: a vision for the future (Study pamphlet number 345 containing opening and closing presentations at a conference on Christianity and Democracy in South Africa, 10–12 July 1996). Potchefstroom, South Africa: Potchefstroom University for Christian Higher Education, Institute for Reformational Studies.

Van der Walt BJ and Venter JJ (1998). Religion and society: a review of the Truth and Reconciliation Commission Hearings, East London, 17–19 November 1997 (Study pamphlet number 361). Potchefstroom, South Africa: Potchefstroom University for Christian Higher Education, Institute for Reformational Studies.

Van Vugt WE and Cloete GD (eds) (2000). *Race and Reconciliation in South Africa: a Multicultural Dialogue in Comparative Perspective.* Lanham, MD: Lexington Books.

Van Zyl S (1999). An interview with Gillian Straker on the Truth and Reconciliation Commission in South Africa. *Psychoanalytic Dialogues*, 9(2): 245–74.

Waller MA and Spiegler MD (1997). A cross-cultural perspective on couple differences. In: *When One Partner is Willing and the Other is Not* (ed. BJ Brothers), pp. 83–98. New York: The Haworth Press.

Weeks GR and Hof L (1995). *Integrative solutions: Treating common problems in couples therapy.* New York: Brunner/Mazel Publishers.

Weeks GR and Treat S (1992). *Couples in Treatment: Techniques and Approaches for Effective Practice.* New York: Brunner/Mazel Publishers.

Worrell Haslam C and Erdman P (2003). Linking systems and attachment theory: a conceptual framework for marital violence. In: *Attachment and Family Systems: Conceptual, Empirical, and Therapeutic Relatedness* (eds P Erdman and T Caffery), pp. 193–211. New York: Brunner-Routledge Publishers.

Worthington EL (2001). Unforgiveness, forgiveness, and reconciliation and their implications for societal interventions. In: *Forgiveness and Reconciliation: Religion, Public Policy, and Conflict Transformation* (eds RG Helmick and RL Petersen), pp. 171–92. Philadelphia, PA: Templeton Foundation Press.

Chapter 3

Reconciliation as compromise and the management of rage

Peter Zachar

There is considerable overlap between individual psychotherapy for trauma-based disorders and truth and reconciliation commissions. In the case of the South African Truth and Reconciliation Commission (TRC), this overlap is reflected in how the commission was described by its proponents. I am specifically referring to the proponents' reliance on language drawn from psychotherapy to justify the work of the commission. In addition to terms such as victim and perpetrator, the commission's proponents used language such as unfinished business, overcoming denial, coming to terms, resolving issues, and healing (TRC, 1998; Rotberg, 2000; Villa-Vicencio, 2000b).

Going beyond shared metaphors for truth commissions and psychotherapy, I will argue that a legitimate purpose of TRCs is to manage both individual and societal rage and that the experience of rage is related to a desire for justice. The types of justice I will discuss include restorative justice, retributive justice, and distributive justice. In combination with both psychological resources for managing rage and preferences for deontological, consequentialist, and virtue ethics approaches to morality, these models of justice influence one's beliefs about the value of truth commissions.

3.1 Restorative justice as forgiveness—virtuous—healthy

As suggested by Elizabeth Kiss (2000), the South African TRC, with its ethic of forgiveness, aimed at establishing restorative justice. Restoration becomes a legitimate goal when inexcusable harm to an individual or group has occurred and social—civil contact has been severed. An understandable response of a person who has been inexcusably harmed is rage. Forgiveness involves getting beyond rage and restoring emotional cohesiveness and balance. The stronger the rage, the more difficult is the act of forgiveness. The same is true if restoration refers to re-establishing civic cohesiveness: rage exacerbates social divisiveness.

Rage can be understood as an emotional state that goes beyond anger. Anger is an emotion of separation in which the target of the anger is put at a distance. Anger is related to an experienced threat and also related to a need to establish control and mastery over the situation (Tavris, 1989). In distinction from anger, in rage the perception of coexisting goodness and badness is lost and the perpetrator is seen as all bad.

Research in scientific psychology has demonstrated that positive and negative states of emotion, rather than being opposite ends of a single bipolar continuum, are independent. According to Watson and Tellegen (1985), these two emotional states can each be represented by a separate bipolar continuum. One bipolar continuum consists of positive emotions such as euphoria on one end and lethargy-fatigue on the other. The other continuum consists of negative emotions such as distress on one end and calmness on the other. Rage, therefore, does not involve a lack of positive emotion—that would be a state of impotent anger often seen in depression. In contrast to depression, rage is a high energy state. Rather than an absence of positive emotion, in rage, the beneficent aspect of positive emotions is overshadowed by a state of hyper-aroused anger with respect to the perpetrator.

Getting beyond rage is a psychologically difficult thing to do, but it is one of the virtues for which Nelson Mandela is most respected. There are several ways to manage feelings of rage in order to get beyond them. Sometimes perpetrators can be seen as not fully in control of their actions and influenced by external forces such as political power. For example, being subject to political influence was a requirement for amnesty in South Africa; sadistic acts that could not be attributed to political objectives were not eligible for amnesty. In other cases, perpetrators can be seen as influenced by internal forces from their past, such as having been victims themselves. The idea, here, is that a previous experience of victimization has been psychologically internalized and is affecting current behavior from within. It is easier to empathize with a former victim who becomes a perpetrator than it is with a perpetrator who has no history of victimization. Finding the victim in the perpetrator is an important tool used by psychologists who have to work with perpetrators and adopt an empathic attitude toward them. In other cases, a power asymmetry between victims and perpetrators can be reversed, specifically by the victims coming to perceive perpetrators as weak and flawed.

In whatever way rage is diminished, it becomes easier to see potential good in perpetrators, or at least to see that they are more than only bad. The bad does not go away; rather, it is understood in a larger, more cohesive context. Forgiveness, as the truism goes, is not about forgetting—and the bad is still bad, but it is not *all bad*. This is a process that takes time. From a psychological standpoint, forgiveness is a healthy outcome—something to be sought—but it has to occur naturally and can't be forced.

In an ethical system that respects moral virtues, forgiveness itself is conceptualized as a virtue. According to proponents of virtue ethics, virtues represent moral characteristics, i.e., virtues are internal states that make morally appropriate behavior more probable. A virtuous person does good because that is who he or she is. Virtue ethicists, therefore, typically hold that we should develop good moral habits so that doing the right thing becomes customary for us (MacIntyre, 1981; Pence, 1991).

In contrast to a character-based virtue ethics, deontological approaches to inculcating moral behavior are principle-based. Proponents of deontological ethics, such as Kant, view morality as grounded in a set of rational principles that we have a duty to obey. We willingly confirm to the moral law because it is the law—being moral isn't about doing what we want to do (MacIntyre, 1981; O'Neill, 1991).

The detachment offered by a principle-based approach enhances the establishment of moral convictions, and these convictions can be useful. At some point in the South African process, almost every group seems to have been upset with, disappointed, and opposed to the procedures of the commission. The commission went forward all the same–in part due to the commitment of true believers in forgiveness such as Mandela and Tutu. Defending a TRC from skepticism and wide ranging criticism is aided by the presence of people who believe that forgiveness is a moral imperative, something we must do.

Convictions can also be criticized for their inflexibility. One criticism of the South African truth commission, and especially of Desmond Tutu, was that forgiveness was presented as a duty or a moral obligation and as something that people must adopt in order to be good and virtuous persons (Gutmann and Thompson, 2000; Ndebele, 2000). In a deontological system, those who behave badly are weak for having failed to follow the rules; in a virtue system, they are bad people. In the mix, they are both weak and bad. Ironically, the victims of the perpetrators can themselves be made to feel 'weak' and 'bad' because they are very angry. Here is the complaint in the words of a young black woman:

> What really makes me angry about the TRC and Tutu is that they are putting pressure on me to forgive . . . I don't know if I will ever be able to forgive. I carry this ball of anger within me and I don't know where to begin dealing with it. The oppression was bad, but what is much worse, what makes me even angrier, is that they are trying to dictate my forgiveness.

> Villa-Vicencio (2000a, p. 201)

I am focusing on restorative justice and the value it places on forgiveness, and especially the problems related to obligatory forgiveness. The complications that result from combining an ethic of duty with an ethic of virtue are compounded by the psychological gloss of the modern era. If forgiveness is also understood to be a psychologically healthy development in those who experienced harm, then those who inflexibly maintain themselves in a state of rage beyond a reasonable period are potentially not only lacking in virtue, are irrational, and even sinful, they are pathological. The association between sinfulness and psychopathology is an old one, and our moral notion of what counts as 'bad' plays a more important role in how we currently conceptualize psychological health and illness than is often acknowledged in psychiatry, as noted by Sadler (2005). One possible prescription for curing the 'pathology' of rage is forgiveness.

There are several problems with prescribed forgiveness. One of the more evident problems is that it encourages the repression and denial of what should not be denied. For example, at my university the psychology department sponsors a Holocaust Memorial Program every spring. As part of the program we bring in survivors and other witnesses such as camp liberators. They tell the audience what they saw and what they experienced. Afterwards they take questions from the audience. There is always a similar theme running through the audience's questions. They ask the survivors if any German soldiers helped them, or if any townspeople helped them, or it they had forgiven the Nazis. These are reasonable questions, but psychologically the audience appears to be seeking answers that will make all the bad things they just heard about seem less bad. If they are less bad, they are also easier to forget. Prescribed forgiveness could rationalize denial. It is always a bit of a shock for the audience when one of the survivors, who was at Auschwitz and who lost his entire family there, tells them that he has not forgiven the Germans, or God—if there is a God. The survivor then states that he does not want to forgive. In contrast to prescribed forgiveness, this man's refusal to sugarcoat these events always felt 'healthy' to me.

A second problem is that prescribed forgiveness of atrocious harms could lead to shallow forgiveness. An individual may conform to an external imperative to behave according to some moral standard, even if that standard is being followed primarily for the sake of appearance, or if it is being done because 'Forgiveness is what good and decent people do.' With 'dutiful' forgiveness, the emotional work of forgiveness is short-circuited. When this happens, permeating resentment and passive-aggressive behavior become more likely. Resentment leaking from multiple pores is not the kind of thing that is going to satisfy the psychologically minded thinker who, in accord with a characterological or virtue approach, believes that rage has to be worked through emotionally. Working through rage can involve integrating a full range of positive and negative emotions about a person into a cohesive whole, or it could involve compartmentalizing the rage about a person in such a way that it does not permeate one's life. In whatever way the rage is metabolized, the bad does not have to be denied in order to maintain a cohesive state of mind, and the lingering resentment is reduced.

A third problem with prescribed forgiveness is that rage, although distressful and disruptive, can be a legitimate part of learning to deal with trauma, tragedy, and mistreatment. In cases where rage replaces a passive acceptance of abuse, it is a psychological advance. There may even be occasions in psychotherapy when a client feels compelled by her or his conscience to forgive a perpetrator, and the therapist instead implements a series of interventions to help the client to explore her or his rage. In a sense, the therapist gives the client permission not to forgive.

3.2 **Retributive justice and vengeance**

In contrast to forgiveness-based restorative justice is retributive justice—the justice of vengeance. It is an alternative response to atrocity-based trauma. Seeking retribution is also a way of dealing with rage, but instead of contextualizing extreme anger in a broader emotional framework (i.e., forgiving), it invokes the defense mechanism of undoing. In undoing, someone acted wrongly and now the scales of justice have to be balanced. It is a common coping strategy for wrongdoers, often seen in the urge to apologize for actions or words that they regret. Undoing is usually defined narrowly as a conscience-based attempt to make up for one's own bad thoughts or actions, but the notion of 'undoing' also captures the intent of retributive responses to the bad actions of another. You killed and will now be killed. You tortured and now will be tortured. You took my money, now I will take yours. Your eye for my eye, your tooth for my tooth.

Psychiatrists have termed this broader kind of undoing *turning of passive to active*. In cases of sexual abuse, using the defense mechanism turning of passive to active is a possible route whereby former victims become perpetrators. They do to another—often compulsively—what was done to them. In cases of physical and psychological aggression, when the target of the harmful act is a former perpetrator and the agent is a former victim, it is called personal retribution.

Although turning of passive to active is an important psychological mechanism, it is important to note that there is no single psychological state that underlies acts of vengeance. For example, if someone is taught by his culture that honor can be satisfied only by seeking vengeance, he may initiate an act of vengeance out of principle rather than rage. Yet, like method acting, enacting the social role of vengeance-seeking might lead one to adopt an emotional state of rage. Socially enacted rage can even be perceived as a virtue.

Psychologically considered, the more that retribution is fueled by rage, the more primitive it is. 'Primitive' in this sense refers to a split psyche where good and bad are not integrated. Conservative political philosophies even offer a strategy for 'civilizing' vengeance (Cassell, 2004; Pojman, 2004). The theory is that rage is removed when the polity reserves the right of vengeance for the group rather than the individual. Vengeance becomes rational retribution. Those working from a more liberal tradition are likely to view such principle-based retribution with suspicion due to the presence of virtual rage. By virtual rage I mean a cognitive rage—a state that lacks the intensity of passion, but can become passionate very quickly. The liberally minded thinkers would point out that a principle-based retribution is often focused on identifying with and assuaging the negative emotions of the righteous victim even when it is clothed in rational language about the moral order, and if the propriety of retribution is challenged, the rage becomes less virtual.

Readers will debate whether or not retribution is primitive and what counts as a civilized response to wrongdoing. People do need to be held accountable for their actions, and invoking some kind of punishment rather than letting them go free can not reasonably be called 'immoral.' There is also a concept called 'moral hatred.' Moral hatred is a term referring to legitimate feelings of intense anger toward a Himmler or a Stalin (Murphy and Hampton, 1988). In this vein, Nkosinathi Biko (2000) has suggested that, in some cases, amnesty perpetuates society's ability to deny the horrors committed. He notes that, with amnesty, the criminal nature of horrific acts is minimized. Biko suggests this is a mistake. Considerations such as these have led Gutmann and Thompson (2000) to observe that the proponents of TRCs have to provide reasons for sacrificing punishment if they are to justify their existence.

3.3 Restorative justice as reconciliation: undoing with dignity

A hallmark of consequentialist ethical systems is compromise. I am here defining consequentialism as something broader than classical utilitarianism. Consequentialism is the view that, in evaluating what actions are the right actions, we should pay attention to the consequences of actions (Pettit, 1991).

Those actions that promote the good are justified. (Classical utilitarianism is a consequentialist theory that states that 'the good' is pleasure.)

Actions often have multiple consequences, both positive and negative. Consequentialists usually accept moral ambiguity without complaint and understand that deciding what counts as a good and moral act requires balancing competing priorities. They try to maximize good outcomes and minimize bad outcomes, but the balance is never perfect. In seeking a balance, consequentialists may consult general principles as a guide to values, and they may also believe that virtue-based approaches are useful methods of training.

Congruent with a consequentialist approach, it is fair to say that the South African TRC aimed at finding a compromise between an ethic of retribution and an ethic of forgiveness. The compromise is civil reconciliation. Borrowing a phrase from Martha Minow (1998), reconciliation is what lies between vengeance and forgiveness. This is also a type of restorative justice. Rather than forgiveness, this type of restorative justice involves the defense mechanism of undoing as a way to manage rage, but it is less vengeful than retribution.

In an oft-quoted but rarely referenced phrase, Freud is claimed to have said that the person who first threw a curse rather than a spear at his enemy was the true founder of civilization (Gay, 1988). I would take this idea further than Freud. Maybe throwing a curse was an important step, but using social pressure to elicit an apology would have been a more essential step. Cursing someone rather than throwing a spear at him or her allows coexistence, but getting an apology would make the additional event of social cooperation more probable. As Villa-Vicencio (2000a) notes, reconciliation falls short of forgiveness, but it still restores enough of a working relationship for cooperation to occur.

One of the core justifications given for the public hearings in South Africa was that the dignity of the victims had been taken away and that public testimony by the victims and the perpetrators restored dignity to the victims and reduced the dignity of the perpetrators (Minow, 1998; Boraine, 2000). In this case, reducing the dignity of the perpetrators by means of public confessions and even apologies was not an end in itself, but a plan for restoring the dignity of the victims.

The dignity that is bought at the price of another's humiliation is a narcissistic dignity. Narcissistic strategies tend to enhance one's own esteem by devaluing others. These strategies create positive emotions about the self by making what social psychologists call downward comparisons, i.e., I'm great because I'm better than you (Bogart et al., 2004). This kind of self-esteem enhancement is probably part of the attraction of apartheid-like system to its beneficiaries. In response to systemic social atrocity, returning dignity to the victim often involves reducing the dignity of the perpetrator—or at least reducing his or her sense of superiority in some way. Narcissism-deflation is an undoing. The playing field is leveled and the probability that victims and perpetrators can relate to each other as citizens possessing the same basic scheme of civil rights is increased.

Restorative justice as reconciliation via restoring dignity and re-establishing the social participation of all groups in society is a difficult process to manage. In order for it to work, the perpetrators should both participate in the undoing and, hopefully, demonstrate genuine sorrow and regret. If they are unrepentant, it is likely that rage will be intensified, as will calls for retribution. The perpetrators also have to accept that they failed morally in committing a crime against humanity or an individual, they have to face public exposure of that crime, and they have to tolerate their own negative feelings about themselves. Tolerating these things is emotionally difficult.

In the worst case scenario with respect to reconciliation, perpetrators begin to see themselves as victims, begin to feel rage, and become self-righteous and dismissive of the charges. This was evident at both Nuremberg and in South Africa, exemplified in Goering's unrepentant arrogance regarding what he considered 'Allied hypocrisy' and Botha's contemptuous refusal to acknowledge his own mistakes and to apologize. Victimhood can be a socially powerful role, and adopting indignation is one way that perpetrators may cope with the negative evaluation of others. Perpetrator self-righteousness understandably fuels calls for retribution on the part of those who were earlier convinced to foreswear it. A sad fact about human history is that rage fuels rage on both sides of an issue.

Another aspect of the utilitarian compromise in South Africa involved reparations. Reparations are a more concrete form of undoing where something is given in order to replace what was earlier taken away. Although it is possible to claim that reparations are only symbolic, I would argue that these compromises are psychologically important—meaningful rather than meaningless symbols. Reparations often involve issuing death certificates, building monuments, funding educational programs or naming new schools, holidays, government buildings and roads. These kinds of public affirmations on the part of the community can hopefully teach future generations about core civic values.

Sometimes the symbolic kind of undoing is not enough and comes to be criticized as useless. In these cases, reparations can evolve into a call for giving money to individuals. Monetary reparations are complicated, but they have a dual target of lessening victim rage and easing perpetrator guilt. This kind of reparation has a more retributive tone to it, especially if individual property is forcibly redistributed. Reparations as monetary payments may even be defended in the name of distributive justice or a fair distribution of social goods, with many different theories of just distribution possible (cf. Nozick, 1974; Dworkin, 1981; Rawls, 2001). Social goods that were stolen can be returned over a period of time rather than all at once. Those victims who might prefer retribution but understand that retribution is impractical because the perpetrators still have political power, might accept monetary reparations as a compromise.

3.4 **Telling secrets**

In addition to shared metaphors such as resolving issues, working through anger, and healing, another parallel between psychotherapy for trauma-based disorders and TRCs is that secrets are told. In the typical dysfunctional family, members are not supposed to tell outsiders what goes on inside the home. The code of silence is even more restricted in sexually abusive relationships where the victim is not supposed to tell other family members about the abuse (Sink, 1988). This dynamic can manifest itself in any kind of small group, including churches, clubs, businesses, governmental offices, and academic departments. And like in families, conflicting feelings of fear and love-appreciation that tend to develop about the abuser(s) help maintain the silence.

Although it is obviously different when practiced on a social scale, a similar code of silence appears to have been operating during the Nazi Holocaust and the Argentine dictatorship. Secret trials and secret torture also occurred in Stalin's Russia, Castro's Cuba, and the South African apartheid system. Although no simple equation with the previous events just listed should be made, it has also been charged that there has been secret torture at the US Naval Base on Guantanamo Bay (Jehl, 2005). Conflicting feelings of fear and loyalty are also involved in the silence that follows.

In an oft-quoted phrase, Michael Ignatieff claims that telling the truth makes it very hard for those who would prefer to deny the reality of horrible events—yet it is central to the program of dignity restoration.

> All that a truth commission can achieve is to reduce the number of lies that can be circulated unchallenged in public discourse. In Argentina, its work has made it impossible to claim, for example, that the military did not throw half-dead victims to the sea from helicopters. In Chile, it is no longer permissible to assert in public that the Pinochet regime did not dispatch thousands of entirely innocent people

> Cited in Boraine (2000, pp. 151–2).

Relaying stories about what happened requires emphasizing some events and minimizing others. The events are not listed like numbers in a statistical data set; rather, they are ordered into a particular narrative told by an individual or a group. Stories are more meaningful vehicles of information transmission, so they are readily retold. When the harms done to the victims are dramatized by public testimony, the resulting stories told by a society about its history are more likely to take those events into account.

A philosophical complication of this kind of truth telling when practiced on a social scale is that events are supposed to be recalled in narrative form and the narratives are supposed to have a moral connotation. This can be called interpretive truth in contrast to forensic truth (Boraine, 2000). If forensic truth involves recounting facts, interpretive truth adds personal and social meanings. For example, on December 1, 1955 a black woman in Montgomery, Alabama refused to give up her seat on a city bus and was arrested. That is forensic truth. A story about the suffering caused by racial segregation and how Rosa Parks came to symbolize a nation's refusal to abide by the principles enshrined in its constitution is interpretive truth.

The complication is that when people are in the middle of events, agreeing on the appropriate moral context is rarely possible. Particularly unamenable to consensus is how much atrocity to attribute to the questionable actions of perpetrators and where to attribute responsibility. Events can evoke negative emotional responses such as fear and anger, and those emotions influence the development of moral indignation. The moral context is especially difficult to define when powerful people are the objects of moral scrutiny. If some citizens invest hope in those holding power, while others oppose them, and if the associates of the powerful are publicly advocating fear and rage, there will be not be consensus within a group regarding the moral context of current events.

Disagreement regarding what moral context a society should adopt for understanding current events does not apply only to what are later labeled atrocities, such as segregation or the Holocaust. It also applies to events such as wars, impeachment hearings, and debates over public policy. Not being able to agree on moral context is a continuous problem. Historians and social critics could probably list past and present examples of deep discordance within a community from all eras and all political persuasions. Post hoc, there are many instances of people looking back and wondering how they or their predecessors could have been so mistaken. The widely popular prosecutions, 30 years after the event, of those who carried out the Sixteenth Street Baptist Church bombing in Birmingham, Alabama are recent examples.

If they are going to have an immediate emotional relevance, TRCs have to occur close to the events in question, long before a consensus about moral context can be constructed. The administrators of TRCs have to decide what events to highlight and how to order them. Witnesses will not always tell the same truth, and disagreement about moral context will usually offer even the most extreme perpetrators an opportunity to question the entire process.

In these kinds of situations different voices have to be afforded attention, particularly voices from outside a particular society itself, including other governments, news agencies, scholars and what Crocker (2000) calls International Civil Societies such as the United Nations. Pushing the comparison with psychotherapy a little further, I suggest that moral conflicts in a community and psychotherapy share more than language. They also share some practices for correcting perceptions that are based on a limited perspective. External agents such as the UN may be better able to adopt the kind of objectivity that therapists are asked to adopt in psychiatry and psychology, an objectivity that understandably eludes those who are emotionally involved in the events under discussion.

3.5 **Justice and democracy**

The notion of conflicting perspectives on the purpose and value of truth commissions calls to mind John Rawls' (2001) idea of a reasonable overlapping consensus. Rawls was interested in understanding how people with different religious, philosophical, and moral viewpoints can agree on what counts as a just basic structure for a democratic society. Rawls said that people do not have to agree on these principles for the same reasons and that a political conception of justice in a democracy has to be one that people with different and conflicting world views can accept. For this kind of consensus, the principles will tend to be both global and vague rather than concrete and applied.

The notion of a reasonable overlapping consensus can also illuminate the processes involved in the establishment and justification of TRCs. Rawls' analysis suggests that the multitude of arguments supporting the establishment of TRCs will always form a patchwork of positions rather than a single and logically coherent justification. We should not expect that everyone has to agree to establish a TRC for the same reasons.

For example, deontologically inclined proponents of restorative justice might believe that forgiveness is better than vengeance, that no one should be left out of society, and that it is good in itself for perpetrators and victims to reconcile. In theory, deontological proponents would view forgiveness and reconciliation as something that we ought to do. That is, they are moral duties. TRCs would therefore be their preferred vehicle of justice.

Consequentialists might also believe that, on the whole, restorative justice is a higher form of justice than retributive justice and would view TRCs as the best solution, but they would be more willing to admit exceptions. For example, in attempting to promote the greater good, they might be less reluctant than the deontologist proponents to use the threat of retribution as a tool to motivate public confessions of perpetrators. They would also readily acknowledge that truth commissions are not a good thing if they inflame rage or lead to widespread re-traumatization. Although the mantra 'never again' and the truth are closely allied, some victims may prefer not to seek vengeance, but the full truth of what happened has, for them, emotional consequences that are barriers to reconciliation. Deciding how much truth and for whom requires finding a delicate balance.

Virtue ethics proponents of restorative justice (which they might call social justice) should be the most comfortable with using psychological metaphors and focusing on the emotional aspects of reconciliation and forgiveness. They will be inclined to acknowledge both suffering and rage. Virtue ethics proponents might also be more inclined to consider how the events are affecting the developing moral perspectives of the children in society, and to see the events as an opportunity for moral education. They would seek not only a more civil society, but a more moral one, by which they mean a kinder one.

Anyone who prefers retributive justice and views it as a moral imperative is unlikely to accept TRCs. This would be true if the proponent of retribution adopts a deontological approach or a virtue-based approach. Proponents of retribution can accept truth commissions only on consequentialist grounds, and then only as a compromise. Some proponents of retribution may recall events such as the implementation of Jim Crow laws after Reconstruction or the rise of fascism after the Treaty of Versailles and realize that punishing perpetrators too harshly eventually leads to an unwanted social backlash. They might accept reconciliation to prevent that backlash. Other proponents of retribution might believe that telling the truth about what happened could prevent such acts in the future, and for those reasons might be willing to forego immediate retribution in favor of reconciliation.

The analysis of the issues offered here suggests that TRCs will have mixed and unsatisfying results over the short term. There are too many competing moral intuitions and too many conflicting psychological dynamics to neatly reconcile. Psychologically, competing moral intuitions (deontology/rules versus consequences/practicalities) probably exist within the same person in addition to existing between persons, complicating issues further. As Gutmann and Thompson (2000) argue, expecting a robust consensus on the purpose and value of a TRC is both illiberal and undemocratic. Democratic consensus in practice involves establishing temporary coalitions where agreement on

specific issues is rea...
We can share politi...
This kind of loc...
views. Shifting coa...
easier for citizens to ...

As there are fewer ...
agement of rage is ...
there should be in...
missions. For wha...
the structure of so...
having been benefic...

There are also dis...
Increasing agreemen...
a lived realization of ...
forget, or they never ...
eastern USA claim ...
sented it, and that bla...
claims of those wh...
college fraternity h...
Prince of England do...
far we have traveled ...
made possible a dist...

The horrors, howev...
petrators, but also by ...
US, segregation is par...
grandparents but ca...
come to be seen as in...
sides, truth commissi...
subject of intense ...
unfortunate correlate...

... re political opponents).
... se goals for different reasons.
... re agreement on moral world
... ments also makes it
... ferences.

... ining alive and the man-
... individual experiences,
... and value of truth com-
... ents that become part of
... by future generations as
... ts in this sense.

... ard to a future consensus.
... h a cost: specifically, loss of
... he injustices committed. People
... ear some citizens of the south-
... ign than historians have pre-
... re of as part of the family. The
... similar. Costume parties where
... lux Klan outfits and the young
... enign interpretation, reflect how
... orrors and how that distance has

... by the descendants of the per-
... many young black people in the
... something that happened to their
... to them. The freedoms hard won
... nd of forgetting occurs on both
... events they study will not be the
... such an easy consensus has some

Acknowledge...

In addition to its o... ... arlier version of this chapter
was read at Annua... ... Philosophical Association,
Eastern Division an... ... The Association for Moral
Education, all in 2... ... rak both provided helpful
suggestions for impro...

References

Biko N (2000). Amnesty and denial. In: *Looking Back Reaching Forward* (eds C Villa-Vicencio and W Verwoerd), pp. 193–8. Cape Town: University of Cape Town Press.

Bogart L, Benotsch EG, and Pavolovic JD (2004). Feeling superior but threatened: The relation of narcissism to social comparison. *Basic and Applied Social Psychology*, **26**: 35–44.

Boraine A (2000). Truth and reconciliation in South Africa: The third way. In: *Truth V. Justice: The Morality of Truth Commissions* (eds RI Rotberg and D Thompson), pp. 141–57. Princeton, NJ: Princeton University Press.

Cassell PG (2004). In defense of the death penalty. In: *Debating the Death Penalty: Should America Have Capital Punishment* (eds HA Bedau and PG Cassell), pp. 183–217. New York: Oxford University Press.

Crocker DA (2000). Truth commissions, transitional justice, and civil society. In: *Truth V. Justice: The Morality of Truth Commissions* (eds RI Rotberg and D Thompson), pp. 99–121. Princeton, NJ: Princeton University Press.

Dworkin R (1981). What is equality? Part 1: Equality of resources. *Philosophy of Public Affairs*, **10**: 185–246.

Gay P (1988). *Freud: A Life for Our Time*. New York: WW Norton & Company.

Gutmann A and Thompson D (2000). The moral foundations of truth commissions. In: *Truth V. Justice: The Morality of Truth Commissions* (eds RI Rotberg and D Thompson), pp. 22–44. Princeton, NJ: Princeton University Press.

Jehl D (2005). Some Republicans seek prison abuse panel. New York Times 22 June. Available from http://www.nytimes.com/yr/mo/day/ [Accessed 22 June 2005].

Kiss E (2000). Moral ambition within and beyond political constraints. In: *Truth V. Justice: The Morality of Truth Commissions* (eds RI Rotberg and D Thompson), pp. 68–98. Princeton, NJ: Princeton University Press.

MacIntyre A (1981). *After Virtue*. South Bend, IN: University of Notre Dame Press.

Minow M (1998). *Between Vengeance and Forgiveness: Facing History after Genocide and Mass Violence*. Boston, MA: Beacon Press.

Murphy JG and Hampton J (1988). *Forgiveness and Mercy*. Cambridge, UK: Cambridge University Press.

Ndebele N (2000). Of lions and rabbits: Thoughts on democracy and reconciliation. In: *After the TRC: Reflections on Truth and Reconciliation in South Africa* (eds W James and L van de Vijver), pp. 143–56. Athens, OH: Ohio University Press.

Nozick R (1974). *Anarchy, State, and Utopia*. New York: Basic Books.

O'Neill O (1991). Kantian ethics. In: *A Companion to Ethics* (ed. P Singer), pp. 175–85. Cambridge, MA: Blackwell Publishers.

Pence G (1991). Virtue theory. In: *A Companion to Ethics* (ed. P Singer), pp. 249–58. Cambridge, MA: Blackwell Publishers.

Pettit P (1991). Consequentialism. In: *A Companion to Ethics* (ed. P Singer), pp. 230–40. Cambridge, MA: Blackwell Publishers.

Pojman LP (2004). Why the death penalty is morally permissible. In: *Debating the Death Penalty: Should America Have Capital Punishment* (eds HA Bedau and PG Cassell), pp. 51–75. New York: Oxford University Press.

Rawls J (2001). *Justice as Fairness: A Restatement* (ed. E Kelly). Cambridge, MA: Belknap/Harvard University Press.

Rotberg RI (2000). Truth commissions and the provision of truth, justice, and reconciliation. In: *Truth V. Justice: The Morality of Truth Commissions* (eds RI Rotberg and D Thompson), pp. 3–21. Princeton, NJ: Princeton University Press.

Sadler JZ (2005). *Values and Psychiatric Diagnosis*. New York: Oxford University Press.

Sink F (1988). Sexual abuse in the lives of children. In: *Abuse and Victimization across the Life Span* (ed. MB Straus), pp. 82–106. Baltimore, MD: The Johns Hopkins University Press.

Tavris C (1989). *Anger: The Misunderstood Emotion*. New York: Simon & Schuster.

The Truth and Reconciliation Commission of South Africa: Truth and Reconciliation Commission of South Africa Report. (1998). Volume 5. London: Macmillan Reference.

Villa-Vicencio C (2000a). Getting on with life: A move towards reconciliation. In: *Looking Back Reaching Forward* (eds C Villa-Vicencio and W Verwoerd), pp. 199–209. Cape Town: University of Cape Town Press.

Villa-Vicencio C (2000b). Restorative justice: Dealing with the past differently. In: *Looking Back Reaching Forward* (eds C Villa-Vicencio and W Verwoerd), pp. 68–76. Cape Town: University of Cape Town Press.

Watson D and Tellegen A (1985). Toward a consensual structure of mood. *Psychological Bulletin*, **98**: 219–35.

Chapter 4

Political reconciliation, the rule of law, and post-traumatic stress disorder

Colleen Murphy

4.1 Introduction

Political reconciliation refers to the process of building healthier relationships among citizens formerly estranged as a result of civil conflict or repressive rule. It remains one of the most important, and most theoretically neglected, challenges facing such citizens when their society transitions to democracy. In this chapter, I discuss why one critical aspect of the process of building healthier political relationships involves the restoration of mutual respect for the rule of law. I then suggest that psychological research on post-traumatic stress disorder (PTSD) provides valuable resources for understanding how successfully to restore such mutual respect. At the same time, knowledge about the impact of the rule of law on political relationships can potentially enrich the psychological research on PTSD.

Theoretical challenges

Political reconciliation is theoretically challenging. In the literature on transitional justice, which discusses the moral challenges facing societies in transition to democracy, there is no consensus either on how civil conflict or repressive rule damages political relationships or on what the characteristics of healthy political relationships among democratic citizens are. For example, there is disagreement about whether it is necessary for citizens to overcome resentment in order to be reconciled. Advocates of restorative justice claim that to develop healthier political relationships is to overcome resentment. In their view, resentment damages political relationships. Critics of restorative justice claim that to build healthier political relationships is to reach consensus on the rules that will govern behavior. Lack of communal norms for behavior, not resentment, damages political relationships. It is difficult to assess either view because authors rarely offer an argument for why we should think of reconciliation in the ways they suggest.

Practical challenges

Political reconciliation is practically challenging partly because of such theoretical disputes. Disagreement about the characteristics of healthy political relationships makes it difficult for policy makers to assess the effectiveness and moral justifiability of processes designed to promote political reconciliation, like truth commissions and criminal trials. A process of reconciliation is effective if it contributes to the development of the core features of healthy political relationships. Gauging the effectiveness of such processes, then, depends on a prior understanding of the key features of healthy political relationships.

Facing skepticism

Because it remains unclear precisely what the process of building healthier political relationships entails, it is also difficult for policy makers, politicians, or academics to respond to skepticism among citizens about reconciliation. Very often there is deep ambivalence among citizens about both the possibility and moral justifiability of reconciliation in the aftermath of institutionalized injustice or systematic violence. Given past violence as well as present anger and distrust, many are skeptical about whether it will be possible for citizens to learn to relate in healthier ways. Even if possible, citizens frequently are skeptical about the morality of reconciliation. For such skeptics, the appropriate moral response to certain egregious wrongs is to sever one's relationships with those responsible, whereas reconciliation entails the restoration of relationships. Without a clear notion of what political reconciliation entails, it is futile for policy makers and politicians to respond effectively to such skepticism by demonstrating the possibility and justifiability of reconciliation. This makes reconciliation even more practically challenging, because both kinds of skepticism undercut the willingness of at least some citizens to do the work required for reconciliation to be successful.

Overview of the argument

It is beyond the scope of this chapter to develop a complete account of healthy political relationships and the criteria by which to evaluate the success of processes of reconciliation. In this chapter, I focus on one aspect of healthy political relationships: mutual respect for the rule of law. The rule of law establishes a stable framework for the interaction of citizens by specifying the expectations citizens and officials should make of each other. The breakdown of the rule of law, characteristic of civil conflict and repressive rule, damages the relationships among citizens and officials, I claim, by violating these expectations. Such violations contribute to widespread distrust, resentment, fear, and a sense of betrayal among citizens.

I argue that there are similarities between the breakdown of the rule of law at the societal level and PTSD at the individual level, and that these similarities have important implications for our understanding of what makes processes of reconciliation effective. Systematic violations of the rule of law are consistent with the kinds of trauma that lead to PTSD in individuals. Like violations of the rule of law, traumatic events violate the expectations of individuals. Just as distrust, resentment, and fear are effects of the breakdown of the rule of law, rage and a deep, general distrust of the social world are symptoms of PTSD. This suggests, I claim, that important parallels exist between the processes that successfully enable individuals to cope with PTSD and the processes that successfully help a society in transition restore the rule of law and cope with the legacy of its breakdown. Consequently, to understand how to restore mutual respect for the rule of law and respond to the legacy of distrust, resentment, and fear, we can draw on the psychological research on PTSD.

There are five sections in this paper. In the first two sections I focus on the account of the rule of law developed by Lon Fuller. The first section discusses the requirements of the rule of law. The second section focuses on the breakdown of the rule of law. In the third section, I turn to the concept of PTSD and outline its central features. The fourth section examines two ways in which the concepts of PTSD and of the breakdown of the rule of law are analogous. I then discuss how this analogy sheds light on our understanding of how to promote political reconciliation by restoring the rule of law. The final section discusses the interaction in practice between PTSD and the breakdown of the rule of law.

4.2 The rule of law

Healthy political relationships

Before discussing the rule of law, I first want to explain what I mean by 'healthy political relationships.' 'Healthy,' according to the Oxford English Dictionary, refers to 'possessing or enjoying good health; ... so as to be able to discharge all functions efficiently' and 'conducive to or promoting health or wholesomeness.' The definition of 'health' is 'spiritual, moral, or mental soundness or well-being' and 'well-being, welfare.' Using these definitions of 'healthy' as a guide, a relationship is healthy if it promotes the well-being of the participants in the relationship. A healthy relationship also enables each participant successfully to fulfil her role or function as required by the

particular relationship in que...
between a parent and chil... is ...
fulfill the responsibilities t...
relationships both to con... ...
enable each participan... ...
relationship in question m... ...
individuals. That is, the res... ...
must not undermine the w... ...
successfully.

My particular interest in thi... ,
other words, I am concerned wit...
capacity as citizens and, at times, ...
political relationships, then, p...
responsibilities attaching to the ...
occupying these roles contribu...

In this section, I describe one ...
ships among citizens in a democ...
define what respect for the rule ...
pose facilitated by the rule of law ...
and officials have of one another ...
tematic fulfillment of these expe...
maintained. Finally, I explain wh...
sidered an aspect of healthy pol...
value and its contribution to the ...

healthy relationship
...rent and the child can
...ive role. For healthy
... participants and to
... by the particular
... well-being of
... particular roles
...o fulfill such duties

...al relationships. In
... individuals in their
... account of healthy
... rights, duties, and
..., making clear how
...lth, of individuals.

...ny political relation-
... the rule of law. I first
...plain the general pur-
...ctations that citizens
... law and why the sys-
... the rule of law to be
... f law is properly con-
...y examining its moral

Eight requirements of th...

In the literature in legal philoso...
represent the standard concept...
Fuller identifies eight requireme...
must be general, specifying rules ...
kinds. Laws must also be b...
citizens know what the law requ...
individuals ought to behave in ...
that occurred in the past. La...
tory. One law cannot prohibit ...
the impossible. The demands law...
constant. Finally, there should ...
enforcement by officials. A...
a variety of ways, including ...
sonal power' (Fuller, 19...

...rinciples of legality
... The Morality of Law,
... (1969, pp. 46–90). Laws
...ting behavior of certain
...ty of laws ensures that
...ective, specifying how
... prohibiting behavior
...ust be noncontradic-
...nts. Laws must not ask
...ld remain relatively
...clared rules and their
...ce may be destroyed in
... the drive toward per-
...ine the standards for

acceptable and prohibited behavior. Conformity to or violation of those rules by citizens should dictate the official treatment citizens receive. So, for example, police should only arrest individuals they believe to have acted illegally.

The eight principles of the rule of law specify necessary conditions for legal rules to be able effectively to govern the conduct of citizens. According to Fuller, law is 'the enterprise of subjecting human conduct to the governance of rules' (Fuller, 1969, p. 105). In Fuller's view, a legal system performs a very particular function in society: it facilitates the ability of citizens to interact with one another successfully. In his words, law 'is basically a matter of providing the citizenry with a sound and stable framework for their interactions with one another' (Fuller, 1969, p. 210). The role of government is to protect and enforce this framework. When a society respects the rule of law, legal rules outline guidelines for the behavior of citizens. Government officials establish and enforce these standards. When the rule of law is upheld, citizens develop common expectations with respect to how they themselves and others should act and these expectations are regularly fulfilled.

Citizen expectations of officials and each other

For Fuller, the claim that law shapes the particular expectations that citizens and officials make of each other is not simply a conceptual claim. Instead, Fuller asserts that citizens and officials who live in a society that purports to govern by law see legal rules in the way just described. That is, citizens and officials attach certain meaning to legal rules. Published laws become the particular standard by which citizens judge their own actions and the actions of others. Laws provide the substance of the general and specific expectations citizens have concerning the ways that they and others should behave.

If the law states that government buildings are supposed to remain closed on declared public holidays, then citizens expect government officials to abide by the law and keep government buildings closed on appointed holidays. This would be a specific expectation of citizens. The content of this expectation is shaped by particular rules. This specific expectation is also influenced by a general expectation citizens have of government officials, namely that officials will act in accordance with or on the basis of declared rules. According to Fuller, at the heart of the rule of law is the principle that 'in acting upon the citizen... a government will faithfully apply rules previously declared as those to be followed by the citizen and as being determinative of his rights and duties' (Fuller, 1969, p. 210). Fulfillment of this general principle becomes particularly important in the context of law enforcement. It implies that government officials should punish citizens only if they violate the public standard for behavior that published rules outline and should punish citizens *because* they violated that standard. In a society that governs by law, this is what citizens expect and this expectation is regularly fulfilled by government officials.

In many contexts, neither citizens nor officials are aware of the meaning they attach to legal rules and of the particular expectations they have of other citizens and officials. In such contexts, officials assume that most citizens will obey the law and that disobedience will be the exception, not the rule. Citizens assume that officials will act in accordance with and will enforce only declared laws. The expectations we develop on the basis of these assumptions become part of the social background we can take for granted when deliberating about how to act. Fuller uses the example of the election to illustrate the many, often implicit, expectations citizens make of each other and of officials in a society that successfully governs by law. He writes,

> Our institutions and our formalized interactions with one another are accompanied by certain interlocking expectations that may be called intendments, even though there is seldom occasion to bring these underlying expectations across the threshold of consciousness. In a very real sense when I cast my vote in an election my conduct is directed and conditioned by the anticipation that my ballot will be counted in favor of the candidate I actually vote for. This is true even though the possibility that my ballot will be thrown in the wastebasket, or counted for the wrong man, may never enter my mind as an object of conscious attention. In this sense the institutions of elections may be said to contain an intendment that the votes will be cast faithfully, tallied.
>
> Fuller (1969, p. 217)

As noted above, the formulation of specific expectations is influenced by the general expectation that officials will obey the constraints imposed by the rule of law. Very often, the commitment such constraints impose are 'so taken for granted that, except when things go wrong, there is no occasion to talk or even to think about it'(Fuller, 1969, p. 218).

Violations of expectation and citizen outcries

Evidence of the existence of these often implicit expectations surfaces when things go wrong and our expectations unfulfilled. Return to the example of an election. When a society purports to rule by law, then elections should not be rigged by ballots not being counted or ballots being counted in favor of a candidate different than the candidate for whom an individual voted. In a democracy, declared rules stipulate that government officials should assume office if chosen by the majority of citizens in an election. To fail to count ballots is to ignore the requirements imposed by officials implied by such declared rules. It violates the requirement that the preferences of the people, as expressed in ballots, should determine who becomes a government official. Citizens criticize officials who corrupt elections. Their reaction intuitively makes sense against the background set of expectations they have of how citizens and officials ought to behave, as required by the rule of law.

Successful legal systems and shared responsibility

The example of the fraudulent election highlights the fact that the success with which a legal system regulates behavior depends crucially upon the activities of officials. According to Fuller, every legal system is 'the product of a sustained purposive effort' (1969, p. 106) and 'maintaining a legal system in existence depends upon the discharge of interlocking responsibilities of government toward the citizen and of the citizen toward government' (p. 216). For a legal system effectively to regulate behavior in practice, officials must outline a standard of behavior that citizens are capable of following and that is actually enforced. The requirements of generality, publicity, and non-retroactivity ensure that citizens know about and are capable of following the law. Lawmakers must also enforce the declared rules. The requirement of congruence ensures that citizens are held accountable for following, or failing to follow, the standard articulated in law.

However, maintaining a legal system also depends upon the actions of citizens. Citizens have a responsibility to obey the rules that officials declare and enforce. For a legal system to function, citizens generally must obey the law. Disobedience must be the exception and not the norm. Where disobedience is widespread, it is futile for officials to declare rules to govern behavior. By hypothesis, such rules will be ignored by citizens and not be taken into account when they deliberate about how to act. After a certain point, disobedience can become too widespread for law enforcement officials to counter. Law enforcement efforts then become ineffective and legislative efforts futile.

The place of justice in the rule of law

The continual existence of legal institutions depends upon a sustained commitment by both citizens and officials to fulfill the responsibilities outlined above. However, neither citizens nor officials are automatically willing to discharge their responsibilities. According to Fuller, citizens and officials maintain their support for a particular legal system so long as they continue to believe that the legal system is operating as it should. A legal system is operating as it should when citizens and officials systematically respect the requirements of the rule of law and when the legal system administers justice. The commitment of legal systems to the pursuit of justice is reflected in the oath of judges everywhere. As legal philosopher David Dyzenhaus notes, 'judges everywhere claim that their duty is . . . to administer justice' (Dyzenhaus, 1998, p. 34).

It may seem odd to include the administration of justice in the notion of how a legal system should operate, because the requirements of the rule of law are strictly formal. The requirements are silent about the content that particular laws must have. Why think, then, that there is a connection between governing by law and administering justice? Indeed, many legal philosophers question the moral value of the rule of law because of the formal nature of the requirements. Shouldn't citizens revise their criteria for judging when a legal system is operating so as to exclude the demand that it administer justice?

Formal justice

In my view, there is in fact a connection between governing by law and administering both formal and substantive justice. The principle 'treat like cases alike' captures formal justice. Such justice requires that rules be applied fairly and impartially. The congruence requirement of the rule of law reflects this formal notion of justice. But in practice, respecting the requirements of the rule of law constrains the actions of officials, rendering unlikely the legislation and administration of substantively unjust laws. Thus, respect for the rule of law promotes more than formal justice. In Fuller's words, 'governmental respect for the internal morality of law [the requirements of the rule of law] will generally be conducive toward a respect for what may be called the substantive or external morality of law' (Fuller, 1969, pp. 223–4). Respecting the requirements of the rule of law encourages officials to pass laws whose content is also just. In another paper, I offer an extended argument to defend Fuller's claim that respect for the rule of law is conducive towards substantive justice (Murphy, 2005). Here I want to sketch the outline of that argument.

Substantive justice

The key to understanding the connection between respecting the requirements of the rule of law and the pursuit of substantive justice lies in appreciating the kind of governance ruling by law mandates. The rule of law ensures that a government publicly pursues its policies and makes known its practices. The rule of law guarantees open governance. Consequently, when it governs by law, a government opens itself up to international and domestic scrutiny of its policies and practices.

The open endorsement and pursuit of unjust policies makes a government vulnerable. It risks being perceived internationally as a pariah, facing international isolation, sanctions, and military intervention. It also risks becoming illegitimate in the view of its own citizens. Thus, there are incentives for a government to avoid the open pursuit of injustice. As the rule of law guarantees open governance, such governments have an incentive to violate the rule of law in order to avoid openly pursuing injustice.

At the same time, a government risks becoming an international pariah and losing its legitimacy among citizens if it violates the rule of law. Respect for the rule of law is increasingly becoming a criterion for legitimacy and good standing internationally and domestically. The only solution for governments that want to pursue injustice without alienating the international community or its own citizens is to maintain the façade of the rule of law but to not actually respect the requirements of the rule of law in practice.

When you carefully examine the practices of governments that have pursued or are pursuing gross injustice, you see that this is precisely what such governments do. Very often governments have seemed to respect the rule of law while pursuing injustice. This is often claimed of Nazi Germany, Argentina during the Dirty War, and South Africa under Apartheid. Despite appearances, however, none of these societies systematically respected the rule of law while pursuing injustice in fact. All three societies systematically violated the rule of law.[1] Consider South Africa under Apartheid and Argentina during the Dirty War. In both cases, there was frequent incongruence between declared rules and official practice. Torture was illegal in both Argentina and South Africa, yet torture against 'subversives' and anti-apartheid activists was systematic. Government officials in Argentina denied responsibility for the disappearances of citizens, which was illegal, and South African officials denied the existence of death squads, which were illegal. Both existed. In South Africa, there was also a fundamental contradiction between the principles of a common law legal order and apartheid. Common law heritage includes a commitment to protect the fundamental rights and freedoms of individuals (Dyzenhaus, 1998, p. 15). Consequently, judges were 'at one and the same time being asked to articulate and give effect to equitable common law principles, and to uphold and enforce discriminatory laws: at one and the same time to be an instrument of justice and at another to be an instrument of oppression' (Dyzenhaus, 1998, p. 15). As Dyzenhaus argues in his critique of judges under apartheid, respect for the rule of law required judges to make explicit this contradiction so that the government could recognize that a commitment to apartheid entailed a rejection of the common law legal order.

---

[1] Fuller discusses the systematic nature of violations of the rule of law in Nazi Germany in *The Morality of Law*. I discuss the cases of Argentina and South Africa in 'Lon Fuller and the Moral Value of the Rule of Law'.

Rationalizing injustices

Sometimes government officials cynically manipulate citizens and the international community while privately acknowledging the unjust nature of their ends. However, often this is not the case. Instead, officials rationalize their participation in injustice or deny that what they are doing is unjust or unjustified. Such denial and rationalization is psychologically important because, as I will discuss in greater detail in Section 4.3, individuals have a fundamental need to believe that they are decent and moral. This belief is easier to maintain when one does not need to justify one's unjust actions to others.

An additional problem with the openness of governance required by the rule of law, then, is that it makes it more difficult for officials to deny, to themselves and to others, that they are acting unjustly. Openness establishes conditions for individuals and governments to be held accountable for their actions. Given how important it is for individuals to believe that they are decent and the very real risks the pursuit of injustice poses for governments, a government that in practice respects the rule of law will be unlikely to pursue unjust policies.[2] The content of the regulations legislated and enforced in a society that rules by law will be moral and the legal system be just when citizens and officials systematically fulfill the expectations required of them.

Respect for the rule of law and healthy political relationships

I have been arguing that there is reason to think that Fuller was right when he claimed that respect for the rule of law promotes justice in practice. This link between the rule of law and justice also sheds some light on why mutual respect for the rule of law is a component of healthy political relationships. Healthy relationships contribute to the moral and mental well-being of individuals. Fulfillment of the responsibilities required by political relationships does not undermine individual well-being. That the rule of law constrains the pursuit of injustice shows one way that it contributes to healthy political relationships. It ensures that the duties demanded of citizens are fair and reasonable in their content. Thus, when a society governs by law, the content of the actions required or prohibited by law will not be incompatible with protecting the health of those who obey legal requirements.

---

[2] My argument defends the claim that there is an incompatibility of the pursuit of *systematic* injustice and the rule of law. It is possible that particular immoral or unjust laws be passed in accordance with the requirements of the rule of law. Respect for the rule of law does not guard against every injustice.

There are additional ways in which mutual respect for the rule of law contributes to the health of political relationships. Specifically, the rule of law structures relationships among citizens and officials that are reciprocal and respectful of agency. I end this section by describing first how the rule of law structures relationships in this way and then discussing why relationships structured in this fashion are healthy.

Reciprocity and respect for agency

Mutual respect for the rule of law guarantees reciprocal fulfillment of responsibilities. For Fuller, the existence of moral duties depends partly on the behavior of others. In other words, it is fair to expect me to fulfill my duties only if those judging my behavior fulfill their reciprocal responsibilities. Fulfillment of one's own citizen responsibilities is a necessary condition for one to be able legitimately to demand actions from others. Reciprocity is realized through mutual respect for the rule of law. When a society governs by law, 'Government says to the citizen in effect, 'These are the rules we expect you to follow. If you follow them, you have the assurance that they are the rules that will be applied to your conduct' (Fuller, 1969, p. 40). In Fuller's view, government officials have the moral right to demand that citizens obey the law only if legal rules outline a standard that citizens acknowledge, are capable of following, and that is actually enforced. The requirements of the rule of law ensure that this is the case.

In addition, implicit in the rule of law is the view that an individual 'is or can become a responsible agent capable of understanding and following rules and answerable for his defaults' (Fuller, 1969, p. 162). When officials respect the rule of law, they treat citizens as responsible and self-directed agents. Citizens are judged based on standards of behavior that they had a real opportunity to follow. Officials assess the behavior of citizens based on a clear, publicly knowable standard. Thus, it is the decisions and actions of individuals, and not the whims of officials, which determine the legal treatment they receive.

Reciprocity and respect for agency are important because they embody two ways of recognizing the dignity of individuals. By treating individuals as agents and respecting reciprocity, we acknowledge through our actions that individuals have a value that constrains how we can legitimately treat one another. One constraint is that we cannot make demands on others regardless of what we do. Another constraint is that we cannot react to others in a way that disregards what they have done; other's actions or omissions necessarily affect our responses to them. Acknowledging and respecting such limitations reinforces that individuals are the source of moral claims and, as agents, should not merely be acted upon. When officials and citizens mutually respect the limitations on their behavior set by the rule of law, they respect others and treat others as agents. This contributes the well-being of citizens by reinforcing their belief in their value and agency.

4.3 The breakdown of the rule of law

In the previous section, I examined the requirements of the rule of law and argued that mutual respect for the rule of law is a constitutive element of healthy political relationships between citizens and officials. In this section, I focus on the breakdown of the rule of law and discuss how systematic violations of the rule of law damage the political relationships among citizens and officials.

When violations of the rule of law are systematic, officials in practice no longer govern by law. Declared rules no longer guide the interactions among citizens or the actions of law enforcement officials. Consider a society in which police brutality against members of racial minorities is common, though illegal. In such a society, members of minority groups will develop expectations about how officials will respond to their actions based on the experiences of other minorities rather than on the basis of declared official rules. Such incongruence between declared rules and the actual practices of law enforcement officials undermines the meaningfulness of declared rules; such rules no longer provide a reliable basis for forming expectations about the behavior of officials.

Violations of the rule of law and substantive injustice

One consequence of systematic violations of the rule of law is an increased likelihood that substantive injustice will be pursued. When officials flout the congruence requirement, they act differently from the way that declared rules permit or prohibit. This means that citizens and the international community cannot look to the written law to determine what policies are being pursued or in which practices officials are engaging. As I discussed in the previous section, when officials do not have to account for or defend their actions, either to the international community or to themselves, they are more likely to engage in manifestly unjust forms of treatment.

Undermining of reciprocity and respect

Violations also weaken the reciprocity and respect for agency at the core of healthy political relationships. In repressive regimes, officials frequently violate the rule of law and yet continue to demand that citizens obey the law.

In such cases, political relationships are no longer reciprocal. Officials continue to expect obedience by citizens, despite the lack of fulfillment of their reciprocal responsibilities as government officials. Officials fail to recognize that their actions undermine the legitimacy with which they can demand such obedience.

Officials in such cases also fail to treat citizens as self-directed agents and to respect their autonomy. Recognition of the agency of others dictates that official treatment of citizens is determined on the basis of the actions of citizens. When the rule of law is systematically violated, then the whim of officials, rather than the actions of citizens, determines the official treatment that citizens are likely to receive. In such circumstances, the exercise of agency is frustrated. The life of citizens goes according to the caprice of officials rather than on the basis of their own actions.

Disrespect for agency and denial of reciprocity fail to recognize the dignity of individual citizens. Such actions send a message that citizens do not deserve better treatment and that citizens are not the authors of their own lives. This message can be damaging to the well-being of citizens in that it damages their self-respect, pride, and other self-regarding virtues. There are additional ways that violations of the rule of law damage relationships. Systematic violations of the rule of law by officials foster distrust, resentment, and a sense of betrayal among citizens. I want to end this section by examining these additional ways that violations of the rule of law impact political relationships.

Erosion of distrust and rise of alienation

Violations erode the trust of citizens in, and alienate them from, the judicial system and law-enforcement officials. When government officials violate the congruence requirement of the rule of law, it is unsurprising that distrust develops. It is difficult to trust politicians who lie or law enforcement officials who harm and brutalize citizens instead of protecting them from harm. Officials who violate the rule of law undermine the confidence with which citizens can look to the written law to determine what officials expect of them. Citizens who know about specific discrepancies between written law and official action have little reason to believe that other written or publicly espoused policies reflect the practices of state agents.

When lawmakers fall far short of the rule of law, citizens feel betrayed. As Fuller notes, a basic principle of the rule of law is 'that the acts of a legal authority toward the citizen must be legitimated by being brought within the terms of a previous declaration of general rules' (Fuller, 1969, p. 214). In cases of incongruence, officials betray this principle. The actions of law enforcement officials are not authorized by previously declared rules. This betrays the expectations that citizens have of officials when they live in a society that purports to govern by law. The discovery that one has been betrayed is painful and disorienting. Being on the receiving end of betrayal can lead to existential despair and even madness.

Resentment, rage, and increased violence

Systematic violations of the rule of law also cause citizens to feel resentment. Resentment builds when officials expect citizens to fulfill certain duties, like obedience to law, despite the failure of government officials to fulfill their reciprocal expectations or duties. Resentment among citizens increases when government officials punish those who disobey the law, yet similar violations by government officials go unpunished. This resentment is reasonable. It is also potentially a source of instability. The more citizens resent their leaders, the more likely they are to erupt in rage and violence and, consequently, the more difficult it is for officials to control them.

The breakdown of the rule of law damages political relationships in a myriad of ways. The rule of law characteristically breaks down in societies where there is repressive rule or civil conflict. For such societies, the restoration of the rule of law is part of the process of reconciliation, or of (re-)establishing healthier ways for citizens and officials to relate. Mutual respect for the rule of law is a key feature of healthy political relationships between citizens and officials.

Many politicians and human rights activists working in transitional societies try to facilitate the process of reconciliation. One objective of this paper is to highlight the role that research of psychologists and psychiatrists on PTSD can play in enriching our understanding of what kinds of processes in fact foster reconciliation. In the next two sections, I discuss what PTSD is and look at two significant parallels between the breakdown of the rule of law and PTSD. In the final two sections, I explore the implications of these similarities for our understanding of how to promote reconciliation.

4.4 Post-traumatic stress disorder

In what follows, I outline key characteristics of the events that are PTSD-inducing as well as the symptoms of PTSD. This information is important for understanding the parallels and interaction between PTSD and the breakdown of the rule of law, which is the topic of the next section.

Traumatic events

One key to understanding PTSD is appreciating why certain events are traumatic. Such appreciation requires a grasp of the framework of beliefs and expectations that individuals rely upon to comprehend and act in society. Psychologist Janoff-Bulman (1985, 1989, 1992) has developed a particularly influential account of beliefs individuals commonly hold. For my purposes, it is necessary only to discuss two kinds of such beliefs. One concerns the nature of the self. The other has to do with the nature of the world.

Agency and the desire for safety

Janoff-Bulman claims that individuals typically believe that they can effectively exercise their agency and that they have value. An agent is someone who can pursue and realize her goals successfully. A belief in the effectiveness of agency entails a belief in the ability to predict the likely consequences of various actions. This ability is essential for agency because the successful pursuit of one's goals depends upon the capability to judge the appropriate action to take in specific situations. Such judgments and comparison of different courses of action are possible only if an individual can predict the probable results of different courses of action.

According to Janoff-Bulman, individuals care about their safety and want to ensure their safety through their actions. Because they believe in their agency, individuals also believe that they can, through their actions, reduce the risk of being harmed. This is what Janoff-Bulman labels the self-controllability belief (Dekel *et al.*, 2004, p. 409). The more an individual believes she is acting in safety-promoting ways, the greater she thinks she is reducing the likelihood of harm to herself. In Janoff-Bulman's words, '[T]he degree to which one views oneself as engaging in the right behaviors (e.g., precautionary, appropriate behaviors) minimizes one's vulnerability to negative outcomes' (Dekel *et al.*, 2004, p. 409).

Belief that the world is meaningful and good

Individuals also commonly believe certain things about the world. Specifically, most individuals believe that the world is meaningful and good. A belief that the principle of desert operates in the world or that the world is just connects these two beliefs. In other words, good things happen to good people and bad things happen to bad people. The operation of desert in the world confirms the agency of individuals because we can predict that if we act well, then good consequences will follow. Thus it is unsurprising that 'The belief in a just world enables the individual to confront the physical and social environment as if it were stable and orderly. It is a belief that individuals are reluctant to give up, and evidence that the world is not really just can be extremely distressing' (Joseph *et al.* 1997, p. 79).

Invulnerability

Individuals often develop a sense of invulnerability because of the conjunction of the beliefs in our agency and decency and in the justness of the world. If we are basically good people, then our actions are basically good (or at least well-intended) and so good consequences should follow from our actions. This is especially true when we take measures to ensure our safety. Thus, 'although we may recognize that crimes, accidents, and illnesses occur to a large portion of the population, it is also possible to believe simultaneously that these misfortunes will not happen to us' (Joseph *et al.*, 1997, p. 79).

Traumatic stressors

It is against this background understanding of common beliefs that we can make sense of the nature of traumatic events. A traumatic stressor is an experience 'outside the range of usual human experience and that would be "markedly distressing" to anyone' (Shay, 1994, p. 5). There are two primary characteristics of traumatic events. First, typically there is a threat to or infliction of physical injury or death upon an individual (Joseph *et al.*, 1997, p. 51). Events of this kind that tend to be PTSD-inducing include natural disasters (such as tsunamis, earthquakes, volcanic eruptions), technological disasters, combat, being a victim of a crime (burglary, assault), sexual assault, childhood sexual abuse, political violence (Joseph *et al.*, 1997, p. 51). '[A]n event...that involved actual or threatened death or serious injury, or a threat to the physical integrity of self or others' (Joseph *et al.*, 1997, p. 13) can be traumatizing for individuals who experience, witness, or confront them.

The second aspect of a traumatic stressor is subjective in nature and centers on how an individual reacts to the traumatic event. An event that involves the threat or infliction of bodily harm is PTSD-inducing if individuals experience the threat or harm in a particular way. If an individual feels 'fear, helplessness, or horror' in the face of experiencing, witnessing, or confronting the threat or harm, then it is more likely she will have post-traumatic stress reactions (Joseph *et al.*, 1997, p. 13).

Effects of trauma

Traumatic experiences call into question the validity of the fundamental beliefs of individuals described above. To illustrate, consider rape. For an individual who has been raped, it is difficult to reconcile her experience with either her belief that she is a decent person or her belief that the world is meaningful and good. If she is a good person, then the rape might seem to provide evidence that the world is not always just and good things do not happen to good people. If the world is just and people do get what they deserve, then the rape might seem to provide evidence that she is not a decent person or has value.

The violation of these deeply held beliefs and expectations by traumatic events can have a profound effect on individuals. When an experience is traumatizing, individuals develop characteristic symptoms. The focus of the research and practice of psychologists and psychiatrists is upon understanding and treating the symptoms of PTSD. There are three general types of symptoms I want to mention.

The first general symptom is that an individual re-experiences the traumatic event. This re-experiencing may occur in dreams, vivid flashbacks where it feels like the event is 'recurring,' as well as 'intrusive' distressing recollections of the events. Individuals may also have a physical reaction or 'intense psychological distress' if exposed to something that to them symbolizes or resembles an aspect of the traumatic event. A related, second symptom is that individuals have extremely intense reactions to people or places associated in their mind with the traumatic event. Examples of such reactions would include outbursts of anger. Alternately, individuals may find it difficult to sleep or concentrate (Joseph *et al.*, 1997, p. 13).

The third general symptom of PTSD is the 'persistent avoidance of stimuli associated with the trauma and numbing of general responsiveness (not present before the trauma)' (Joseph *et al.*, 1997, p. 13). Individuals may try to avoid thinking about or being around particular people or places associated with the event. They may try to suppress any emotional reactions to such people or places. In other words, individuals may try to cultivate a sense of detachment from particular people or places.

Making 'sense' of trauma

According to the influential psychology theorist Mardi Jon Horowitz, these characteristic reactions reflect the difficulty individuals have making sense of their traumatic experiences. Individuals have an internal drive to make all of their beliefs consistent. Traumatic experiences provide information 'which is incompatible with existing [cognitive] schemas' of individuals (Joseph *et al.*, 1997, p. 73). This incongruity is distressing and requires an individual to reappraise and revise her view of the world. In the aftermath of trauma, individuals try to find a way to make their experience cohere with their beliefs about the world and themselves. To prevent emotional exhaustion during this period of integration and revision, individuals react by detaching themselves from the event and the world. The vivid reactions that individuals have when not detached reflect their process of integration.

Sometimes, a traumatic event can undermine the world view of individuals, shattering some of their fundamental beliefs. Individuals vary in the degree and number of assumptions rejected as a result of exposure to the traumatic stressor. According to psychologists Dekel *et al.*,

> The psychological aftermath of a traumatic event is multidimensional and may be manifested by cognitive, somatic, psychiatric, and functional dysfunction. Among long-term sequelae that investigators have observed in victims of traumatic events is the challenging, and even the shattering, of their basic cognitive schemes regarding the world and themselves, including a feeling of invulnerability, the tendency to see the world as meaningful, and the tendency to see themselves as worthy.
>
> Dekel *et al.* (2004, p. 407)

A traumatic event may lead individuals to abandon one of their core beliefs. For example, an individual may no longer view the world as a meaningful or valuable place. This may contribute to a loss in the belief of one's agency. Once the world is no longer seen as a predictable place, it is difficult to feel a sense of control over one's life. In an uncertain world, it is difficult to form reliable expectations, or any expectations at all, about how others will react to one's actions. This in turn may lead to a general apathy towards one's projects or the world.

Losing fundamental beliefs

Losing the belief in the meaningfulness of the world and in our agency can lead to paranoia or fear. Psychiatrist Jonathan Shay (1994) writes, 'Every trauma narrative pierces our adult cloak of safety; it...leaves us terrified and disoriented' (p. 37). After a traumatic event, we may no longer trust or assume that we can effectively reduce our vulnerability through our actions. A natural consequence of this frame of mind is paranoia, constantly being vigilant, no matter what we do to reduce risk, because harm may still come our way at any moment.

Such paranoia may reflect a loss of general trust. Shay works with combat veterans with PTSD. When describing the effects of PTSD he writes,

> Combat trauma destroys the capacity for social trust, accounting for the paranoid state of being that blights the lives of the most severely traumatized combat veterans. This is not a selective mistrust directed at a specific individual or institution that has betrayed its charge, but a comprehensive destruction of social trust. Lies and

euphemisms by the soldier's own military superiors and civilian leaders of course undermine social trust by destroying confidence in language.

Shay (1994, p. 34)

When social trust is lost, individuals can no longer take anything, including the words of others, at face value. Normally, an individual can trust that the meaning of words is undermined when the expectations we make of others on the basis of their words are violated. Such distrust can undermine our capacity for intimacy, which is possible only in a context where you trust the one with whom you are intimate. 'Unhealed PTSD can devastate life and incapacitate its victims from participation in the domestic, economic, and political life of the nation' (Shay, 1994, p. xx).

To summarize, PTSD refers to the characteristic symptoms that individuals exhibit when exposed to a traumatic stressor. A traumatic stressor refers to an experience outside the ordinary that would normally be distressing. Such experiences call into question the fundamental beliefs and expectations of individuals that form part of the cognitive framework they use to navigate in the world. The challenging of these beliefs has a powerful effect on individuals. Symptoms of PTSD include flashbacks, difficulty sleeping, and avoidance of people and places associated with the experience. It can contribute to their abandonment of those beliefs and to distrust, rage, resentment, or detachment.

4.5 Implications for theorizing about the rule of law

In the previous sections I discussed the concepts of the rule of law and of PTSD. In this section, I first discuss structural similarities between these concepts. My objective in exploring these similarities is to show two ways that the concept of PTSD can enrich our grasp of reconciliation by deepening our understanding of the rule of law.

What the breakdown of the rule of law and post-traumatic stress disorder have in common

The breakdown of the rule of law and PTSD-inducing traumatic events share two important features. First, both consist of actions whose occurrence violates the expectations of individuals. Violations of the rule of law contravene the expectations citizens have about how officials or other citizens will act. Traumatic events challenge the validity of beliefs individuals commonly have about the nature of the world and themselves. These beliefs are used as a guideline for forming expectations about what the consequences of our actions will be. These expectations form part of the framework individuals rely upon when deliberating about how to act.

In addition, both phenomena have analogous, profoundly damaging effects. The legacy of the breakdown of the rule of law includes widespread distrust, resentment, and uncertainty among citizens; symptoms of PTSD consist of distrust, fear, rage, and uncertainty. The intense, analogous effects of the violation of expectations in both cases suggests that fulfillment of certain expectations is crucial for societal and individual well-being.

How theories of post-traumatic stress disorder can be a resource in understanding the breakdown of the rule of law

Primary and secondary post-traumatic stress disorder

Psychologists increasingly distinguish among various types of PTSD. These distinctions provide resources for developing a more nuanced perspective on the societal impacts of the breakdown of the rule of law, given the conceptual similarities between the rule of law and PTSD. One distinction psychologists make is between primary and secondary PTSD. What is interesting about this distinction is that it highlights the different ways individuals with various relationships to a traumatic event might be impacted by such an event. Individuals with primary PTSD directly experienced the threat or infliction of physical harm and exhibit certain characteristic symptoms as a result (Figley and Kleber, 1995, pp. 78–9). Secondary PTSD impacts the significant others who learn about such traumatic experiences. Significant others might include spouse, children, friends, colleagues, or helping professionals. Secondary PTSD refers to the characteristic behaviors and emotions that result from the knowledge that a significant other suffered a certain event.

Application to breakdowns of the rule of law

That particular ways of experiencing traumatic events results in distinct effects suggests that the breakdown of the rule of law might not impact everyone in society in the same way. The effects of the breakdown Fuller discussed might be different, or more pronounced, among various groups within society. Consider a society in which torture is systematic, though illegal. Assume that security forces disproportionately target members of a certain ethnic or racial group. Violations of the congruence requirement by security forces will affect members of the targeted group in different ways than it affects members of the non-targeted group. Many members of the nontargeted group may never learn about or have to come to terms with violations during the repressive regime. Like secondary PTSD victims, they may only learn about the breakdown after the fact. In contrast, sympathetic but nontargeted individuals or members of the targeted group live with the daily knowledge of the discrepancy between declared rules and legal practices. Their experience is continually and directly traumatic in a way more analogous to those with primary PTSD. The impact that the breakdown of the rule of law has, then, can vary among different segments of society. Consequently, processes designed to restore mutual respect for the rule of law and deal with the legacy from its breakdown need to be sensitive to the differential effects it may have upon society.

Post-traumatic stress disorder and healing processes

The conceptual similarities between the breakdown of the rule of law and PTSD are of use when thinking about processes of reconciliation. Given that the cause and effects of both are analogous, it is likely that there are structural parallels between their healing processes. Only recently have scholars begun to think systematically about how to judge the effectiveness of processes designed to restore the rule of law and deal with the legacy from the breakdown of the rule of law. Thus, discussions about therapy for PTSD have the potential to contribute to the discussions about processes of reconciliation.

Among psychiatrists and psychologists, there is no consensus on what form of therapy is best when treating individuals with PTSD. Thus, there is no substantive notion of the therapeutic process from which to examine what features might find analogues in processes of reconciliation. However, when thinking about processes of reconciliation, it is instructive to look at the aspects of the therapeutic process currently being debated. The issues about which psychologists are debating suggest questions about reconciliation that need to be, but currently are not systematically being, asked by advocates of reconciliation.

Additionally, there is no agreement among psychologists and psychiatrists about what the goal of therapy should be. There is a minimum consensus that, when therapy is successful, patients should report reduced distress. However, there are competing understandings of what reducing distress entails. Distress may be reduced because, as a result of therapy, individuals are able to work through their anxiety when it arises. Or distress may be reduced because, through therapy, anxiety is no longer part of the current chapter of their lives.

These various conceptions of reduced distress reflect different views of the proper goal of therapy. Some therapeutic approaches set overcoming anxiety as a goal while others aim to help individuals cope with their anxiety. Anxiety is overcome when a patient no longer experiences fear in situations that previously caused anxiety. The outcome of therapy is different if an individual learns to cope with anxiety. In such cases, an individual would continue to experience fear in situations that are anxiety-producing. The difference would be that she learned how to respond in ways that enabled her to deal with her fear in a healthier way.

Underlying debates about the appropriate goal for therapeutic processes are unstated assumptions about what is possible for individuals to achieve. One reason to view the goal of therapy as that of learning how to manage, rather than overcome, anxiety is the conviction that overcoming anxiety is impossible. If an individual will always feel fear in certain situations, then the best she can try to do is learn to respond to these effects of PTSD in a way that enables her to live to the greatest extent possible a normal life.

Application to breakdowns of the rule of law

These questions about the goal of therapy and what is possible in therapy suggest issues that advocates of reconciliation should be debating more explicitly. In the literature, there is not substantial discussion about what the goal of processes of reconciliation should be. Yet there are a number of goals that processes of reconciliation might have. For example, one goal might be to help a society in transition overcome the effects of the legacy of the breakdown of the rule of law, including pervasive distrust and resentment. Another, different goal would be to help a society learn how to cope with the pervasive distrust and resentment.

Just as the resolution of questions about the goal of therapy turns partly on what kind of change is possible for individuals with PTSD, the resolution of debates about the appropriate goal of processes of reconciliation depends on what kind of reconciliation is possible for each society in transition. In a particular case, it may be impossible to surmount the resentment and distrust among citizens. The goal of processes of reconciliation, then, would be to help citizens interact in the healthiest way possible, given their distrust and resentment.

Psychologists also disagree about what method is most successful for realizing the goal of therapy. In particular, there are debates about whether, and to what extent, it is healthy for individuals to re-experience anger as part of their therapy. Becoming angry is seen by some as an important aspect of therapy because this enables individuals to have a cathartic experience. Psychotherapists, for example, are interested in providing a venue for patients to work through their anger. Critics of this school of thought argue that this approach reinforces and entrenches the anger of patients rather than helps them move past it. It is better, they argue, to help individuals move beyond their anger, without requiring that individuals experience a stronger version of their anger. The role of the therapist, on this view, is to help patients see how their anger is poisoning their lives and why they need to set such anger aside in order to be able to move on with their lives.

We should be asking analogous questions about the kinds of processes societies use to foster reconciliation. Should a society strive to establish a context in which catharsis might be achieved? Or should a society work to raise consciousness among citizens about how anger and resentment poison relationships? Was it helpful for Bishop Tutu to praise and hold up as role models victims who expressed forgiveness during the hearings of the South African Truth and Reconciliation Commission? Or should he instead have encouraged victims to express the anger and resentment they felt towards their perpetrators? If voicing anger is a necessary condition for overcoming anger, then processes of reconciliation should be structured to allow anger to be articulated.

Therapeutic relationships and relationships that facilitate political reconciliation

One final debate in psychology that is instructive for understanding and evaluating processes of reconciliation centers around the nature of the therapeutic relationship between the patient and therapist. There is no consensus on what kind of relationship a patient and therapist need to have in order for therapy to be effective. In particular, therapists disagree about how deeply the patient should trust the therapist and why such trust is important. We might ask similar questions about those who should conduct processes of reconciliation. (Why) is it necessary for the individuals in charge of processes such as truth commissions to be trusted within society? (Why) is it valuable or necessary to have an outside, third party, like the therapist, to facilitate such processes?

In this section, I have argued that the breakdown of the rule of law and of PTSD share a similar structure. Both involve the violation of certain fundamental and important expectations. In both cases, the effects of such violations include deep distrust, resentment, and other negative psychological effects that impair the ability of individuals or society to function in a healthy way. I have suggested that these conceptual similarities have two interesting implications. First, they provide a way for distinguishing more carefully among the various effects of the breakdown of the rule of law. Second, debates about PTSD suggest a framework for examining the efficacy of different kinds of processes of reconciliation.

4.6 Implications for post-traumatic stress disorder

In the previous section, I explored implications that the conceptual similarities between PTSD and the breakdown of the rule of law might have for understanding the nature of and remedy for the breakdown of the rule of law.

In this section, I focus on the frequent interplay between the breakdown of the rule of law and PTSD in practice. Systematic violations of the congruence requirement of the rule of law are also typically PTSD-inducing events. After looking at this interaction, I consider how this recognition might enrich our understanding of PTSD.

Breakdowns of the rule of law are post-traumatic stress disorder inducing

Frequently, the official actions that violate the congruence requirement of the rule of law are also potential traumatic stressors. Governments rarely publicly sanction actions that are likely to draw international or domestic criticism. However, repressive governments characteristically rely upon terror, understood as 'the arbitrary use…of severe coercion' (Linz, 2000, p. 100) in order to frighten citizens into compliance. So, while declared rules rarely sanction torture or extra-judicial killing, in practice torture and extra-judicial killing are often systematic in repressive regimes. Argentina during the Dirty War is a paradigmatic case of such official, though illegal, practices. When describing what happened to the desaparecidos, or disappeared, Marguerite Feitlowitz writes, 'suspected "subversives" were kidnapped from the streets, tortured in secret concentration camps, and "disappeared". Victims died during torture, were machine-gunned at the edge of enormous pits, or were thrown, drugged, from airplanes into the sea' (Feitlowitz, 1998, p. ix). The disappeared faced threatened or actual infliction of bodily injury or death and lived in uncertainty and fear. Their experience fulfilled both criteria for traumatic stressors.

Direct and indirect effects

Recognizing that the same event can be part of the process of systematically violating the rule of law and a PTSD-inducing traumatic stressor puts particular traumatic events into social context and helps us make sense of observations of psychologists working with survivors of political violence in a society with ongoing or recent political violence or repressive rule. Such psychologists recognize that the effects of torture and killing extend far beyond the victims and their immediate family and friends. They recognize, in other words, that political violence has societal ramifications. As Elizabeth Kornfeld writes about Chile,

> Violations of human rights cannot be viewed exclusively from the perspective of isolated individual abuses. Their implications are much more extensive, for they describe not only a system's response to conflict, but a general ambience of political threat, both of which lead to an atmosphere of chronic fear. Those violations have

implied a strong threat affecting everyday life in Chilean society... Insecurity, vulnerability, and fear were widespread feelings among people, whatever their actual political involvement. Fear, which is normally a reaction to a specific external or internal threat, became a permanent component of everyday personal and social life. This constant state of fear, while affecting more directly those people who identified themselves as possible targets of political repression, did not leave the uninvolved unscathed.

Kornfeld (1995, p. 117)

The framework of the rule of law helps us make sense of why and how individual traumatic events can impact members of society who have no direct or significant relationship with those who were harmed or threatened with such harm. The rule of law draws attention to the broad, shared expectations that a legal system cultivates and the way that those shared expectations can be undermined or maintained by the actions of officials and citizens. When a particular official tortures a citizen illegally and the official's action is part of a larger systematic effort, then the official's individual action contributes to the ongoing officially sanctioned process of creating an uncertain environment for citizens. These systematic actions undermine the reliability of the shared expectations citizens develop based on declared rules. Thus, the systematic actions of officials undermine the confidence with which citizens can look to declared rules to determine what official treatment they are likely to receive if they perform certain actions. The social environment becomes unpredictable as a result.

Creating an environment of uncertainty undermines the ability of citizens to act effectively as agents. Citizens can no longer reliably decide which actions to take to ensure their safety. Such decisions depend on calculations of the consequences of different courses of actions. Calculations are difficult to make when one can no longer predict the likely consequences of different courses of action. When they can no longer act as agents, it is difficult for citizens to believe in the efficacy of their agency. This belief is normally part of the cognitive schema of individuals; undermining this belief threatens the very framework individuals rely upon when navigating in the social world. Thus, the rule of law highlights the broader, indirect effects that traumatic events that are also violations of the rule of law might have on the general relations or dealings among citizens and the general atmosphere within society.

Research implications

This interaction between the breakdown of the rule of law and PTSD-inducing events suggests interesting considerations for the research on therapy for PTSD. The validity of an answer to particular questions, such as what it is possible for individuals to achieve in therapy, might be context-specific. The achievable goals of therapy might be different depending on the political context. If, as I suggested, repressive regimes systematically violate the rule of law in practice, under repressive regimes it is difficult for citizens to develop stable expectations of how officials and other citizens will respond to their actions. In such contexts, it might be impossible for individuals to overcome their anxiety because one cause of anxiety, namely an unpredictable social environment, remains. The possibilities for the goals of therapy might be broader in a stable democratic context in which there is a more stable social environment.

4.7 **Conclusions**

It is common for academics and politicians to call for reconciliation in societies emerging from civil conflict and repressive rule. However, it remains unclear what the call for reconciliation means. In this paper, I discussed one important aspect of the process of reconciliation, namely the restoration of mutual respect for the rule of law. I argued that our understanding of what this process entails can be enriched by looking at the psychological research on PTSD. Not only can academics interested in societies in transition benefit from the research of psychologists, but also psychologists can benefit from the work being done on societal reconciliation. As I suggested in the last section, discussions of societal reconciliation draw attention to the broader social context in which traumatic events occur and highlight the role that this social context might play in influencing what it is possible for individual therapy to achieve.

Acknowledgments

I would like to thank Maureen Adams, Azzurra Crispino, Paolo Gardoni, Katya Hosking, Kathleen Murphy, Nancy Nyquist Potter, Gerald J Postema, Linda Radzik, Ingra Schellenberg, Susanne Sreedhar, and Theodore George for their very helpful comments on earlier drafts of this paper. This paper was presented during a seminar on Lon Fuller at the Law Faculty of McGill University and as part of the meeting of the Society for the Study of Genocide and Holocaust during the Central Division meeting of the American Philosophical Association. During both presentations I received numerous helpful suggestions for which I am very grateful.

References

Dekel R, Solomon Z, Elklit A, and Ginzburg K (2004). World assumptions and combat-related Posttraumatic Stress Disorder. *Journal of Social Psychology*, **144**(4): 407–20.

Dyzenhaus D (1998). *Judging the Judges, Judging Ourselves*. Oxford: Hart Publishing.

Feitlowitz M (1998). *A Lexicon of Terror: Argentina and the Legacies of Torture*. Oxford: Oxford University Press.

Figley C and Kleber, R (1995). Beyond the 'victim': Secondary traumatic stress. In: *Beyond Trauma: Cultural and Societal Dynamics*. (eds R Kleber, C Figley, and B Gersons), pp. 75–98. New York: Plenum Press.

Fuller L (1969). *Morality of Law*. New Haven: Yale University Press.

Janoff-Bulman R (1985). The aftermath of victimization: Rebuilding shattered assumptions. In: *Trauma and its Wake*, Vol. 1 (ed. CR Figley), pp. 15–35. New York: Brunner/Mazel Publishers.

Janoff-Bulman R (1989). Assumptive worlds and the stress of traumatic events: applications of the schema construct. *Social Cognition*, 7: 113–36.

Janoff-Bulman R (1992). *Shattered Assumptions: Towards a New Psychology of Trauma*. New York: The Free Press.

Joseph S, Williams R, and Yule W (1997). *Understanding Post-Traumatic Stress: A Psychosocial Perspective on PTSD and Treatment*. Chichester, UK: John Wiley and Sons.

Kornfeld E (1995). The development of treatment approaches for victims of human rights violations in Chile. In: *Beyond Trauma: Cultural and Societal Dynamics* (eds R Kleber, C Figley, and B Gersons), pp. 115–31. New York: Plenum Press.

Linz, J (2000). *Totalitarian and Authoritarian Regimes*. Boulder, CO: Lynne Riemner Publishers.

Murphy C (2005). Lon Fuller and the moral value of the rule of law. *Law and Philosophy*, 24: 239–62.

Shay J (1994). *Achilles in Vietnam: Combat Trauma and the Undoing of Character*. New York: Scribner.

Chapter 5

When philosophical assumptions matter

Allison Mitchell

5.1 **Introduction**

The notion of truth is of central importance both to academic philosophers
and those persons carrying out the urgent and demanding practical work performed by truth and reconciliation commissions. This shared commitment to
understanding and applying the concept of truth suggests that people engaged
in both types of pursuits may be able to learn from one another.[1] In what
follows, I will explore the relation between the commissioners' conceived procedures and the possible realization of those aims typically associated with
these groups. My main purpose will be to develop a philosophical perspective
on the work performed by truth and reconciliation commissions, a picture
whose value can be measured against the results it generates in the domain of
real lived experience and human action. A pragmatist conception of philosophical inquiry motivates and guides this project: a careful, systematic, and rigorous analysis of the meanings of our ordinary terms and concepts may promote
self-awareness and knowledge of the world that is useful to us within the
context of our everyday lives. Philosophy may help us to identify, clarify, and
reflect upon what counts for us as persons, providing us with understanding
that is both independently and instrumentally valuable. A philosophical
approach to the concept of truth (and related practices or notions) will help
us begin to understand the abstract notion and the central role the practice of
truth-telling plays in many of our lives.

----

[1] Readers seeking to understand the history and contemporary significance of philosophical thought about truth may find Bernard Williams' *Truth and Truthfulness* (2002) and
   Pascal Engel's *Truth* (2002) both accessible and insightful. Julian Baggini (2002, p. 22)
   attempts to diagnose the value placed by commissioners on the full acknowledgment of
   truth in *Making Sense: Philosophy Behind the Headlines*.

Commissioners tend to understand the concept of truth and the activity of truth-telling in terms that may seem perfectly intuitive, uncontroversial, and familiar to us: telling the truth involves making sincere claims about matters of fact that correspond with what really happens (or happened) in objective reality. Yet commissioners endow both the concept and the activity with seemingly incredible significance and power: telling the truth may be (necessary and) sufficient to bring about the kind of idyllic state of affairs we tend to encounter only in imagination—a world in which people (truth-tellers, naturally) coexist peacefully without the felt threat of future conflict. While many of us would confirm the intuitive value of truth and truth-telling, we may not be able to say exactly why the truth matters to us. If we are unused to thinking about truth-telling in instrumental terms, then we will want to proceed with caution in determining just which ends may be brought about through its practice. Likewise, we will want to specify the sense in which those ends are 'brought about,' generated, or promoted. Publicly perceived as necessary, significant, and powerful bodies, commissions can have a profound impact on the recovery of national unity while at the same time encouraging individuals to move forward with lives that may have been interrupted by physical pain, psychological terror, or gross political injustices. Anyone who appreciates the obvious significance of the commissioners' work will seek assurance that their procedures are the ones best suited to the attainment of their stated aims. If we can locate more effective ways to confront the past and promote peaceful coexistence, then we will want to clarify and recommend such alternative procedures.

5.2 **Overview of the argument**

The aims most commonly expressed by people involved in the work of commissions are twofold: reconciliation in the sense of peaceful coexistence, and the prevention of future injustices modeled upon past patterns of abuse. Of course, not every commission prioritizes these ends, and different commissions may understand the nature of the ends in quite different ways.[2] Nevertheless, the frequent expression of these two aims makes them suitable for a general investigation into the relation between commissioners' procedures and ends. My own project begins with the question: does truth-telling

---

[2] Neither Argentina nor Sri Lanka state reconciliation (in any sense) as one of their aims: Argentinians resisted peaceful coexistence in the conditions that were current at the time, and the Sri Lankans sought to document the disappeared in order to recommend reparations for their remaining family members (Hayner 2002, pp. 160–1).

in the sense specified by commissioners promote their stated aims? Intentionally and meaningfully ambiguous, this question admits of two possible readings: first, does the way in which people involved in the work of commissions understand the activity of truth-telling suggest the possible or likely realization of their desired ends? In other words, should we expect these groups to succeed in light of their own understanding of their work? This question about the nature of and relation between abstract concepts (or conceptions) suggests the usefulness of philosophical analysis. Second, regardless of how they conceive of their procedures and ends, do commissions tend to succeed (as a matter of fact) in bringing about the kind of better social world they recommend? This second question concerns the nature and significance of tangible results, and so is a matter for empirical study. Although I will concentrate mainly on the first question, I assume that a clear understanding of procedure will have obvious practical value for the identification and successful realization of commissioners' goals. Over the course of this chapter, I will develop and illustrate how an intuitive realist picture of the world expressed by commissioners, alongside a picture of their role as impartial investigators, restricts the range of practically realizable goals. Then I will suggest an alternative picture of the commissioners' work that opens up the possibility of achieving a more ambitious set of aims. A provisional thesis guides my subsequent remarks: while impartial investigation into matters of fact may be necessary and sufficient for reconciliation, the achievement of moral agreement about those facts will be necessary (if insufficient) for the realization of the broadest possible range of aims. In order for their procedure to promote their desired ends, commissioners will need to develop and express a partially shared understanding of the moral significance of past events.

5.3 Uncovering assumptions

A philosophical perspective on the relation between commissions' procedures and ends must be empirically informed in order to be relevant and useful. In developing a picture of the work these groups perform, I will use the written mandates published by a variety of commissions to identify and describe those shared pre-theoretic assumptions about truth and objectivity that cast doubt upon the realization of their stated aims. By 'shared pre-theoretic assumptions' I mean to describe those (often implicit) beliefs shared by persons prior to or independent from any philosophical reflection or theorizing. Throughout, I will use the case study of South Africa as a starting point to develop very general suggestions about the necessary and sufficient conditions for the achievement of reconciliation and the prevention of future injustices.

This particular group's conception of the relation between its procedure and aims is standard and thus serves as a constant point of reference in our consideration of other commissions.[3] Clearly, the procedure and results of the South African commission will reflect, to some extent, the specific demands associated with confronting and overcoming apartheid; for this reason, we must not apply indiscriminately the insight provided by the case of South Africa to other nations. Yet we require a concrete example to lend our philosophical claims empirical legitimacy, and the South African commission is particularly well-suited to this function. For their well-crafted and extensive written mandate contains a clear statement of procedure and desired outcomes alongside a detailed view of their possible relation. Moreover, the unprecedented size and reach of this group's work, combined with its variety of functions (e.g., granting amnesty, searching premises and seizing evidence, subpoenaing witnesses, running a witness-protection program, developing and implementing mental health services) and the unqualified assumption that truth-telling both promotes reconciliation and contributes to the prevention of future injustices, suggest the usefulness of South Africa as a case study of the relation between commissions' procedures and goals. Both Hayner (2002, p. 156) and Ash (2000, p. 308) remark on the South African commission's explicit and unwavering faith in the movement from truth to reconciliation.

Commissioners tend to express the following picture of the general process underlying their particular projects: truth-telling within the context of an organized and public conversation provokes a widespread catharsis and generates an accurate and shared view of objective reality, grounds reconciliation in the sense of peaceful coexistence, and contributes to the nonrepetition of past patterns of abuse. Wilkins (2001, p. 93) and Ash (2000, p. 308) support this basic picture of the commissioners' conceived procedures and ends. One's immediate response to this conception of the relation between procedure and ends may range from mild skepticism to outright disbelief. How could the activity of truth-telling by itself give rise to such a remarkable chain of effects? What must the commissioners assume about the world in order for them to put this philosophical view into practice? How are these assumptions philosophically and/or practically significant? Answering these further questions requires us to look very closely at this picture of the relation between procedure

---

3 A selection of written mandates is available through the 'Truth Commissions Digital Collection' published on-line by the United States Institute of Peace. Background information on (and detailed analysis of) recent truth commissions can be found in Patricia Hayner's *Unspeakable Truths*. The procedures and aims of South Africa's Truth and Reconciliation Commission can be found on the group's official website.

and desired aims, focusing on the philosophical assumptions that make the empirical tasks practicable. We may classify the assumptions in terms of three categories: the first one will contain 'metaphysical' assumptions, or claims about the constituents of ultimate reality; the second category will contain 'epistemological' assumptions, or claims about the nature of knowledge and our methods of acquiring it; the third category will contain 'linguistic' assumptions, or claims about the meaning and reference of the terms in our natural language. We will see momentarily that people involved in the work of commissions are required to make controversial assumptions in all three categories.

Underlying the commissioners' picture of their work are some familiar common sense, ordinary, or 'everyday' assumptions about language, truth, and objectivity that constitute a view we may describe critically as 'intuitive realism.' This choice of terminology reflects both the traditional philosophical view that it most resembles as well as the strong intuitive pull of this widely shared position. Intuitive realism consists of the following particular assumptions: first, in order for the process of truth-telling to contribute to knowledge of objective reality, the commissioners must assume (pre-theoretically, and implicitly) that telling the truth involves making sincere claims about matters of fact that correspond with what really took place during a clearly specified period of history. We could interpret this assumption linguistically, as a claim about the meaning of the phrase 'truth-telling' or the nature of the practice it designates. Yet the claim is more sophisticated than this definitional interpretation suggests: it says something, moreover, about the relation between language and truth. This secondary linguistic assumption surfaces out of the commissioners' recognition of truth as a norm of enquiry: in order to view their work as contributing to an accurate view of the past, the commissioners must understand victims' and perpetrators' true beliefs as corresponding with objective reality, the facts, or what really took place. Once again, this assumption is more complicated than a linguistic reading implies: it involves a further claim about the nature of ultimate reality. This secondary metaphysical assumption is directly relevant to the practicability of the commissioners' tasks: the commissioners assume that the subject matter of witnesses' beliefs is a mind-independent realm about which they can secure and express verifiable information. Here, a mind-independent realm is one whose existence and nature does not depend upon persons' thoughts about it. In this sense, persons providing testimony to commissioners are making claims that must be sensitive to objective reality. With this trio of assumptions in place, the commissioners are required to make a final assumption about their situation as investigators. This final epistemological claim reveals the commissioners' faith in the adequacy of their procedure: the commissioners recognize their capacity to verify the truth of witnesses' claims through the use of certain fact-finding procedures, organizing the results with the aid of a standard information-management model. This standard approach to the management of information is based on a detailed tabulation of specific acts via a database. Hayner (2002, pp. 80–5) provides a detailed description of this widely used model and asks whether such a context-insensitive model is suitable for the management of value-laden information. These assumptions constitute the philosophical view that in part determines the successful application of the commissioners' model work.

We may acquire a better perspective on intuitive realism by introducing a final set of terms and then placing the commissioners' view alongside its more sophisticated philosophical counterpart.[4] If intuitive realism is the view that true statements capture what happens in objective reality, then philosophical realism designates a family of views that are committed to the real existence of things that are independent of us. Most of us are realists with respect to physical facts: we do not believe that the number of planets in the solar system, or our own physical size and shape, are a function of what we happen to believe or want at the time of investigation. Likewise, most of us are epistemic realists, because we believe that we can secure and verify knowledge concerning a mind-independent realm of objects. Perhaps fewer of us are naturally committed to a particular philosophical theory of truth, or a view about the meaning of the term or the nature of the concept. People involved in the work of commissions are, however, committed to a position that philosophy calls the correspondence theory of truth: this view states that a claim is true if it corresponds to the way things are in objective reality. The challenge for the truth and reconciliation commissioners, in light of their intuitive realism, will be to develop a conception of their procedure that suggests its usefulness in bringing about desirable ends.

We must appreciate that this commitment to intuitive realism brings with it very serious practical implications. Any commissioner who endorses such a world view will be engaged in work that has no connection to his aims or goals. Let us imagine, for the moment, that the commissioners did not assume that witnesses' true claims corresponded with objective reality; in this case, they would not be able to identify reconciliation and the nonrepetition of past

---

4 Readers lacking a background in philosophy (in particular, contemporary Anglo-American analytic philosophy), or people seeking a fuller exposition of the concepts discussed in this paper, may find the following reference texts helpful, interesting, and widely available: *The Shorter Routledge Encyclopedia of Philosophy* and the (web-based) *Stanford Encyclopedia of Philosophy*.

patterns of abuse as possible and appropriate aims for their work.[5] In fact, they would be unable to locate any tangible results at all for their work: if we are in a position to wonder whether our claims describe a world that exists independently of our conception of it, then we will have to doubt similarly whether any new description of reality could promote or even suggest a concrete, tangible, or practically valuable alteration in our shared circumstances or experiences. We must assume that the world we describe (and in so doing seek to confront and change) is mind-independent before we can expect our descriptions to have any kind of practical impact on the unfolding of those events experienced by all of us. Our sincere claims about what took place must latch on to or describe objective reality if (the understandings gleaned from) those statements are going to have any kind of bearing on the world outside of us. Now, if the commissioners interpret truth-telling as a matter of making sincere claims about objective reality, then they must confront an unfortunate if inevitable feature of our epistemic situation as inquirers. The view that a range of beliefs purports to represent how things are, and the related suggestion that their subject matter is objective, opens up the possibility that some of our beliefs are false. If our methods for acquiring beliefs are unreliable, or if they are imperfectly implemented, or if relevant evidence is not available to us, then we may develop false beliefs. Persons are fallible in the sense that they make claims that are always subject to analysis, criticism, and reformulation in light of new information concerning how things are. Hookway (1995, p. 48) develops this notion of fallibilism in a more general discussion of objectivity in ethics. This uncontroversial philosophical point about knowledge acquisition should be familiar to anyone who has tried to learn a new sport, or navigate around a foreign land, or develop meaningful and sustained relationships with other persons. Victims and perpetrators of politically motivated crimes will be particularly fallible for a variety of reasons: lapses in memory may surface out of the long stretch of time between trauma and remembrance, post-traumatic stress may cause disturbances of memory, a fear of retaliation may provoke silence on certain matters, and the prospect of material compensation may encourage the fabrication of stories. Hayner (2002, pp. 148–9) considers

---

[5] Commissioners express different (and sometimes conflicting) understandings of reconciliation (Hayner 2002, pp. 154–5). Ordinary usage suggests the restoration of friendly relations, or else the cultivation or illustration of compatibility. Yet commissioners most commonly interpret the notion to mean 'peaceful coexistence'. Hayner's (2002, pp. 162–3) more sophisticated interpretation of the concept encourages its application both to retrospective testimony and interpersonal relations.

in greater detail the significance of these challenges to the reliability of testimony. As retrospective testimony is ultimately unreliable, historical truth will be difficult to establish. Ash (2000, p. 314) confirms the unreliability of retrospective testimony and the difficulty of establishing historical truth. In so far as the commissioners' aims depend for their realization upon an accurate record of the past, the unreliability of testimony may serve as an inevitable, forceful, and permanent barrier to the success of these groups.

Returning for the moment to the commissioners' conception of truth-telling, we can place the definitional claim alongside our fundamental fallibilism and see whether an inconsistency or contradiction results. Indeed, here we encounter our first reason to doubt seriously the suitability of commissioners' procedures to the achievement of their goals: if telling the truth involves making claims that correspond with historical matters of fact, and if the correspondence relation creates a gap between statements and the world such that witnesses' claims may not, in fact, capture (or indeed, have any relation to) what really happened, then reconciliation and the nonrecurrence of past patterns of abuse will be left ungrounded. These twofold aims require for their successful realization an absolutely infallible inquirer whose sincere claims about matters of fact are always true descriptions of the world. Now, we all appreciate that such an ideal knower is empirically impossible; moreover, we proceed with our projects despite and in full recognition of our capacity to develop false beliefs. Nevertheless, setting aside for the moment the unrealistic requirement of an ideal knower, a closer consideration of the commissioners' philosophical assumptions leaves us with compelling reasons to doubt the capacity of the commissions' conceived procedure to promote their twofold aims.

We can focus on just one of the commissioners' pre-theoretic assumptions, in order to appreciate the remaining concern about the possible success of these groups. Returning to the commissioners' picture of the general process underlying their particular projects, we should notice immediately a fundamental and overarching assumption about the significance and power of truth-telling. Echoing George Santayana's famous insight that those who forget the past are doomed to repeat it, commissioners often maintain controversially that confronting the past (through truth-telling) will promote reconciliation and prevent a recurrence of evil. We must test the assumption that telling truths about what really happened will promote peaceful coexistence and that achieving and expressing a clear view of past injustices will prevent future ones. Even if witnesses unfailingly told the truth, an understanding (or its expression) simply cannot by itself promote a certain state of affairs. For this reason, commissions simply cannot by themselves be responsible for creating a better social world, or enhancing the mental health of individual persons, nor should we expect them to do so. We may explain this unfortunate yet unavoidable and partial powerlessness in a variety of ways. First, commissioners claim to focus on statements of fact rather than statements about value; they conceive of themselves as information-gathering bodies primarily, groups engaged in reflection about value (if at all) secondarily.[6] Here we should challenge whether a morally neutral procedure could help us understand and bring about a social world that better expresses our values and priorities. Second, commissions tend to rely on a 'balance of probabilities' or 'preponderance of evidence' standard in reaching their conclusions of fact, i.e., a conclusion is established when there is more evidence to support rather than deny it (Hayner, 2002, p. 232). A shared understanding of such weakly established 'facts' may not bear upon the future because it fails to reflect the past. Our interpretations of the past will have to fully and accurately describe (rather than partially capture) what happened in order to be useful for our empirical purposes. Third, moral agreement about past events simply may not apply to future situations: difficult episodes in history may be irreducibly particular in the sense that whatever general conclusions we derive from them will not find new cases for application. For example, we may have difficulty conceiving the mere possibility of another terrorist attack like the one waged recently on America; such a fundamentally particular atrocity defies the imagination and seems utterly unrepeatable. Another Holocaust may seem similarly inconceivable, a radical and unique failure of humanity that gave rise to unspeakable pain and horror. Finally, even if sufficiently similar cases present themselves at a future point in time, we may choose to understand them differently precisely because our original understandings failed to prevent a nonrecurrence of past abuses. In other words, we may discard rather than reapply an understanding on the basis that it did not guide us well in our practices.

---

[6] Actually, these groups have a much less straightforward and strikingly ambivalent approach to matters of value: for example, they insist on the impartiality of a procedure that involves not only the collection of facts but also the assignment of blame and potentially severe legal consequences to people identified as blameworthy perpetrators of horrific crimes. A concern with the notions of fairness, historical accuracy, and the truth is evinced in many aspects of their procedure; their shared aims reflect their valuation of peace and community. This strong sense of ambivalence may be a hidden demand of reconciliation: if groups with seriously divergent moral perspectives are attempting to confront the past together in the interest of creating and sustaining a wider community, this task could be better facilitated if people set aside their distinctive evaluative perspectives and instead focus on their common personhood.

5.4 **Revising the aims**

Critical reflection upon the commissioners' conceived procedure suggests the possibility (and perhaps likelihood) that the practice of truth-telling could contribute to the achievement of a more realistic or practicable set of aims. In particular, work carried out by commissioners may be rehabilitative insofar as it publicly acknowledges past abuses, responds to the specific psychological and material needs of witnesses, and outlines institutional responsibility and reforms. Public proceedings can advance understanding and reduce animosities between ethnic, regional, and political groups who lack knowledge of other groups' sufferings. Disclosures of fact and admissions of guilt can be psychologically significant for victims of politically motivated crimes, many of whom have experienced years of silence or denial on the part of their governments. Having the full truth told publicly may provide perpetrators with a sense of relief and victims with a sense of justice. Moreover, the public expression of blameworthiness and remorse may indicate a willingness on the part of perpetrators to engage, once more, in civil society. In this sense, the act of remembering can have a strong moral force. Such moral force is closely connected to the very public nature of the proceedings. As Hayner (2002, p. 228) points out and both Cooper (2001, p. 213) and Crocker (2001, p. 286) confirm, the impact and reach of a commission will increase significantly if the proceedings are publicly accessible.

Finally, while receiving compensation does not lessen the pain associated with past abuses or rectify wrongdoings, reparations for state crimes often signify a government's commitment to the rehabilitation of society and can make everyday life less difficult for victims. In fact, the most significant contributions a commission can make to societal healing, within the context of this narrow set of aims, may be its assessments of institutional responsibility and recommendations for reforms. Wilkins (2001, p. 94) insists strongly and convincingly that the achievement of reconciliation is crucially dependent upon such recommendations regarding institutional reform. Nations that rely on commissions during transitional periods often have institutional deficiencies that inhibit or prevent recovery without insightful aid from outside observers. Now, this less ambitious set of aims (i.e., public acknowledgment of matters of fact, material compensation for victims, recommendations for institutional reforms) is recommendable for two strong reasons: it is both practicable and consistent with the commissioners' intuitive realist world view. Another virtue of embracing a less ambitious set of goals is that such a move respects the difficulty of achieving hoped-for ends and challenges 'the abilities of any short term process to satisfy . . . huge and multifaceted demands' (Hayner, 2002, p. 251).

5.5 The importance of establishing a shared moral understanding

We will want to distinguish provisionally between historical investigation and reflection about value, or between fact-finding and the establishment of a shared moral understanding, in determining how the commissioners can best achieve this revised set of ends. The commissioners tend to confuse impartial historical investigation with reflection about our values and priorities, conceiving their procedure in terms of morally neutral fact-finding while at the same time expecting their work to contribute to a better social world. Their emphasis on the impartial collection, organization, and reporting of facts probably reflects a commendable desire for historical accuracy in recording very serious events. Without accuracy, these groups could not achieve those aims specified within the context of their mandates. Yet conceiving of their work in value-free terms is problematic for two reasons. First, preserving the illusion of moral neutrality requires commissioners to ignore the sense in which all truth-telling and fact-finding is informed variously by different conceptions of value. Decisions about the relevancy of data, the suitability of an approach, and the best form of presentation reflect value judgments about what deserves our critical attention and what beneficial purpose its analysis would serve. The very decision to create and run a truth and reconciliation commission reflects a prioritization of understanding, forgiveness, peace, and community. Second, conceiving of their procedure in value-free terms may restrict the range of relation of truth-telling to reconciliation.

Now we have the philosophical groundwork in place to raise our central question about the relation between abstract conceptions of procedures and aims. We want to determine the truth-value of the following hypothesis: that the collection, organization, and recording of facts (in so far as telling the truth publicly encourages individual psychological healing) may be both necessary and sufficient for the social state of reconciliation. Although the commissioners' belief in a logical connection between truth-telling and the achievement of their aims is at best controversial and at worst false, we should not ignore the psychological force of hope, faith, and ungrounded belief in the success of the procedure. We could understand the motivation for assuming or expressing a philosophically empty (or controversial) logical connection in terms of the significance attached to the concept of truth as well as the potentially therapeutic value of public storytelling and acknowledgment. The assumption expresses a more fundamental Enlightenment hope or belief that the pursuit and attainment of knowledge will promote a more peaceful and humane world. A strong desire for the commissions to be successful, alongside a shared commitment to the stated aims may, by itself, promote peaceful coexistence and contribute to the avoidance of future atrocities. Moreover, we cannot let our philosophical concerns overshadow or diminish the fact that most people involved in the commissioners' process defend its value and insist that it works. Our philosophical doubt should resurface, however, in response to the claim that the committees can be successful in the total absence of reflection about human value.

Guaranteeing or even promoting the nonrepetition of past forms of abuse seems to require more than impartial fact-finding on the model of scientific inquiry. Clearly, agreement about historical matters of fact is insufficient for the prevention of future injustices: two people may agree about what happened in the past, yet disagree wildly about the moral significance of past events. Let us imagine that a perpetrator of torture and multiple homicides appears to give testimony before the South African commission, while family members of a particular victim wait expectantly in the audience to hear his version of events. The perpetrator provides an accurate and detailed description of the circumstances surrounding the victim's death but is completely remorseless and unapologetic. Although the family is grateful to learn what happened to their deceased relation, they react in horror and with disgust to the murderer's total lack of personal accountability and regret. Next let us imagine that the commission decides that the perpetrator is guilty from a moral point of view, but the politically motivated nature of the crime, combined with his willingness to give public testimony, means that they will grant the 'murderer' amnesty. Everyone agrees about the matters of fact surrounding the death, yet nobody agrees about its moral significance. Examples like this suggest that the achievement of moral agreement about matters of fact, brought about by the cultivation of a partially shared understanding of what constitutes right and wrong action accompanied by a shared vision of a better social world, will be a necessary (if insufficient) condition for the achievement of the broadest possible range of aims.

What would such moral agreement look like? What would its realization require? We can at least begin developing a sketch of this state of affairs and hope that further investigation will fill out the details. Minimally, such an agreement would consist of three parts: first, it would specify a set of morally reprehensible actions that took place during the relevant period; second, it would provide a reason (or set thereof) to interpret them as blameworthy; finally, it would involve an explicit and unwavering commitment to the overarching values expressed in the work of commissions (e.g., understanding, forgiveness, community). In order fully to confront, acknowledge, and move beyond a difficult past, people need to agree not only that certain events took place, but also that certain persons involved in them behaved well or poorly. Moreover, individuals who are committed to sharing a better social world will need to apply moral concepts like 'honorable' or 'blameworthy' to actions in similar ways and for similar kinds of reasons. Commissioners must attempt to develop and express a shared and self-consciously value-laden interpretation of the past and vision of the future if they want to progress in the way they describe. One would be correct to worry that such agreement would be difficult or even impossible to obtain. If we have endowed commissions with duties that lie outside the realm of their responsibility, then we have done so with the purpose of understanding the connection between conceived procedure and desired ends. The procedural adjustments required by the prioritization and cultivation of moral agreement should leave us content to aim for the narrower and more realistic set of ends.

5.6 The importance of moral reflection to commissioners

The achievement of a better social world requires a commitment on the part of nations, governments, and citizens to understand and challenge their present pre-theoretic assumptions while developing and defending a clear moral vision of past events and future possibilities. Recognizing the difficulty of establishing truths about what really happened during a traumatic period in history, and appreciating the sense in which social–scientific investigation without moral reflection cannot prevent a recurrence of the past, commissioners must develop a sense of themselves as engaged in reflection about what matters to them as persons. Commissioners will be engaged in moral reflection in at least three respects: first, they will need to identify and describe whatever values underlie both their procedures and their desired ends. Next, they will critically and self-consciously reassess their significance for everyone involved in the commissioners' work. Finally, commissioners will need to develop and recommend a social vision that respects diversity of opinion without slipping into a crude relativism. In other words, the shared conception of a better social world must accommodate a variety of intuitions about what constitutes right and wrong action without sacrificing a unified, consistent, and practically valuable interpretation of the past and set of recommendations for the future. In short, people involved in the work done by commissions must commit themselves not only to certain values, but also (and perhaps more importantly) to critical reflection about them. Finally, and in view of the fact that not even moral agreement will guarantee peaceful coexistence, nations must not place undue responsibility on truth commissions to secure the nonrecurrence of previous patterns of abuse. Recovering nations should consider any and all factors that could contribute to societal healing, including an end to the threat of violence, the establishment of new communities, the diagnosis and treatment of structural inequalities and material needs, and (perhaps most importantly) the passage of time. On this note, Hayner (2002, pp. 163–5) encourages nations and their citizens to understand and take seriously whatever factors (independent from the work of commissions) may contribute to their ultimately desirable ends.

5.7 **Assessing the proposal to reconceive the project of truth and reconciliation commissions**

We have yet to consider the practical implications of our view that moral agreement will be necessary (if insufficient) for the realization of the broadest possible range of goals. Such a position has potentially serious and wide-ranging practical implications: the commissioners will need to replace the process of disinterested, impartial, scientific observation with whatever tasks are involved in cultivating moral agreement about historical facts. This reconception may involve choosing different persons to serve on commissions, collecting and organizing information in new ways, and making different kinds of recommendations. For example, people might be hired or elected on the basis of their capacity to shift perspective and identify with heterogeneous points of view, or their ability to mediate between conflicting moral orientations, or their capacity to reconcile discordant stories and identify which facts stand in need of a shared moral understanding. Commissioners will need to discard their standard information-management model in favor of one that does not sidestep concerns about value, or else develop an approach that is appropriate to the requirements of moral agreement.

We may respond to a trio of possible objections to our philosophical perspective on the work of commissions by way of conclusion. First, someone might insist that we cannot so quickly or clearly distinguish between social-scientific investigation and reflection about value, insisting on the basis of this contrast that moral agreement is required for the achievement of the commissioners' dual aims. After all, we have underlined the various ways in which fact-finding is not a morally neutral endeavor, outlining some of the general values expressed in the decision to establish and run such a body. Nevertheless, the commissioners' tendency to maintain a conception of themselves as impartial investigators alongside an understanding of their procedure as morally neutral forces us to draw some kind of distinction between science and ethics in order to illustrate the strangeness of using an allegedly value-free procedure to achieve value-laden ends.

Second, one might object that moral agreement is either practically unrealizable or else may be undesirable in certain situations. Of course, we can list a variety of contexts in which securing moral agreement may seem less important to a person than maintaining his own distinctive moral identity or outlook: a US soldier disobeys orders given by his military superiors to torture and humiliate Iraqi prisoners, a passionately atheistic teenager refuses to recite the daily pledge of allegiance at her high school, or a recovering alcoholic declines the customary glass of champagne at his supervisor's retirement party. Our motivation may be less altruistic and simply a matter of stubbornly refusing to consider a wider community and instead choosing selfishness. Even if we do decide to prioritize agreement in our reflection upon and conversations about right and wrong behavior, we may still find that agreement is unrealizable. The sheer variety of human responses suggests that the harmony of desires and interests required for unforced agreement may never obtain within a community. Yet the aim of national reconciliation already implies a strong prioritization of agreement over individual integrity; persons must be open to serious changes of mind or heart if they want to achieve social solidarity. A unified and shared vision of the past, present, and future will most certainly require some people to set aside their personal beliefs, assumptions, or intuitions about what it means to live well. The achievement of moral agreement should not be confused with consensus about the form and content of a life well lived.

Finally, and most seriously, one might object that the achievement of moral agreement about matters of fact remains ultimately insufficient for reconciliation and the nonrepetition of past patterns of abuse. Victims and perpetrators may succeed in reaching a shared understanding of the past and yet fail to secure peaceful coexistence or prevent future conflict. Underlying this objection is the unfortunate, unavoidable, and all too frequently unacknowledged truth that no mode of confrontation with the past can guarantee a certain kind of future; we could know everything there is to know and reach consensus on all moral matters, and yet still be susceptible to future conflict on a grand scale or to the repetition of patterns of action that we are unable to predict, influence, or control. On behalf of the people whose lives are impacted directly (and often seriously) by the work of commissions, let us seek to avoid the sacrifice of hope to the rigors of disinterested analysis.

References

Ash T (2000). *History of the Present: Essays, Sketches, and Despatches from Europe in the 1990s.* London: Penguin Press.

Baggini J (2002). *Making Sense: Philosophy Behind the Headlines.* Oxford: Oxford University Press.

Cooper D (2001). Collective responsibility, 'moral luck', and reconciliation. In: *War Crimes and Collective Wrongdoing* (ed. A Jokic), pp. 205–15. Oxford: Blackwell Publishing.

Craig E (2005). *The Shorter Routledge Encyclopedia of Philosophy*. Oxford: Routledge Press.

Crocker D (2001). Transitional justice and international civil society. In: *War Crimes and Collective Wrongdoing* (ed. A Jokic), pp. 270–300. Oxford: Blackwell Publishing.

Engel P (2002). *Truth*. London: Acumen Press.

Hayner, P (2002). *Unspeakable Truths: Facing the Challenge of Truth Commissions*. NY: Routledge Press.

Hookway C (1995). Fallibilism and objectivity: science and ethics. In: *World, Mind, and Ethics* (eds. J Altham and R Harrison), pp. 46–67. Cambridge: Cambridge University Press.

The South African Truth and Reconciliation Commission. *Truth: The Road to Reconciliation*. April 2003. http://www.doj.gov.za/trc. Truth commissions digital collection. May 2005.

J Cornelius. The Jeanette Rankin Library Program at the United States Institute of Peace. http:\\www.usip.org/library/tc/tc_supdoc.html

Stanford Encyclopedia of Philosophy. September 1995. E Zalta. The Metaphysics Research Lab, Centre for the Study of Language and Information, Stanford University. http://plato.stanford.edu

Wilkins B (2001). Whose trial? Whose reconciliation? In: *War Crimes and Collective Wrongdoing* (ed. A Jokic), pp. 85–96. Oxford: Blackwell Publishers.

Williams B (2002). *Truth and Truthfulness*. Princeton, NJ: Princeton University Press.

Chapter 6

How much truth and how much reconciliation? Intrapsychic, interpersonal, and social aspects of resolution

Deborah Spitz

6.1 Introduction

A therapist and patient approach truth and reconciliation as personal matters, explored through the creation of an individual narrative. For individuals who have experienced a traumatic event such as rape, however, the issues of truth and reconciliation are social and political as well, because a severe social injustice has occurred. Psychotherapeutic experience suggests that for patients who present with histories of trauma, telling and understanding and retelling in the creation of a narrative may not be enough to bring about healing. The psychiatric literature on post-traumatic stress disorder has, understandably, focused more on symptom management and on the relationship between patient and therapist than on societal aspects of healing (Davidson, 2003). This chapter draws on psychotherapeutic work with patients struggling with trauma, to explore the limits of narrative and to inquire what processes beyond psychotherapy alone might foster closure. I argue that psychotherapy can provide a place to identify and clarify past events, and to explore feelings and psychological consequences of those events, but that it cannot provide reconciliation. This chapter will examine why.

6.2 Historical background

Influenced by Freud's shift in focus from trauma to intrapsychic conflict as the etiology of neurosis, traditional psychotherapy has offered a personal, nonpolitical, nonsocial resolution to the problems experienced by patients. Dora, one of Freud's (1953) celebrated patients, might now be referred for family therapy (where her problem would be considered in the context of social issues and family dynamics) or to a support group (where the problem would be formulated more in social and political terms), but in Freud's day she became a psychoanalytic patient whose problems were formulated psychologically in terms of fantasy, conflict, and repression. Psychoanalysis and psychotherapy use the process of 'remembering, repeating and working through' to help patients resolve the issues that plague them. Through clarifying past experiences and fantasies, re-experiencing affects attached to those experiences that might have been walled off, and examining transference issues within the therapeutic relationship, psychotherapy offers the hope that, by repeated tellings of a story, a patient may gain insight and obtain relief through the emergence of more mature coping strategies and defenses. These are intrapsychic changes within the individual and do not address social issues of restitution, redress, or justice.

6.3 Trauma and psychotherapy

For patients who have experienced trauma such as rape, this intrapsychic model falls short. Why? First and most simply, in rape there has been a violation of social norms as well as a personal violation. This violation challenges psychological capacities, such as the ability to handle intense affect and conflict and, at the same time, ruptures interpersonal trust and trust in the social world. The social world and its institutions, its legal structures, its implicit guarantees of safety and respect, fairness, accountability, and justice, are all called into question. The violated person no longer feels at home in the social world—if indeed she ever did—but rather feels alienated from it. Secondly, in the trauma of sexual assault, the psychological issues of conflict and repression are usually far less important than feelings of shame, and with shame comes not only anxiety about revealing oneself and one's history but also a sense of separation from others. Rebuilding a connection with others is a social process, requiring others to acknowledge that a violation occurred, that this violation was serious rather than inconsequential, and that the violated person's response was not bizarre or out of keeping with the event that prompted the response. Shame worsens when others do not acknowledge that a serious violation has occurred, when others imply that what happened was trivial or allege that the violated person's response was extreme, peculiar, and unreasonable. These issues can begin to be addressed directly in individual therapy. But the therapist is one person hearing the story and cannot always or fully represent the kind of social response that the injured person requires in order to heal. The therapist may be an exceptional ally, but the patient may view the therapist's values as unique and different from—and therefore unrepresentative of—those of the broader society. Third, for some patients there is a need for redress. This need moves the work of repair away from the confidentiality of psychotherapy and into social and political arenas. Only outside of psychotherapy can the patient confront a perpetrator with an accusation or appropriate anger. Outside of therapy are the legal system and political institutions which represent the values of the broader culture and define the formal social response to a particular traumatic event. Psychotherapy in these cases is only one part of a larger process of reconciliation, which involves issues of redress and justice; I address the larger process in Section 6.4 (see 'Reconciliation with the social world').

There are several caveats to offer in this consideration of rape and the psychotherapy of trauma. Rape is a particular kind of trauma, an assault involving power and violence inappropriately tied to sexuality. Important distinctions can be made between rape and other traumatic events; for example, some nonsexual violence may not necessarily aim to humiliate the victim, and many violent acts engender more anger rather than shame. However, some of the issues raised in this discussion have relevance to other types of trauma as well. The victim's sense that the world is no longer predictable, the destruction of her sense of justice and fairness, and the questioning of her own perceptions are common themes in many types of trauma, including traumatic experiences with natural disasters. It is beyond the scope of this discussion, however, to consider the complexities of rape when used as a weapon of war, when the humanity of individuals is deliberately and manifestly ignored not only by individual perpetrators but by institutions and governments themselves. I attempt to deal here with the disruptive experience of rape within a society where rules of morals and justice forbid sexual violence, yet social practices do not follow those rules. The following example illustrates some important issues that emerge in the psychotherapy following such an assault. Identifying information and many details have been changed to protect the patient's confidentiality.

Patient example

This 25-year-old female scientist presented to me after discharge from an inpatient unit where she had been hospitalized after an overdose. She was ambivalent about psychotherapy, having had several unsuccessful attempts at psychotherapy in the past. She had a long history of presenting a falsely reassuring picture of herself to others, whether parents, colleagues or friends. This helped her cope with anxiety but left her feeling that no one really knew or loved her, and she herself was uncertain about which of her feelings were authentic. She had many symptoms of distress including panic attacks, self-injurious behavior, dissociation, and fluctuating depressive symptoms. She was mistrustful of relationships and at times felt angry with those who tried to help her. At her initial evaluation with me, she met criteria for the diagnosis of borderline personality disorder, post-traumatic stress disorder, and recurrent major depressive disorder.

The therapy

Initially we spent our sessions clarifying her feelings about her relationships with friends and her family, her negative feelings about her body, and her work. Then, after reading a newspaper article about gang rape, she revealed to me that as a teenager she had been brutally beaten and raped by a group of male students in high school. She told no one about the assault at the time. She believed her parents sensed that something bad had happened to her but that they didn't want to know about it. Later she put herself in harm's way, aware that she didn't care enough what happened to her. She was raped at a drunken party several years later, and had subsequently entered into a physically and sexually violent relationship.

She was ambivalent about discussing what she had revealed and was not sure how to view what had happened. At times, she saw rape and injustice everywhere she looked, and she felt vulnerable and desperate. Yet she had told herself to move on and not think about it, and minimizing the event had seemed to work for a number of years. She attempted to define the injury left by the assault. It had not destroyed her, though it seemed to have stopped her psychological development, so that she felt much younger than she was. It had destroyed her sense of trust in the safety of the world. And as she took stock of the world 10 years later, she saw much to reinforce her lack of trust. She struggled to get her bearings as she weighed two incompatible views of what had happened to her. On one hand, it was horrible and extreme; on the other hand, the overtly sexual depictions of women in popular culture and the frequency of rape in the news seemed to indicate that rape was an unfortunate but not uncommon event that did not shock people very much.

The therapist

As a therapist, it was difficult for me to get my bearings as well. In both inpatient and outpatient work, I encounter rape and injustice too often. One of my inpatients was a middle-aged woman who had been hospitalized many times for psychosis after refusing her outpatient medication. She repeatedly came into the hospital mute, neither eating nor drinking. The team finally decided to hold a series of family meetings with the patient, her husband, and their grown daughters to talk openly about what we observed. The patient wished for her husband's love but felt rejected by his extramarital affair. She was afraid to say anything because she knew that her husband had viciously assaulted his first wife and might hurt her too. Consequently, the team came to believe, she expressed her anger and other feelings through being psychotic and mute rather than by speaking out. Another patient, a homeless woman, had been beaten by her father and then by her husband and subsequent men. Before admission, she had lived with a man who gave her cocaine, spent her money until it ran out, and then kicked her out on to the street. Still, she did not want to give up her freedom to sign into a drug treatment program for battered women. My male resident said he was starting to hate men because of their behavior. Another patient, a 50-year-old physician with depression and alcohol abuse, was admitted still grieving over her parent's marital rupture in her childhood, the breakup of her own marriage several years ago, and most recently the duplicity of her husband who hid his money over the years so that he could evade alimony and child support payments. These vivid stories, illustrating the limitations of legal remedies and the complex vulnerability of our patients, tempered the staff's optimism and hope that the political or legal systems could bring a just resolution for our patients.

Both patient and therapist, then, struggle with how to understand traumatic events in the context of the social world. In psychotherapy sessions, my patient and I sat together in the shadow of the gang rape, realizing its repetitive power in the second rape and in her subsequent relationships. The power of rape was palpable to us. But how then to understand that several of the boys who raped and beat her went on with their lives to become doctors and lawyers, presumably not too encumbered by reflection and remorse? If the social world is trustworthy and just, why was my inpatient unit filled with women whose fathers and husbands beat them or frightened them? Surely these social conditions have as much to do with my patients' turbulent course and repeated hospitalizations as do their diagnoses of bipolar disorder or major depression or psychosis. And yet, it is important to seek a way of thinking about the social world that fully acknowledges the terrible personal experiences and their social causes that these patients report, but that also recognizes the constructive resources and potentials of the social world.

Issues in psychotherapy

Every patient brings to therapy a history of prior relationships, a posture of comfort or discomfort with particular cultural values, experiences of trust and mistrust, and an array of skills for dealing with the world; this complex history pre-dates the occurrence of a particular traumatic event that may have prompted the patient to seek treatment. Trauma occurs in the context of the person's characteristics, experiences, and history up until that point: how capable of handling intense affect, how capable of trust, how self-aware. The traumatic event or series of events can often cause the natural development of skills and experiences to falter or stop. It is then a task of psychotherapy to enable those developmental processes to resume. A person who has been reluctant to depend on distant or overly emotional parents may be able gradually to establish a relationship of trust in therapy, and at that point therapist and patient can attempt to disentangle those issues that pre-dated but may have been exacerbated by the trauma, from those issues that relate to the trauma alone. Therapy must examine the patient's dichotomous view of herself as either completely normal or terribly damaged, and must address her shame and sense of disconnection from others and from society. At times, the patient may feel 'flooded', reminded of her traumatic experiences everywhere she looks, and the therapist may have this experience as well. The patient may feel ashamed, disconnected from others, and disconnected from society, questioning where she fits in or if she fits in at all. As she explores her past experiences of power and powerlessness, and of sexuality as distinct from violence expressed through sexual means, she can begin to consider her current or developing desires. These are difficult issues to discuss, and patients often begin by speaking in a numb, disconnected manner, unable or unwilling to feel deep emotions because of the intensity of the trauma they have experienced.

6.4 **What about truth and reconciliation?**

With these issues in mind, I return to the concepts of truth and reconciliation. Judith Herman (1992), in her powerful book *Trauma and Recovery*, describes the historical tension between society's recognition of trauma and our desire to recoil from and forget it, which parallels the patient's own experience of remembering and forgetting. Herman sets out a model for acknowledgement and recovery that directly addresses not only the personal devastation and loss but also the social disconnection that arises in traumatized individuals. She notes that the disconnection caused by trauma destroys 'the victim's fundamental assumptions about the safety of the world, the positive value of the self, and the meaningful order of creation' (Herman, 1992, p. 51). Recovery, for Herman, involves a healing relationship, the assurance of safety, the process of remembrance, mourning, and reconnection, and the ultimate sense of commonality with other human beings.

Reconnection and reconciliation

Reconnection is at once a personal quest and a social process. It involves reconnecting with—and possibly modifying—one's former sense of self before the trauma (if that is possible; clearly for some traumatic events that occur very early in development, it is not), reconnecting with others in social relationships, and reconnecting with the social world beyond friendships alone. Shame distances the patient from self-respect, it distances her from others, and it calls into question her connection with the social world. She feels defiled, separate from the community, and may fear being judged by them. Resolution, then, must address issues at three levels: (1) intrapsychic; (2) relational, between people; and (3) social, the connection between the patient and the social world. The therapist plays a role at each of these levels. Intrapsychically, the therapist can be seen as an extension of the patient's observing ego, helping the patient to rebuild her sense of self. Relationally, the therapist is another person with whom the patient can have a relationship, thereby reconnecting her by extension with some others. Socially, and most problematically, the therapist is a representative of the social world. What does this last role involve? As a representative of the social world, the therapist who acknowledges and empathizes with the patient's experience of violation provides a model of what social validation can be and offers hope that the social world itself can echo that validation.

Meaningful reconnection at any level, personal, relational, or social, requires some kind of reconciliation. Reconnection might involve identifying parts of oneself that one pushed aside (for example, feelings of rage or sorrow underlying the numbing that follows an assault, or memories that one had ignored). But one may encounter these feelings or memories with a feeling of revulsion, shame, or horror; without reconciliation, one cannot accept one's limitations and thereby accept oneself. Because there has been a rupture of confidence in oneself, in other people or with broader society, reconciliation must occur before solid reconnection can take place. To understand why this is the case, we need to consider the kinds of reconciliation that exist. One can be reconciled *to* something, usually something one does not particularly like. (For example, one can be reconciled to a painful experience in life because there is no choice but to accept it.) This kind of reconciliation implies sad acceptance, resignation, or even submission to something or someone. Of course, there are experiences that we usually meet with sad acceptance or resignation, such as death or unexpected loss. However, one can also be reconciled *with* something or someone, which implies willing acceptance, hope, and optimism about the future. At times, psychotherapy attempts to foster reconciliation *to* something difficult that is painful to accept. If patients can speak of their despair and experience their sadness, they may ultimately extend their capacity to tolerate what is painful but unavoidable. This kind of psychotherapeutic work is deeply personal, taking place within the psychological life of the patient and in the interpersonal space between therapist and patient. But reconciliation as resignation will not suffice if the patient is to reconnect credibly with her sense of self, reengage with others and then also meet the social world with affirmation. And as the work of repair moves from the patient's view of herself to reconciliation and possible reconnection with others and with the social world, individual psychotherapy by itself has a facilitating but more limited role. Let us consider each of the three levels of reconciliation and reconnection I have discussed—with oneself, with others, and with the social world.

Reconciliation with oneself

In the process of working with trauma, the patient struggles to find a way to reconnect with her feelings that are numbed, with memories that are confusing, and with the person she once was before she was violated. This involves being reconciled *to* some terrible aspects of her experience but also involves being reconciled *with* herself, accepting herself as someone deserving of care and respect. The patient may have to face disappointment in herself; for example, she may feel that she 'did not fight back hard enough,' even if any fighting could have led to greater danger. Or she may struggle with the issue of complicity. A woman may believe that she unwittingly challenged her attackers by being smart, attractive, articulate, and not cowed in the face of harassment and verbal threats. She may have believed they would not really hurt her. She may have dismissed their verbal menace. Even if she did nothing wrong, there is a tendency to blame herself and for others to blame the victim. As Herman points out, some segments of our society consider that *simply acting as if there is no threat* is provocative and worthy of retaliation (Herman, 1992, p. 69).

In order to consider these things—who one was before a traumatic incident, what happened, what one did or didn't do or feel, and what one feels and believes now—one must face some unsettling truths. My patient now recognizes that she minimized a real danger in the world—that some men and boys harbor rage toward women and will act on it. She has come to understand that a smart and successful woman can provoke a variety of feelings and behaviors, which she may not intend to provoke but which must be recognized. She can no longer be naïve; the world is less safe than she once assumed. If women honestly acknowledge these truths, we feel an altered and more realistic degree of vulnerability. We do not simply assume that others with whom we come in contact share the same values and views. We take more seriously unwelcome comments and looks as conveying a potential yet nevertheless real threat. And if men acknowledge these truths also, they have a different appreciation of how menacing the social world can be in spite of their own personal experience.

Naiveté is no contributing *cause*. My patient's sense that she may have unwittingly challenged the boys who raped her could be felt as a self-reproach, a vestige of self-blame; this is undeserved and surmountable. But her growing understanding of the realities of the world is important as she begins to consider the complexities of reconciliation with the social world.

Reconnection and reconciliation with others

Beyond reconciliation with oneself, the repair of trauma must address the disconnection the patient experiences from others and from society itself. Such reconnection, unless it is only superficial though deeply false, rests on being reconciled *with* particular others and (more complex and more difficult) with the social world. Fortunate people with prior solid and trusting relationships may find their trust challenged by traumatic experiences of coercion, capriciousness, or cruelty. However, patients whose childhood relationships were characterized by abuse or dissimulation may have difficulty trusting anyone at all. For this reason, the role of the therapist as another person with whom to reconcile is especially important. And the therapist must be for the most part dependable, fair, concerned, interested, stable, and honest enough to acknowledge disappointments and failures within the relationship with the patient, if trust is to develop.

But not all others are worthy of trust. Ironically, people who cannot trust others easily at times exhibit the tendency to place far too much confidence in people who deserve little or none, jumping into relationships with little solid evidence of trustworthiness on the part of the other person, only to be bitterly disappointed. One must learn that trust cannot be taken for granted but must develop over time, based on data such as behavior, feelings, and experiences. The patient must recognize that her desire for relationships, and her fear of relationships, may blind her to data she needs to recognize in order to assess psychological and physical safety. She must be clear that some people will not care how she feels. And she must be equally clear that some people will.

A relationship with one individual, the therapist, is not enough. Cultural attitudes—for example, that 'uppity' women deserve to be punished—are more effectively challenged by a group of others who themselves have been victims of violence, than by one therapist alone. There is power in a group, whether a therapy group or a network of supportive people, that no one individual can confer. And clearly the therapist cannot convincingly stand in for a pluralistic society with conflicting values and beliefs. Just as relationships with certain others cannot possibly merit trust, certain patterns in the social world render reconciliation very difficult.

Reconciliation with the social world

How can one be reconciled *with* the social world, and not simply reconciled *to* it, after a traumatic event? Michael Hardimon suggests that Hegel's notion of being at home in the social world can help to answer that question. He notes,

> According to Hegel, people—modern people, anyway—are *at home in the social world* if and only if
>
> 1. the social world is a home;
> 2. they grasp that the social world is a home;
> 3. they feel at home in the social world; and
> 4. they accept and affirm the social world.
>
> Hardimon (1992, p. 181, emphasis in original)

Hardimon goes on to say,

> Being at home in the social world (and hence reconciliation) is both an objective and a subjective matter. It is not wholly subjective, since there is an objective condition the social world must meet—that of being a home—if people are to be at home there... But being at home in the social world is not wholly objective either, since there is a set of subjective conditions people must satisfy in order to be at home (conditions 2 through 4).
>
> Hardimon (1992, pp. 181–2)

We can only be reconciled with the social world if that reconciliation is warranted; that is, if the social world itself is worthy of respect, balances the needs of individuality and community, and reflects at least some of our values and our beliefs. Rigidity or hostility in important social structures or widely held cultural attitudes (for example, that women are partly responsible for rape by being out alone at night) can preclude full reconciliation. And hostile institutions (such as legal systems that protect the powerful or that do little to protect the privacy of the victim) that fail to meet the objective conditions required for reconciliation *should* and *must* preclude reconciliation.

Because we are social beings, some kind of reconciliation with the social world is a necessity of life. To do this, one need not accept and affirm all aspects of the social world. In a pluralistic society such as our own, there are subcultures that can offer refuge when other social structures seem unbending or hostile. In order for the social world to feel like a home, one must find a part of that world in which one agrees with the norms and values exhibited in the practices of a social group. For many who have experienced rape, a group of peers can affirm a sense of connection with others and with a subgroup within society, such as feminists or rape activists.

It remains, however, for both therapist and patient to contend with the realistic biases and limitations of the greater social world as it exists. This patient never filed a report with the police, believing that the social prominence of the families involved would bring on retaliation and hostility but little justice. We cannot know whether prosecution would have been successful. When I first heard the story, I wished that the incident had been reported, but then I realized that I had no idea what the legal outcome might have been—vindication or simply further exposure to ridicule and humiliation. The social tolerance in the United States for violence toward women in words, pictures and behavior makes it difficult to have confidence that a sexual assault will be punished. That privileged people who committed a horrifying violation are now continuing in their protected lives undermines our sense that there is justice and alienates us from the social world. My own knowledge of the violence and cruelty in the lives of my inpatients, and the limited interventions that are possible, modulates my hopes for fairness in the social world. The solution is not acceptance, but social change.

The role of psychotherapy in these situations is limited but still important. It is to clarify that the political and social changes necessary *cannot* be formulated as psychological problems. So, to go back to the inpatient unit, when the husband of my mute patient wants us to 'fix' her, we must clarify to both of them what is psychosis and possibly treatable with medication, and what is a family problem of infidelity that this allegedly psychotic woman sees with clear eyes and a sad heart. We have to speak this truth.

6.5 Truth and reconciliation

What role does truth play in reconciliation? Being truthful is a prerequisite for reconciliation, both in the sense that the patient must be honest with herself and in the sense that the therapist must be truthful with the patient. If there is dishonesty between the patient and another person, or between patient and therapist, then mutual trust is undermined and reconnection cannot be genuine. If the patient harbors reservations that are never discussed—ways in which the therapist has disappointed or failed the patient for example—whatever trust exists in the relationship is limited and only confirms the patient's sense that no real connection can take place. Furthermore, the therapist who claims to be trustworthy must in fact *be* trustworthy. If the therapist is not trustworthy but pretends to be, and the patient pretends as well, we have only a recapitulation of prior abusive situations where unsatisfactory or truly terrible events were framed as acceptable. And if the social world is in fact not a home though its inhabitants acknowledge it to be a home, there is again only a false resolution and no possible reconnection or reconciliation. So there are many possibilities of false resolutions that have to do with submission, resignation, or reconciling oneself *to* a bad relationship or an unsatisfactory social world, where there is neither justice nor honesty. Genuine resolution, in contrast, requires changes on all three levels discussed in Section 6.5 (see 'Reconnection and reconciliation'): intrapsychically within the patient, relationally between the patient and other people, and socially, between the patient and the social world. This requires that the social world be sufficiently just that it can address injustices such as rape. Psychotherapy can help an individual come to a complex set of truths about what happened. It must identify certain unpalatable truths about the person herself, about others, and about the social world so that it is clear where responsibility lies. Because there are some social practices that are awful, yet common, like rape, recognizing these truths may render reconciliation with the social world difficult indeed. Facing these truths in psychotherapy, or with other like-minded people, may be a precondition for doing something to rectify the social situation, which lies outside the domain of psychotherapy and in the domain of political and social activism.

References

Davidson RT, ed (2003). *Focus*, 1(3): 237–333.

Freud S (1953). Fragment of an analysis of a case of hysteria (1905). In: *Standard Edition of the Complete Psychological Works of Sigmund Freud* (ed. J Strachey), VII, pp. 3–122. London: Hogarth Press.

Hardimon MO (1992). The project of reconciliation: Hegel's social philosophy. *Philosophy and Public Affairs*, 21(2): 165–95.

Herman J (1992). *Trauma and Recovery*. New York: Basic Books.

Chapter 7

Beyond virtue and the law: on the moral significance of the act of forgiveness in Hegel's *Phenomenology of Spirit*

Mary C. Rawlinson

> This was what interested me most about them: not the dead—what can you really say about a million murdered people whom you didn't know—but how those who had to live in their absence would do so.
> *Philip Gourevitch (2000)*

A terrible truth of human life is that we must live with those who have wronged us and with those whom we have wronged. In the early months of 2005, four young Ugandan women, abducted eight years earlier from their boarding school by the Lord's Resistance Army, escaped and returned home. During their time with the rebels, they served as sexual slaves to rebel commanders and became killers themselves. Everyone who was captured was made to kill in the first week of their captivity. The women recount how shortly after their abduction, they were ordered to beat to death one of their classmates who had been captured with them (Thernstrom, 2005). The rebels beat them until they beat the girl to death. One woman tells of beating to death a 10-year-old boy shortly after her own capture, when she herself was only 14. Other children who were abducted were made to return to their villages and kill their parents, relatives, and neighbors, sometimes mutilating them first by cutting off their noses, ears, or genitals, or plucking out their eyes. The four young women, who were 22–24 years old at the time of this writing, were relatively lucky in that they have been accepted by their families and allowed to return to their villages, though they are shunned and taunted and face ruined futures.

The International Criminal Court at The Hague intervened in Uganda and, in 2005, issued arrest warrants for the rebel leaders. Many war victims and local leaders urged the Court to delay the warrants in favor of a period of amnesty. They argued that local Acholi rituals of confession and forgiveness were more likely to secure a future for their people than the application of law and the condemnation of the rebels. They feared that the threat of prosecution would cause the rebels to continue the violence and believed that amnesty would be more likely to end it. Through a public confession and appeal for forgiveness, they argued, the rebels could be reconciled to the community, so that it could move forward. Such strategies of reconciliation have been employed in South Africa and Rwanda and, indeed, are ancient elements in many African traditions (Lacey, 2005).

With respect to Uganda, the position of the local leaders and war victims privileged the future over the past, and reconciliation over justice, judgment, and punishment. More important than treating the rebels as war criminals, subjecting them to a judicial procedure that would detail and prove their crimes, and inflicting punishment on them, they argued, is the need for the community to find a way forward. The leaders and victims argued for an alternative process of confession, forgiveness, and reconciliation, not for the sake of the rebels but in order to establish a social space in which being together as neighbors restores the future of each individual. Their call for confession and forgiveness in the name of the future of the community assumes that the reintegration of the guilty is necessary to the restoration of each victim's own agency and future.

Less dramatic examples of the way in which the future of a victim depends on reconciliation with a wrongdoer can be found easily in daily life. A husband abandons his wife for a younger woman, yet they must continue to collaborate in the raising of their children. A mother makes a promise to her child and fails to keep it, yet he remains dependent on her. A supervisor encourages an associate in a project and then fails to back him up, yet they must go on working together. A friend betrays my confidence, yet our affection remains dear to me. An injured party who seeks revenge and refuses to forgive courts further injury in the loss of the relationship itself. What seems to be required is not so much judgment, justice, and punishment, but reconciliation—the restoration of the relation that sustained both individualities.

The arguments of the Ugandan leaders and victims, as well as these daily examples, suggest that each individual's agency or future, can only be sustained by a complexity of social relations. Reconciliation proves necessary as a response to injury and harm, because the one who has been injured cannot be himself or return to his own agency apart from those social relations.

Moreover, these arguments and examples suggest that reconciliation is only possible if the opportunity to forgive is created by the remorse of the perpetrator. The victim has been shorn of his agency and made an object of use, to be disposed of at will, whether by violence in the extreme or by lies and manipulation in daily betrayals. The opportunity to say 'I forgive' restores the victim to the position of agency within the social relation and makes the perpetrator, who now waits for forgiveness, dependent on him.

Among philosophers in the Western tradition, Hegel is unusual in making forgiveness the core of his analysis of moral judgment as well as social life. Most philosophers rely on a concept of rights derived from a social contract, as well as on a concept of justice as equity or fairness in analyzing moral harm. Contemporary approaches to genocide, torture, and other forms of organized violence against classes of persons reflect this heritage by identifying commissions on human rights as the appropriate forum for their adjudication and declarations of human rights as the appropriate articulation of what has been transgressed. In the analysis of ethical life and moral philosophy that forms the heart of the 'science of the experience of consciousness' laid out in his *Phenomenology of Spirit*, Hegel turns instead to the act of forgiveness as the point of orientation for ethical action and moral thinking (Hegel, 1979; references in the text hereafter are to paragraph numbers). In his account, both social life and the individuality of the single consciousness are sustained on the basis of the act of forgiveness.

Hegel's analysis provides a philosophical elaboration of the insight of the Ugandan leaders and victims: that forgiveness proves socially and personally sustaining only because it is itself the result of collaboration. The reconciling power of forgiveness depends upon the act *being elicited* rather than being produced spontaneously by a single consciousness. Forgiveness, in so far as it is a socially constitutive force, responds to the truth as laid forth in another's act of confession. It requires a narrative of the transgression *before others*. The abject truthfulness of the confession solicits from the judging consciousness a generous suspension of both the moral law and the legal code by which the perpetrator would be held to account for his transgression. The confession, though necessary, hardly restores the loss, and forgiveness constitutes moral generosity. Unlike mercy, it is not dispensed from above by a superior judge, but circulates freely among the members of a *socius*. Only in a spirit of generosity can the injured one let go the wrong, resist the instinct to settle accounts, and forgive the other in the name of their shared life. Beyond the moral law and legal code, the act of forgiveness can reconcile the parties and restore the sociality that sustains each one, but only on the basis of a narrative that genuinely captures the transgression.

In the course of this analysis, Hegel also identifies a persistent error that is associated not only with the inadequacies of rights and 'legal status' as conceptions of moral agency and responsibility, but also with terrorism and its mass murders and other transgressions. Terrorism results when the single individual believes in the immediate identity of his will with the universal and, therefore, in his absolute right to impose his will directly on an evil world, without the mediation of others through social forms and institutions. Hegel links terrorism to *dogmatism*, to the adherence to oneself as a source of moral truth, rather than to action before and with others. Terrorism results when the particular consciousness valorizes its own virtue or its own law over the exchanges of social life. ('Consciousness' in Hegel's analysis refers to the single empirical human being in its entirety, not merely to mental or psychological capacities. The destiny of consciousness is to become self-conscious, to become aware of its own awareness or knowledge of its own knowing. In the course of his analysis, Hegel considers the whole range of experience from the sensuous and sexual to speculative reason. The *Phenomenology* traces the genealogy of consciousness as it develops through its various essential forms.) The hard-headedness with which these forms of consciousness terrorize the world is matched only by their hard-heartedness: their unwillingness to forgive and to be freed from revenge by letting the other go free. Hard-headedly sticking to an inner virtue or a formal law, these figures hard-heartedly engender terror, a war of each one who adheres relentlessly to his virtue or law against the other hard hearts.

7.1 Hegel's project: the critique of dogmatism and the necessity of narrative as the reconciling power

Hegel's *Phenomenology of Spirit* takes the form of an autonarrative novel organized by the difference between the narrator and the hero, 'natural consciousness.' It is the story of how the hero becomes the narrator. Addressing natural consciousness in the certainty of its immediate experience, the narrator, 'we, philosophical consciousness,' challenges the hero to say what he means: the ordinary individual is challenged to express in language—*to say*—the certainty that suffuses specific aspects of experience in his everyday life—*what he means*. As the hero attempts to say what he takes to be the truth of his experience, he discovers that he is not who he thought he was and, in this way, he produces a new and more comprehensive account of himself. As the narrative project progresses, the hero becomes an increasingly dense and rich complexity of ways of knowing or apprehending and more and more capable of saying who he is without denying or subordinating essential elements of his experience. Moreover, he discovers that his own narrative activity implies a complexity of social relations. He discovers that, as the narrator of his own experience, he is already operating in the first person plural. The narrative of the *Phenomenology* describes this transformation of the single consciousness, which believes that it exists on its own, into 'we, philosophical consciousness,' the one who knows himself to be real only as the member of a *socius*.

By interrogating itself, through the attempt to 'say what it means' or narrate its own experience, consciousness discovers all the possible figures of experience within itself. Each figure of consciousness—ordinary perception, scientific reason, the citizen, the family, the man of faith—contributes to the complex truth of consciousness. At the same time, each figure gives way to a more comprehensive one that supercedes and preserves it, until consciousness reaches 'that point where knowledge need no longer go beyond itself because nothing is other to it' (Hegel, para 80). As a genealogy, the multiplicity of shapes forms a necessary and complete system. To the extent that consciousness remains afflicted by an alien alterity, a form or feature of experience that it does not understand as constitutive of its own being, its development is incomplete.

From the perspective of the hero, this 'progression of shapes [*Gestalten*]' or 'thought positions [*bestimmten Gedanken*]' constitutes a 'highway of despair.' He undergoes 'many deaths of many selves' (Hegel, para 15, 32, 78). Taking as the whole what is only a part or aspect, natural consciousness finds repeatedly that the identity it has claimed cannot be sustained in the narrative project and that a new shape of identity, reconciling the previous shape with that to which it opposed itself or which it took to be inessential, is required. His attempts to say what he means, to articulate his experience, reveal that his hard-headed 'one-sidedness' is not sustainable. So often disabused of what it thought it knew, it loses faith in its endeavors.[1]

The narrator redeems the loss, suffering, and despair of the hero by reconciling the oppositions that afflict his experience. The narrative supercedes each shape, each specific determination, by incorporating them within a developmental history: the seed or germ of the hero's experience results in the fruit of the comprehensive narrative perspective. The truth of the single consciousness turns out to be its collaboration in a social form. From the point of view

---

[1] I am indebted to the work of Terry Pinkard for an understanding of the importance of the concept of sustainability to Hegel's method. 'One's character, one's self-identity, is constituted in part by the norms that one takes to be imperative for oneself, and these norms are social in the sense that they can only be sustained by those participating in the various practices continuing to regard themselves as bound by those norms and continuing to subject each other to them' (Pinkard, 1995, p. 73).

of the narrator, the hero is 'only an instance.' In the fraternal orders of science, politics, and philosophy, 'natural consciousness' is but a 'moment' in the enterprise of truth. To think, not from one's own perspective, but from that of the whole and, thus, to think of one's self as only an instance of the general figure of the scientist or citizen or friend, for example, is to become the philosophical narrator, the one who sees each part in its place in the whole system of parts and who can produce the narrative whole itself. Saying what he means, the narrative project of philosophy, requires the hero to see his single consciousness as belonging to a world of others and to recognize himself in supra-individual institutions and forms.

Those hard-headed positions that assert the independence of the individual—his self-sufficiency—are not sustainable in experience itself. Both virtue's faith in its own 'inner voice' and reason's faith in its own law-giving procedures produce the 'one-sidedness' that gives rise to personal and social instability, and to terrorism. Neither is adequate to sustain the sociality that turns out to be essential to the existence of each single human being.

Neither virtue nor law-giving reason 'says what it means.' The narratives of virtue and law contradict the very experience that the hero meant to voice. They err, not by being false, but by absolutizing what is only a moment of experience. Hegel's critique of virtue and law focuses on the reconciliation of two related oppositions by which these shapes are afflicted: on the one hand, the single consciousness [das Einzelne] opposes itself to the others, and, on the other, it opposes the truth of its own interiority to the untruth of the actual world.

The 'onesideness' of these shapes produces a triad of errors:

1 *The certainty of immediacy.* Sometimes this error takes the form of a belief in the certainty of what is given. Thus, in sensuous certainty, consciousness identifies truth with the immediacy of being in sense-experience. The truth is the 'This, Here, Now.' After all, no one, except perhaps a philosopher or a madman, doubts in any practical way the certainty of immediacy, that the table or book that I see before me is really there. Yet, if I try to say what I mean, if I try to articulate the truth of this immediate certainty, I find it slips my grasp. The 'now' exists only in relation to other nows, to the temporal continuity of the past and future. The 'here' exists only in relation to what is 'there,' and changes as I move. The 'this' exists only in relation to a whole network of other objectivities. What appears to be given as an immediate certainty is, in fact, the result of a complex of mediating relations.

2 *The sophistry of the essential/inessential distinction.* Sometimes consciousness errs by identifying itself with an aspect of experience, as if it were the

whole, rather than a constitutive element. Employing what Hegel calls 'the ruse' of the essential/inessential distinction, consciousness will take now one, now another aspect to be the truth of the whole, when in fact each is necessary. In perception, for example, consciousness identifies truth first with the properties of the object, as if those properties were merely given in the thing. A collection of properties, however, is not yet a thing. Hence, consciousness finds it necessary to insert its own perceiving as constitutive of the thing. The unifying, categorical activity of consciousness represents the sensuous multiplicity in the unity of *the* thing. But consciousness is not just the unifying 'I think which accompanies all my representations.' It is also a multiplicity of senses. So, now it is the thing that appears to be intrinsically unitary, and its multiplicity is laid at the door of consciousness. In this 'sophistry of perception' the abstract unity of the concept of the thing, on the one hand, and the multiplicity of the senses and sensuous properties, on the other, are alternately taken to be the truth of both consciousness and the thing. If the thing is essentially a unity, its multiple sensuous properties are inessential and appear only in virtue of the interference of consciousness' own senses. If the thing is essentially a sensuous being, its unity is contributed by the synthetic activity of consciousness. Correlatively, consciousness is first identified with the multiplicity of its senses. Then, its synthetic activity is taken to be what is essential about it, and its senses rendered inessential. This sophistical 'toing and froing' always results from the failure of natural consciousness to recognize that each moment is essential and its inability to figure out a way of articulating their belonging-together.

3 *The faith in the 'beyond.'* Finally, consciousness' error of taking the part for the whole sometimes results in the bifurcation of itself and the world into separate beings, one essential or true and the other inessential. Thus, the 'understanding' or the 'unhappy consciousness' of religion distinguishes between the world of appearance and a supersensible world that is its truth. Similarly, these figures distinguish between the empirical self of sensuous experience and an intelligible self that belongs to a world 'beyond' experience. The resolution of this dichotomy in the world and the self can only be projected into another time and place, as an abstract regulative ideal, thought but not experienced. It depends upon a salvation on the other side of death. This faith locates truth in the 'beyond' at the expense of the actual world, so that the others with whom I actually live can be sacrificed to it.

This triad of errors—the certainty of immediacy, the sophistry of the essential/inessential distinction, and the faith in a 'beyond'—all exhibit the same logical form. In each case, consciousness takes as absolutely true what is in fact only a moment, an aspect of truth. It embraces a part as the whole and, in doing so, divests some immediacy of the mediating relations that sustain it. Hence, the certainty of the 'now' evaporates as soon as I try to express it, just as the confidence of perception is spent in its sophistical oscillation between the one and the many, and just as the knowledge of the understanding or religious consciousness is, in fact, only a faith that cannot be validated except 'beyond' experience. In each case, the effort to hold fast to a moment, as if it were the truth, cannot be sustained in the course of the narrative project.

And, just as the different moments within any given shape of consciousness are each essential and must be thought and expressed, not immediately, but in relation to one another, so too the various shapes of consciousness belong together in the temporal dimensions of the narrative of philosophical consciousness. Narrative, unlike the profession of faith or the logical proposition, is the rhetorical form in which consciousness can say what it means. Regarded from the side of the single consciousness, as it is in the *Phenomenology*, Science consists in '. . . his acquiring what thus lies at hand, devouring his inorganic nature, and taking possession of it for himself' (Hegel, para. 28). Through narration, by saying his experience so as to represent its different epochs and figures as a developmental history, the single consciousness overcomes dogmatism's fatal error of sticking only to one 'determinateness.' In the narrative of his development, each figure of consciousness or way of knowing that the single consciousness has embodied finds its proper place in relation to the others. Saying what he means, the hero 'takes possession' of immediacy, what 'lies at hand,' rendering himself for himself an 'acquired property' [*ein erworbene Eigentum*]. Taking possession of himself through narration, the single consciousness comes to see that the oppositions which afflicted his experience are only apparent: 'distinctions which are no distinctions' (Hegel, para 28). In this narrative process, each shape, each moment takes its place among the others, quietly retiring its dogmatic claim to truth.

Hegel takes this transmutation to be an acquisition and an enowning, not a loss or process of alienation, but the way by which the hero comes into his own. It is a loss only of what is not sufficiently real to sustain itself anyway. And a loss only from the point of view of the individual who is not yet adequately transmuted and, hence, still blind to the truth of his existence as a moment of the whole. The development of his individualism itself depends on his position as a node in a network of relations. The narrative, even his own personal narrative, who he is to himself, finds its voice in the first person plural. The 'I' is always already a 'we.'

Thus, as Hegel himself regularly reminds the reader, the goal of the *Phenomenology of Spirit* is nothing less than the production, out of a collection of underdeveloped particulars, of the material unity of a social voice, a 'we.' Within the 'we' of philosophical consciousness—the narrative voice—each single consciousness knows itself to be at once both an instance of the whole series of shapes comprising the truth of consciousness and only a moment of a corporate form. Thus, through the collaborative work of narrative, each part is reconciled to itself and to the whole: each aspect of each shape of consciousness, each shape of the series, each single consciousness with the others whose story is also its own, 'Our own act,' the act of 'we, philosophical consciousness.' Each moment demands its due, and the error of sticking hard-headedly to one determination or hard-heartedly sacrificing actual social relations to an abstract future or to an image of others as 'alien' cannot sustain itself before the power of narration. Thus, Peter Singer has argued that the Nazis 'did not dare to be open about what they were doing to the Jews . . . If it had been possible to ensure that every page of Nazi history were written as it happened, and offered for discussion to the German people, it is hard to believe that the Holocaust would have taken place' (Singer, 2004, p. 137). Such actions simply would not have been sustainable within the community's self-narration.

Hegel's analysis requires that the narrative must belong to each and all and must include all the moments and aspects of experience. In principle, nothing can be excluded. To the extent that any single consciousness or any aspect of experience remains other to it, the narrative is incomplete. Hegel's own narrative deserves criticism with respect to the difference of gender, for he denies to women a genuine agency and voice in the public sphere, relegating them to the privacy of the family where they tend the body. Similar criticism might be directed at his valorization of European culture. Nevertheless, these criticisms would follow from his own injunction that the narrative of experience is incomplete as long as anything is defined as 'the other' or 'inessential' and prevented from contributing its voice to the story.

Correlatively, the elaboration of social forms that are adequate to sustain the life of consciousness will require ' a struggle among people and groups over, among other things, what kind of narrative best elucidates the implicit norms of a practice and over who fits into that narrative and who does not' (Pinkard 1995, p. 87). Narrative is essential to reconciliation in societies such as South Africa or Rwanda that have been traumatized by civil violence, violence inflicted upon each other by those who live together in the same place. Narrative is essential not only because of the necessity of the story as a condition for confession and forgiveness, but also because the mere act of the collaborative narration itself puts the opposing forces into a social relation that supercedes the opposition between groups and the exclusion of the other from moral regard. Conversely, the refusal to engage in collaborative narration is an essential element of tyranny and terrorism. 'Power largely consists in the ability to make others inhabit your story of their reality, even if you have to kill a lot of them to make that happen' (Gourevitch, 2000, p. 181). In his analysis of the genocide in Rwanda, Philip Gourevitch, notes repeatedly the way in which the recovery of a future for this society was impeded, not only by the continued presence of armed militia ready to resume the slaughter, but also by the denial that any genocide had occurred. In fact, it was the lack of recognition of the facts of the genocide that enabled the international community to pursue policies that aided the perpetrators (Gourevitch, 2000, p. 325). Moreover, it was the denial on the part of the perpetrators themselves of what had taken place that undermined the 'special genocide law' providing amnesty or reduced sentences for those who confessed their crimes (Gourevitch, 2000, p. 339). This failure of narration went hand-in-hand with the inability to restore the social relations that could sustain a future for the country.

Collaborative narration involves the *acknowledgment* of the other, not a speaking *for* him, but a speaking *with* him. Moreover, it is not a conversation in which we might exchange our points of view while keeping our positions separate and intact. Collaborative narration depends upon the recognition that the other belongs to the same story as I, that the story is neither his, nor mine, but ours. Husbands have often spoken for their wives, or the developed world on behalf of the developing world, but collaborative narration requires that he who has been speaking cede the narrative position to the other. The acknowledgment of the other implies listening to the other and speaking with him, even if it is only to tell the story of our disagreement and conflict. Arundhati Roy suggests that it is just this failure to acknowledge the other as one who speaks in his own right about our social relations that lies at the heart of recent terrorist attacks:

> Terrorism as a phenomenon may never go away. but if it is to be contained the first step is for America to at least *acknowledge* that it shares the planet with other nations, with other human beings, who, even if they are not on TV, have loves and griefs and stories and songs and sorrows... The American Way of Life is simply not sustainable. Because it doesn't acknowledge that there is a world beyond America.

> Roy (2002, pp. 207, 298)

The insertion of the other into the narrative space is, at the same time, his insertion into the social space, and this collaboration is essential to each and all. It may be that there are times when one needs to speak for the other, but that cannot be done until one has spoken with the other and the other has had the opportunity to speak for himself. Otherwise, one is always speaking in his place, and he has no place within the social relations that the narrative sustains. And, Roy's point, like Hegel's, is that a narrative that does not sustain us all will not sustain any of us in the end.

7.2 **The critique of virtue and law**

Hegel's analysis of forgiveness appears quite late in the course of the *Phenomenology*, after a long critique of forms of virtue and reason's moral law as insufficient to sustain the 'we' of social life. It culminates the analysis that began with a myth of the origin of society in the relation of mastery and slavery. Thus, it is an answer to the question of how human beings might live together without domination in 'mutual recognition.'

Both the 'man of virtue' and the rational subject of the moral law exhibit the 'one-sidedness' that makes social relations unsustainable. Each repeats the triad of errors characterizing the natural consciousness that does not yet realize itself as a moment of a social whole:

- ◆ Both locate moral value in the self's own intentions, as over against the mediation of its relations with others. In doing so, the 'man of virtue' renders the other a suspect alien interiority and a 'Fiend' to be combated. The rational subject of the moral law takes the other to be an abstract 'legal person' devoid of the determinations of life, thus covering over the real inequities of actual social relations.

- ◆ Both take action to be inessential to the constitution of the moral subject, privileging the 'beauty,' self-consistency, or purity of the will. In the case of virtue, this takes the form of an adherence to a 'divine inner voice,' while reason relies upon its own formal principle of universalizibility. In either case, the moral subject is assumed to be fully constituted prior to its action, which is merely an effect.

- ◆ Both locate the realization of moral value in a world 'beyond' the actual. Both assume that moral agency is realized within the individual, but that in the public world of action it is 'merely *implicit*, merely *postulated*.' It belongs to a world that remains hypothetical.

Virtue

As a necessary moment in the experience of consciousness, virtue contributes to the formation of ethical practice and moral thinking. It installs the essential idea of the singular human being as responsible for his own action and judgment. Nevertheless, it exhibits the hard-headedness of natural consciousness in mistaking an aspect or part for the whole of moral experience. Virtue's 'one-sidedness' consists in sticking steadfastly to interiority as the site of moral truth. It appears in Hegel's analysis as a series of figures—the law of the heart, the knight of virtue, the spiritual zoo, absolute freedom, the beautiful soul, conscience—which is defined by a consistent failure to recognize the sociality and publicity of moral life.[2]

Hegel locates virtue historically in the Enlightenment's 'faith' in the 'pure insight' of reason. Hegel condemns its struggle 'against the impure intentions and perverse insights of the actual world' as 'twaddle' and a 'penetrating infection' or 'disease' (Hegel, para 538, 545). The virulence of his criticism arises both from his view of Kantian moral philosophy as a dangerous 'perversion' of the genuine sociality of ethical practice and from the historical example of the French Revolution, in which virtue's rhetorical logic and the explicit worship of reason yield the Terror.

Insofar as it focuses on intentions that are 'placed altogether beyond anything actually done' (Hegel, para 619), Kant's moral philosophy constitutes a 'dissemblance' or 'duplicity' (Hegel, para 616).

- On the one hand, Kantian reason claims for itself the capacity to make moral judgments and elaborates explicit procedures for doing so. Moral judgment depends only upon the operation of 'healthy reason' itself, upon its own independent test. On the other hand, it is to apply universally, so that the independence of its own test has already been superseded by the assumption that its conclusions belong to all the others as well.

- On the one hand, reason secures the validity of its judgment by limiting its scope only to a purity of intentions, established by an absolute allergy to the body that acts. Its judgments do not apply to its actions, and refer only to the rational consistency or purity of its own soul. On the other hand, its judgments articulate imperatives of action, and its abstract purposes or intentions can be translated into action only through the sensuous nature, which it supposedly has purged. In articulating principles of action, it assumes that the impulses of that body will conform to reason, 'for moral action is nothing else but consciousness realizing itself, thus giving itself the shape of an *impulse*' (Hegel, para 622; emphasis in original). Thus, it oscillates between the view that moral intention is essentially opposed to empirical motives and the insistence that they are in absolute conformity.

---

2 There are significant differences among these figures, particularly the degree to which each one understands itself as an action; however, my analysis focuses on the structural analogy among them, the persistent valorization of interiority and intention over sociality and action. It is this 'one-sidedness' that constitutes them as a series.

♦ On the one hand, moral consciousness insists on the 'great gulf' between the realms of freedom and nature (Kant, 1987, p. 35). It insists on an absolute difference between the intelligible world of the moral law where the purity of intention and self-consistency of the will are guaranteed and the empirical world of action. Moral action arises from this abyss, and consists in the impossible project of making the latter accord with the former. On the other hand, the moral law can be established as valid only on 'one condition:' that there be a 'future world' in which the gulf is overcome and nature conforms to the world of freedom and moral consciousness. Hence, the assumed difference was never absolute, as their conformity was always already given in principle. In this world, consciousness can only act morally based upon the assumption of 'a possible kingdom of ends as a kingdom of nature' (Kant, 1956, p. 104). Yet, the realization of this future world is infinitely deferred. It remains a purely intelligible or supersensible world, opposed to the world of action.

In its 'shiftiness' and 'hypocrisy,' virtue or the 'beautiful soul' claims to be doing its duty and therefore is morally worthy, at the same time that it denies reality to the world in which it acts and derives the value of its intentions from a world beyond experience. Thus, it is a 'hollow' self, filled with empty intentions and empty rhetoric: 'It lives in dread of besmirching the splendor of its inner being by action and an existence; and, in order to preserve the purity of its heart, it flees from contact with the actual world, and persists in its self-willed impotence to renounce its self which is reduced to the extreme of ultimate abstraction…' (Hegel, para 658).

Yet, this 'hollowness' is not without result. The man of virtue opposes the truth and goodness of his own interiority to the hypocrisy and evil of the actual world. He sticks to the interiority of his heart, refusing to recognize either the exteriority of ethical practice and moral judgment or the complicity of his own interiority with the interiority of the other. His 'one-sidedness' renders the other a 'Fiend' to be 'combated,' while he adheres to his own will as if it were something immediately universal, with tyranny and social terror the result. The hard-heartedness of this hard-headedness makes the reciprocities of ethical and moral life impossible. Either it produces no more than 'pompous talk' and 'proselytizing rhetoric' or, when it attempts to act in the name of its 'divine inner voice,' the terror of civil violence.

Hegel's analysis of the rhetoric of virtue is well reflected in contemporary political language, which exhibits both the justification of aggression by characterizing the other as a 'Fiend' and the inversion of language that turns aggression and harm into an intervention on behalf of humanity. Its talk about '. . . doing what is best for humanity, about the oppression of humanity, about making sacrifices for the sake of the good . . .' really serves only to declare that 'the individual who professes to act for such noble ends and who deals in such fine phrases is in his own eyes an excellent creature—a puffing-up which inflates him with a sense of importance in his own eyes and in the eyes of others, whereas he is, in fact, inflated with his own conceit.' (Hegel, para 390).

Genocide regularly involves the demonizing of the victims, as in the case of Nazi Germany, or a narrative of past injustices in which the victims are represented as fiendish perpetrators who deserve to be punished, as in the case of Bosnia or Rwanda. The reliance on this rhetorical strategy constitutes one of the remarkable similarities between the terrorism of religious fundamentalism and that state-sanctioned violence directed against it. Just as perpetrators of 9/11 justified their actions through the representation of the US as the 'Great Satan,' so Bush justifies the US aggression in Afghanistan and Iraq as an assault on 'evildoers.' Moreover, dissent and critique are stifled by the same rhetorical ploy:

> To call someone 'anti-American,' indeed, to *be* anti-American, (or for that matter anti-Indian, or anti-Timbuktuan) is not just racist, it's a failure of the imagination. An inability to see the world in terms other than those that the establishment has set out for you: if you're not a Bushie, you're a Taliban. If you don't love us, you hate us. If you're not good, you're Evil. If you're not with us, you're with the terrorists.

> Roy (2002, p. 278)

Whatever other rhetorical strategies are employed—the circulation of false information, the suppression and denial of facts, the strict control of available images—their success in motivating and sustaining aggression depends upon this logic of 'fiendishness.' It gives rise to a narrative in which, whatever the other has done, it cannot be forgiven and justifies his destruction.

The abstraction from the world of action in favor of a 'divine inner voice' and a perfected future world makes possible as well a rhetoric of inversion that represents the subjection of the other as his liberation. No doubt there was a time in human history when the powerful were frankly aggressive but, in the modern context of law and rights, leaders have regularly found it necessary to justify war as a way of ending war. In announcing the assault on Afghanistan, George W. Bush insisted, 'We're a peaceful nation.' After quoting him in her essay 'War is Peace,' Roy appends a list of the score of nations that the US has been at war with and bombed since World War II. She remarks, 'So now we know. Pigs are horses. Girls are boys. War is peace' (Roy, 2002, p. 217). Iraq in 2005 is not France in 1944, yet the same rhetoric of liberation is deployed to justify military violence. Given the lack of even minimal physical security, the disruption of basic services and infrastructure, the suspension of ordinary routines of work and leisure, and the escalating factionalism of the society, it is hard to imagine how the ordinary Iraqi could embrace his 'Enduring Freedom.' Yet, 'Operation Enduring Freedom' is represented as a mission *on behalf of the Iraqi people*, not merely an episode in the US's own 'war on terror.' The readiness of US leaders to speak for the Iraqi people, to take the place of the Iraqi people in their own narrative, is constantly justified by reference to the abstract virtue of those leaders, the 'peaceful' who make war. The exercise of power over others is regularly derived from the 'virtues' of the American nation: 'The most free nation in the world. A nation built on fundamental values; that rejects hate, rejects violence, rejects murderers, and rejects evil' (Bush, 2001). Moreover, a 'divine inner voice' is repeatedly invoked explicitly to justify war in the name of peace.

Whatever the success of these rhetorical strategies, this virtuous consciousness, having reduced what should belong to the world of action and others to its own interiority, soon discovers that the others also have the law of *their* hearts, which they do not find 'fulfilled' in his. And, these 'others ... turn against the reality he set up, just as he turned against theirs ... now he finds the hearts of men themselves opposed to his excellent intentions and detestable' (Hegel, para 373). Thus, virtue's 'heart-throb for the welfare of humanity,' by rendering the other a 'Fiend,' abstracting from the conditions of action and valorizing its own 'divine inner voice' over the material institutions and practices that might mediate social relations, in fact, produces war and civil violence. In attempting to impose the law of its heart, it

> ... meets with resistance from others, because it contradicts the equally *particular* [*ebsenso einzelnen*] laws of their hearts; and these others in their resistance are doing nothing else but setting up and claiming validity for their own law. The universal that we have here is, then, only a universal resistance and struggle of all against one another, in which each claims validity for his own particular consciousness [*seine eigene Einzelheit*], but at the same time does not succeed in his efforts, and is nullified by their reciprocal resistance. What seems to be public order, then, is this universal state of war, in which each wrests what he can for himself, executes justice on the other particular consciousness and establishes his own, which is equally nullified by the others.
>
> Hegel (para 379, emphasis in original)

In this 'universal state of war' produced by the dogmatism of virtue, the actual world becomes the stage for a '*fury* of destruction,' and 'what is called government is merely the victorious faction' (Hegel, para 591; emphasis in original). Hegel takes as an historical paradigm the successive waves of terror that came to define the French Revolution, in which leaders such as Saint-Just and Robespierre, who made the execution of citizens for no specific crimes of political affiliation a state policy, were themselves executed in turn on the same grounds. Unfortunately, examples of this factionalism are fully plentiful around the globe today. In a plethora of contemporary countries, from Haiti to Bosnia to Uganda, the legitimacy of government has been derived from the exercise of military power on a 'fiendish' opposition, 'justifiably executed' by the faction in power, initiating cycles of violence that often, as in the case of Uganda, make it impossible to separate the victim from the perpetrator, for the one has become the other, leaving no one innocent. The logic of factionalism, in which each one claims an absolute right or 'universal freedom' for his own 'inner, divine voice', produces only '...death, a death which has no inner significance or filling... It is thus the coldest and meanest of deaths, with no more significance than cutting off a head or swallowing a mouthful of water' (Hegel, para 590). Because the legitimacy of government is not referred to the future of the society as a whole, because it is derived from a narrative of past injustice by the 'fiend', because it is not located in material practices and institutions that mediate among individuals, the state reflects only the tides of power and its waves of executions.

Moreover, today the rhetorical logic of virtue determines, as even in states of the developed world that are thought to be well-constituted. In the US and Europe, politics consist in a struggle of opposing factions and exhibits these same rhetorical strategies of rendering the other a 'fiend' and inversion. The activities of political parties are regularly explained in terms of how they serve certain 'special interests' and the idea that they might share a mutual interest in the welfare of the nation is nowhere encountered. The opposing party is not represented as misguided or mistaken, but as a moral threat, as representing the wrong 'values.' The factionalism was so intense in the US in 1995 that a political party could undertake to 'close down the government' in the name of protecting American values. This factionalism destroys the agency of the state. The impossibility of negotiation within this rhetorical logic makes it impossible to go forward on the range of urgent issues afflicting society, from health care to social security to the widening gap between rich and poor.

Thus, factionalism produces a political climate in which 'being suspected takes the place, or has the significance and effect of being guilty, because the government by faction has no legitimate way to establish guilt' (para 591). The condemned's crime is not an act in the world, subject to law and evidence, but an interior state. He is subjected to the annihilation of the ruling faction simply in virtue of being an alien interior. It consists just in the failure to hear the ruling power's 'inner, divine

... . that he may be listening to the voice of his own conscience. While Hegel's ...... al paradigm is the French Revolution, Foucault locates the logic of the ... State in just this threat of 'being suspected.'

> Ultimately, everyone in the Nazi State had the power of life and death over his or her neighbors, if only because of the practice of informing, which effectively meant doing away with the people next door, or having them done away with. So murderous power and sovereign power are unleashed throughout the entire social body ... this is ... a murderous State ... and a suicidal State.
>
> Foucault (2003, pp. 359–60)

In .... absolute terror, no one is safe, as each and every one can become a victim ...... ling faction simply in virtue of being a self and representing an inter...... might contradict the rulers' 'inner, divine voice.' Thus, this terror '...... to *the thinking of oneself* (Hegel, para 592; emphasis in original). ...... of suspicion suffuses politics in the US and Europe where scanda...... tool of power and the representation of the other as having the wrong 'values' is a common strategy. Thus, it was perhaps naïve of John Kerry, despite the facts of his military service and Bush's lack thereof, to be surprised to find himself represented in the 2004 Presidential Elections as less than fit to serve as commander in chief and, even, 'soft' on terror. More terrible examples of the suffusion of society by this logic of suspicion can be found in the practice of informing in the former East Germany or in a variety of dictatorships from Chile under Pinochet to Saddam's Iraq. These societies prove incapable of sustaining a future, because it becomes impossible to maintain any integrity of person or to live alongside one's neighbors without fear.

S... ore terrible is the corollary practice to the logic of suspicion deployed in ...... Rwanda of forcing participation in murder in order to make it imp...... gitimately to suspect anyone, because everyone is guilty.

> 'Eve...... was called to hunt the enemy,' said Theodore Nyilinkwaya, a survivor of the ma...... in his home village of Kimbogo, in the southwestern province of Cyangugu. 'B...... someone is reluctant. Say that guy comes with a stick. They tell him, 'no, ...', OK he does, and he runs along with the rest, but he doesn't kill. They s...... might denounce us later. He must kill. Everyone must help to kill at least one ......
>
> Gourevitch (2000, p. 24)

Thus, like ... young women in Uganda, each member of the society, however he may have been abused and violated, is also a perpetrator of abuse and violence. Each one deserves both restitution and punishment. How can a society go forward and sustain a future when its members are at once victims and victim......

Law

Hegel's critique of law as a concept through which to understand moral experience, like his critique of virtue, directly addresses Kant's moral philosophy, and it analyses the rhetoric as well as the logic of law. The critique demonstrates the same unsustainable oppositions that afflicted virtue, between the single consciousness and the sociality of morality, on the one hand, and the interiority of consciousness and the publicity of action, on the other. Moral reason attempts to express the moral good as maxims of action, i.e., in propositional form. Here again 'healthy reason' runs into the problem of saying something other than what it means. In translating the faith of virtue and the conviction of duty into a plurality of commandments, 'healthy reason' demonstrates, not the necessity, but the contingency of its position. Take, for example, the injunction that 'everyone ought to speak the truth.' Yet, I cannot speak the truth, if I don't know the truth. So, what 'healthy reason' *meant* to say in this commandment is that 'everyone ought to speak the truth according to his knowledge and conviction at the time.' Thus, not only is 'healthy reason' forced to admit that it did not say what it meant and, therefore, did not speak the truth, but also it is forced to recognize the contingency of the commandment. Moreover, if 'healthy reason' insists that the injunction that I ought to know the truth is implicit in the commandment, then it admits that it might not know the truth, which it was supposed to possess immediately as '*healthy* reason' in the inner conviction of duty.[3]

The commandment to 'Love thy neighbor as thy self' runs into similar contradictions. The commandment implies that my love will be good for the other, removing evils and improving his condition, but this requires that I can distinguish between what is bad for him and what promotes his welfare. In short, 'I must love him intelligently. Unintelligent love will perhaps do him more harm than hatred' (Hegel, para 425). Thus, the commandment again proves to

---

[3] Hegel also demonstrates how law repeats the sophistical logic of the thing of perception, oscillating between the determinations of the One and the many, now one and now the other taken as essential. On the one hand, there is only one law, the principle of noncontradiction, which provides a sufficient test in every case. On the other hand, it is necessary to produce a multiplicity of maxims or laws of action, just because the law of noncontradiction has no content of its own and cannot generate a principle of action. From the point of view of reason it is the law of contradiction that is essential and the multiple maxims merely its examples. From the point of view of action, it is the maxims that are essential and the law of contradiction an empty form. Similarly, the law itself is a mere form and does not include within itself the principle of its application. Consciousness may follow it or not, and reason's legislation always has the form of a conditional. [Act *as if* you belong to a 'merely possible' kingdom of ends. *If* you are to think of yourself as free,

be contingent upon the knowing or not knowing of 'healthy reason.' It also assumes that I will have the occasion to act on behalf of the other, which may or may not arise. It takes no account of the fact that the beneficence of the general will in the form of the state is 'so great a power that, if the action of the individual were to oppose it . . . such an action would be altogether useless and inevitably frustrated' (Hegel, para 425). Against this collective action of the state, beneficence is no more than the 'sentiment' of a single and isolated self and, as such, 'as contingent as it is transitory.' The commandment expresses nothing more than the tautology that it is good to do good to the other when he deserves it and bad to harm him when he doesn't.

As mere propositions, these laws simply are inherited by 'healthy reason' or embraced as given immediacies. They have no validity without the supplementation of a narrative that links them to a particular content and a particular occasion. The mere articulation of the law does not relieve 'healthy reason' of the need to make judgments as to what counts as doing good for the other or whether, in fact, he knows the truth. The necessity of judgment always exceeds what can be articulated in the propositional form of the law.

What legitimates these laws in Kant's analysis is the concept of universality: the idea that the moral law applies to each and all. Thus, 'healthy reason' sets up a test for determining which maxims it must embrace: 'Act only on that maxim through which you can at the same time will that it should become a universal law' (Kant, 1956, p. 88). This, however, renders the necessity of universality a mere form, leaving it again subject to the contingency of the content. Take, for example, the question, 'Ought the law of property to be absolute?' (Hegel, para 430). Suppose someone entrusts something to me. Can I not alter my point of view, as I do when I give something away, so that what was his, I now consider to be mine? If I can 'alter the view that it is my property into the view that it belongs to someone else, without becoming guilty of a contradiction, so I can equally pursue the reverse course' (Hegel, para 437).

---

then you must act rationally and in accordance with the principle of noncontradiction. '. . . we must presuppose [freedom] if we wish to conceive a being as rational . . .' (Kant, 1956, p. 116).] Thus, the unity of the law cannot account for the multiplicity of acts that it is said to govern, for it does not contain within itself the necessity of their generation. Finally, the formal test of self-consistency treats the law as a unity, a proposition. Yet, the law, as a maxim of action, has many parts, as the law of property involves the thing owned, the owner, and those who recognize the ownership, and it is in these parts that the law may come into contradiction with itself, that is, in terms of its content, not its form. So, either the law is a unity and as such self-consistent, but formal and empty. Or, it has content, that is, parts, and as such can fall into contradiction, even having satisfied reason's formal test of self-consistency.

Moreover, the idea of nonownership or ownership of goods in common is no more self-contradictory than the law of property. Thus, the 'criterion of law' applied by 'healthy reason' in order to determine moral truth 'fits every case equally well, and is thus in fact no criterion at all' (Hegel, para 429). Again, the necessity of judgment always exceeds the validity of the law. Hegel remarks that 'it would be strange' if the law of contradiction, which establishes only the formal limits of theoretical or mathematical truth, were to yield a greater result in the area of practical action (Hegel, para 431).

Moreover, 'healthy reason,' whether in the form of the lawgiver and or in its activity of testing laws, is guilty of moral 'insolence.' 'Honest reason' cannot validly legislate on its own without the mediation of historically elaborated social forms, and what validates the laws produced by those forms is not 'healthy' or 'honest' reason, but the historical processes and the procedures of the social forms themselves. 'Honest reason's' attempt to base the law on its own 'healthy common sense' is no more than a 'tyrannical insolence which makes caprice into law and ethical behavior into obedience to such caprice' (Hegel, para 434). Similarly, the idea that 'honest reason' could derive what is right from a test it performs on its own divests the moral law of its power to claim us. Insofar as its validity is contingent upon reason's own test, it has no power to compel reason, but must wait to be recognized by it. If the moral good takes the form of law, either reason legislates directly and produces a tyranny or it makes the law contingent upon its own test and eliminates any sense of being compelled by what is right.

Hegel's point is not that the concept of law is unnecessary, but that it is secondary to and an expression of the intrinsic force of moral obligation which derives from the fundamental sociality of human being. It is not the law that makes killing wrong, but the wrongness of killing that justifies the law. The right is something absolute by which we find ourselves claimed:

> It is not, therefore, because I find something is not self-contradictory that it is right; on the contrary, it is right because it is what is right. That something is the property of another, this is fundamental; I have not to argue about it, or hunt around for or entertain thoughts, connections, aspects, of various kinds: I have to think neither of making laws nor of testing them ... since if I liked, I could in fact just as well make the opposite conform to my indeterminate tautological knowledge and make that the law ... I could make whichever of them I liked the law, and just as well neither of them, and as soon as I start to test them I have already begun to tread an unethical path.
>
> Hegel (para 437)

Valid moral laws reflect, not the operation of 'healthy reason' independently legislating or testing laws, but necessary relations that sustain forms of life. The law reflects not a mere 'willing and knowing', but the social forms and relations that are necessary to sustain the single consciousness. Hegel refers to Antigone in this passage and clearly has in mind as paradigmatic the sorts of obligations we find ourselves under simply by being who we are: mother, son, brother. I owe something to my children merely because they are mine, and to fail to meet that obligation is to undermine the very being that I am. The validity of the law of parental obligation derives, not from a rational proof of its self-consistency, but from the actual relations of parents and children and their constitutive role in human identity. Similarly, the validity of the State's authority over me and my allegiance to it is contingent not upon an 'alien decree,' but upon the way in which my welfare depends upon its operations. The clean water that I drink, my security in the street, the metro that transports me, the hospital that cares for me, the schools that educate my children: these are the sustaining elements of my experience from which the validity of the State's claims upon me derive. The laws to which it subjects me are validated, not by a formal principle of duty, but by these sustaining relations that are reflected and articulated in the formal laws, but without which the laws would be mere 'alien decrees.'

Moreover, under the concept of law, Hegel argues, each human being is reduced to the 'sheer *empty unity* of the person' and the social world to a 'sheer multiplicity of personal atoms'(Hegel, para 480; emphasis in original). 'Healthy reason' can claim the law of noncontradiction to be a sufficient ground for moral life only by divesting morality of all life—that is, all determinate content. The other is respected by reason simply because he *is*, but what is respected is not the other, but the formal self-consistency of reason within him. Under 'healthy reason's' moral law each 'person' is required to abstract from the actual conditions of his life and to identify himself with the self-consistency dictated by the law of noncontradiction, which has no content and can produce no content from within itself. (Thus, 'healthy reason' can only *test* the maxims that it finds *already given*.) The moral subject of the law has no name and no history. 'To describe an individual as a 'person' is an expression of contempt' (Hegel, para 480).

Moreover, this generic 'person' is not innocent. The discourse of universality, rights, and equality in which the 'legal status' of the 'person' is elaborated depends upon a mythological account of the origin of human society in a 'state of nature' and in the fiction of a voluntary 'social contract.' It installs 'man' as a generic figure of the human, at the same time that it identifies citizenship with property. In this tradition, 'The true founder of civil society was the first man who, having enclosed a piece of land, thought of saying, "this is mine"' (Rousseau, 1994 Part II, p. 55). The 'rights of man' and the proclamation that 'all men are created equal,' in fact, refer only to certain men of property. As

Anthony Woodiwiss has argued, the historical emergence of 'human rights' . . . is coterminous with the emergence of what are commonly referred to as structural inequalities—that is, with the emergence of forms of inequality that are independent of personal attributes and instead derive from modes of economic, political, and cultural organization. (Woodiwiss, 2005, p. 7).

The actual narrative of these rights of the 'human person' reveals their complicity with the history of property and their production as safeguards of the privilege of property. The mythological accounts of society's origin in a voluntary contract obscure the way in which these rights were instituted precisely in order to establish the validity of ownership and to secure inequities of wealth. The rhetorical strategies of rights—the fiction of the 'state of nature,' the myth of the voluntary social contract, the abstraction of the 'person,' the recreation of man as generic, the ideology of equality, and the institution of fraternity as a figure of the social bond—install a social logic that legitimates inequities of wealth as well as the subjection of certain classes of humans as the servants of that wealth.

A contemporary example of the effect of this language of the person can be found in UNESCO's recent attempt to draft a 'Declaration of Universal Norms for Bioethics.' The document repeatedly invokes the equality of persons, with the effect that the genuine inequalities that frame the ethical urgencies under consideration are obscured. By asserting the 'fundamental equality of all human beings in dignity and rights' UNESCO, no doubt, *means* well, but such a statement *takes the place of* a genuine recognition of structural inequities of power and wealth which insure that many subjects do not enjoy an equality of dignity and rights. A person who cannot vote or drive in her own country, a person who is condemned by her village council to be raped in order to settle a dispute among men, a person whose children die of dysentery in the twenty-first century, for example, is not 'fundamentally equal,' or such equality is empty and amounts to nothing real. This is a classic demonstration of consciousness meaning one thing and saying another.

The power of this rhetoric of the 'rights of man' both to hide and justify inequities of wealth seems to make privilege genuinely blind to itself. How else can one understand James Madison's rhetorical query in his 1817 inaugural address, at a time when women and many men were literally considered property: 'On whom has oppression fallen in any quarter of our Union? Who has been deprived of any right of person or property?' Similarly, gender discrimination was so 'taken for granted' by the framers of the Universal Declaration of Human Rights (1948) that they failed to see any problem in confining the scope of the document to the public sphere, thus ignoring issues such as domestic violence, coerced marriage, or reproductive rights (Woodiwiss, 2005, p. 124).

The narrative of 'man' is not the narrative of each and all. Not only does it hide the genuine inequities of wealth and privilege authorized under the 'rights of man,' but it preempts the alternative voices within which they might find expression. These others cannot take the position of the subject in the narrative of 'man' and must remain spoken about, rather than speaking for themselves. Moreover, the pretension of 'man' to be the generic human person precludes the possibility that the experience of the others, of women and men who do not belong to the Anglo-European tradition of private property, might supply new conceptual figures for thinking about what is universal in human experience. To describe these individuals as 'persons' is an 'expression of contempt,' because this rhetoric displaces their voices in the figure of man, so that the actual narrative of their condition is never heard, as if the narrative of 'man' exhausted all possible meaning and left nothing meaningful to say about human experience.

Thus, virtue gives rise to the rhetoric of the 'Fiend' and a logic of suspicion, while law produces the discourse of 'man' who speaks for and acts on behalf of the others.

Either the other is, as in the case of virtue, an alien interiority to be converted or eliminated or, as in the case of law, the other is rendered an abstraction and merely implied in the formal principle that reason deploys in its own test. What both virtue and law fail to recognize is that moral value resides only in action, for it is action that mediates their irreconcilable differences, both the opposition between the single consciousness and the others, and the opposition between interiority and the world. Action is '. . . a display of what is one's own' in the publicity of the world, 'whereby it becomes, and should become, the affair of everyone' (Hegel, para 417). On the one hand, 'An individual cannot know what he is until he has made himself a reality through action' (Hegel, para 401). Hegel is not suggesting that it always easy to interpret my actions, either for myself or for others; only that, however difficult it may be to read them, it is in action that my capacities and motives are proven. Indeed, action often reveals that our motives were not what we took them to be or that we were not who we thought we were. Perhaps I think I am only being generous by interceding on behalf of a colleague but, in fact, my action subordinates him and makes him seem dependent, and my 'generosity' is only a display of my own power. Or, I may think of myself as a good friend but, when I betray my friend's confidence, I prove otherwise. Or, I may think of myself as having certain capacities and talents but, unless proven in action, they remain at best hypothetical and possibly false. It is by reflecting on our actions that we come to know what our motives and feelings and capacities are.

On the other hand, action converts the interiority of the single consciousness into something public. However, he might attempt to mask his motives, and even succeed in doing so, his action is not only his own, but something also for others. The single consciousness may 'think he acts for himself,' but his action inscribes him as a reality in the actual world and makes him subject to the counteraction and judgment of others (Hyppolite, 1974, p. 294). 'His *actual* existence itself consists only in his being and living in contact with others' (Hegel, para 645; emphasis in original). Action necessarily involves others in the agent's own aims and interests and requires their collaboration.

The actual world, too, ceases to be in opposition to the single consciousness as it was for virtue or legislative reason, for through action what was given becomes a result. Through its action, consciousness 'makes an actuality in place of that which was given' (Hegel, para 359). Actuality is transformed through action, and the world can no longer merely be opposed to the single consciousness as an alien reality, for it is the result of the self's own work.

Action, as the 'transition from a state of not being seen to one of being seen,' (Hegel, para 396) reconciles the single consciousness with himself, who is no longer split between his embodied self and the dark interiority of a purpose or intention that could come to light only in a future world beyond experience. It reconciles the single consciousness to the actual world as the very daylight in which he can display himself. And, it reconciles the single consciousness with the others, for by his action something that might have seemed to be a matter for himself alone is made public and becomes involved with the affairs of others. Through action the single consciousness elaborates projects and interests that concern his entire community. The recognition of the publicity of action promotes a social order in which each understands himself to be acting for the others, as well as for himself. The forms of life in such a society, then, would reflect these shared purposes and collaborative projects, an intertwining of interests and aims. Without these mediating forms, the single consciousness, however well-intentioned, inevitably collides with others, no less well-intentioned.

An act, however, is something particular and cannot, in itself, realize the entirety of the complex web of obligations within which the single consciousness is woven. Action on behalf of one interest or aim necessarily involves a failure to act on behalf of other interests and aims. Your aged mother falls ill. She lives at some distance in another state. Do you leave your husband and small children, as well as your work, in order to care for her? Whatever the decision, some genuine obligation will go unfulfilled. No doubt, a social order that embodied a greater communality of aims and interests would reduce such conflicts, but only a utopian faith could believe that they would be eliminated altogether. That your choice responds to the necessity of an obligation does not erase the fact that it fails to respond to another pressing claim. Guilt, therefore, necessarily attends those actions that result from our choices and values.

> Guilt is not an indifferent, ambiguous affair, as if the deed as actually seen in the light of day could, or perhaps could not, be the action of the self, as if with the doing of it there could be linked something external and accidental that did not belong to it, from which aspect, therefore, the action would be innocent.
>
> Innocence, therefore, is merely nonaction, like the mere being of a stone, not even that of a child
>
> Hegel (para 469).

Hegel considers the question of guilt in relation to the case of Antigone, who chooses to act on behalf of her brother against the decree of the state. Neither the demands of the family nor the authority of the state is qualified in Hegel's analysis. There is no 'light of day' in which the conflict between the two might be seen as false or accidental. To the extent that forms of life exist that recognize the publicity of action, as well as its particularity—the fact that the act is both mine and before others—the social order provides structures that minimize and ameliorate these conflicts. The welfare of my mother or my children would not be an affair for me alone and social structures would reflect that. Even so, guilt remains an essential, not an accidental, feature of action. The single consciousness, then, is always in need of forgiveness.

7.3 The inequality of forgiveness

> One answers before the Other because first one answers to the Other.
>
> Jacques Derrida, *The Politics of Friendship* (2002)

Hegel's analysis of forgiveness appears against the background of an account of conscience or 'judging consciousness.' Despite its interiority, Hegel distinguishes conscience from the other forms of virtue in two ways. First, 'conscience knows that it has to choose and to make a decision' (Hegel, para 643). For conscience, the moral good is neither given immediately as a 'law of the heart,' nor is it procedurally guaranteed by a law of pure duty. Conscience realizes that moral judgment necessarily exceeds the formality of law, as well as any calculation of duties, and it knows it must 'make its *own* decision without reference to any such reasons' (Hegel, para 645; emphasis in original). Secondly, conscience knows that moral life consists both in action and the 'declaration' of the conviction that informs the act. It understands itself to act *before others* and to be required to make its case before others. Conscience is both a 'judging consciousness' and a consciousness subject to judgment.

To the extent, however, that conscience takes *judging itself* as an 'actual deed,' it merely 'utters fine sentiments,' rather than 'proving its rectitude by actions' (Hegel, para 664). If every action that reflects our choices and values involves guilt, as well as interest, then any action can be deemed unworthy. All action is 'charged with the aspect of particularity' (Hegel, para 665) and, as such, reflects as well the contingent ambitions, interests, and priorities of the single consciousness. No action is purely a reflection of duty, any more than any duty is pure, without a complicating relation to other commanding duties. Thus, judging consciousness can always find something in the action to condemn. To the extent that conscience sets itself up as 'knowing well and better above the deeds it discredits, and wanting its words without deeds to be taken for a superior kind of reality,' it is this judging consciousness itself that is 'base,' 'vile,' and 'wicked' (Hegel, para 666). In sticking fast to a figure of virtue or a law of duty, conscience denies the real conditions of moral life: the necessity of making a choice and acting, the way in which that choice is made before others and involves others in the action, the impossibility of acting well in the absence of social forms that support our intertwined interests, the impurity of action that is always interlaced with interest, and the impossibility of realizing in any particular action all the obligations that rightly lay claim to the action.

Confession occurs, Hegel argues, when the consciousness that is judged re-cognizes in the other his own subjection to the conditions of action. The guilty one confesses his guilt, not as 'an abasement, a humiliation, a throwing-away of himself' (Hegel, para 666), but precisely because only recognition from the other in the form of forgiveness can restore him to the sociality that is necessary to sustain him. His confession is a solicitation. By putting himself into language and saying what he has done, the consciousness that is judged makes an appeal to the other. He returns himself to the genuine sociality of action by no longer holding fast to his deed that transgressed it. He surrenders himself to the other, openly recognizing his dependence on and debt to the other, as well as the other's own subjection to the conditions of action. To be forgiven, consciousness must act: it must make a confession, for 'language is self-consciousness existing for others' (Hegel, para 652). His act transgressed the others with whom he, as an actor, must collaborate, and his confession opens the possibility of reconciliation or the restitution of that collaboration.

Moreover, forgiveness is not something that could be earned or deserved. It is not in virtue of promises or explanations that forgiveness is granted, as if it were the result of a bargain or an admission that the deed was not as bad as it seemed. Forgiveness is given not because it is justified or because accounts have been squared; instead, it is precisely a gift, a generosity that can be neither derived nor compelled.

Hegel emphasizes the inevitability that guilt will attend those actions that reflect our choices and values. In his analysis, the one who is judged confesses because he recognizes this inevitable guilt in the other. Hegel's point here, however, is certainly not that we are all guilty in the same way, but that the very possibility of forgiveness only arises because each one is sustained only by the sociality of action and each one knows himself to be guilty in his own way.

Furthermore, forgiveness matters in relation to that which can never be justified or explained, which is in that sense 'unforgivable.' There are all sorts of occasions for apology, from bumping into someone on the bus to running late for an appointment to forgetting to return something that I have borrowed. Not to 'forgive' someone for an accident or for being temporarily overcommitted or for a minor thoughtlessness would be, indeed, churlish, and such 'forgiveness' is generally easily given and at very little cost. Forgiveness matters not so much in these isolated instances as in those cases where the social relations that sustain each one have been violated and rendered impossible. A husband betrays his wife. He lies to her and manipulates her to his convenience and gives to another the enthusiasm, time, and attention that belongs to their relationship. Perhaps he tells stories about her to his friends to justify his behavior or reveals secrets that she entrusted to him alone. How is it possible to forgive so intimate a betrayal that strikes at virtually every condition of life? How is it possible to tell if remorse is genuine? Does it matter if the confession is produced spontaneously or given only in response to being discovered? The confession is genuine only if its purpose is to restore the other's agency by genuinely offering the opportunity to say 'I forgive.' Forgiveness will be forthcoming only in the service of the future of the social bond. Both the confession and the forgiveness embody a risk, for there is no way to tell in advance whether either is genuine. It will be in the name of the sociality that sustained each individuality that the risk is taken and in the actions that result from the risk that the validity of the confession and forgiveness is determined.

In the case of the radical evil of genocide, rape, murder, and other extreme crimes, there can be no question of the confession being adequate to justify the forgiveness. Here, forgiveness remains an 'enigma,' 'exceptional and extraordinary.' It cannot be justified or derived; rather, it 'arrives,' interrupting the ordinary conditions and transactions of life. 'It is even, perhaps, the only thing that arrives, that surprises, like a revolution, the ordinary course of history, politics, and law. Because that means that it remains heterogeneous to the order of politics or of the juridical as they are ordinarily understood' (Derrida, 2002, p. 39).

Forgiveness cannot be exacted by virtue or the moral law. It belongs to no one as a right. The confession solicits forgiveness and, in doing so, opens up the possibility for the victim to say 'I forgive.' It re-positions the one who has been wronged as the narrative voice. Thus, the confession transforms the victim into a subject who speaks for himself, on whose word the victimizer waits. Far from merely reversing the power relations, it reconfigures them, so that the exercise of the victim's power to forgive releases each one from the guilty deed. The unconditioned arrival of the word of forgiveness, which can be neither derived nor commanded, lets each go free.

Even more complex are those cases where victim is also victimizer. Jews who were persecuted by the Nazis fight Palestinians for control of their land and undertake strategies from assassination to torture (cf. Wiesel, 1982). The young Ugandan women who were abducted as children, beaten, and sexually enslaved became murderers and terrorists themselves. Palestinians who have been abused and disenfranchised take up arms and kill, not only soldiers, but also children on their way to school. In Bosnia or Iraq or India, the cycles of violence between factions are sufficiently old and complex that there are many victims and victimizers on every side. Yet, in all these cases, one thing is true: that the Jews and Arabs of the Middle East, the rebels and other peoples of Uganda, the Muslims and Hindus of India, or the Hutus and Tutsis of Rwanda will either forgive one another in order to interrupt the cycles of violence and revenge, so that they may live together, or they will not live at all. It may be possible to bring particular agents to justice, to hold them accountable for their actions and exact punishment, but no settling of accounts, nor juridico-political agreement could ever be sufficiently unambiguous in its 'fairness' to put an end to this violence without the supplementary arrival, unconditioned and underived, of forgiveness on all sides.

In Hegel's analysis, the failure of judging consciousness to forgive constitutes its own 'wickedness.' His analysis applies not so much to victims, for whom forgiveness may indeed be essential to the restoration of their agency and sociality, but to those juridico-political powers that undertake to act on behalf of or in the place of the victimized. Just as Antigone violated the law by sticking fast to her duty to her brother, so Creon sows destruction by refusing to forgive her. His 'hard-heartedness' not only dooms her to death, but also dooms his son in whom the future of the community is embodied.

By refusing to 'put itself into an exchange with the other which, in its confession, had *ipso facto* renounced its separate being-for-self,' judging consciousness condemns itself (Hegel, para 667). Its 'hard heart' denies the necessity of this exchange to the restoration of the conditions of action and sociality on which the future depends. Hegel's thinking here is not very different from the arguments of those Acholi chiefs for whom the future was more important than justice and punishment.

The fabric of social life is sustained not by invoking an abstract equality of persons that is always conveniently projected into a future world in principle 'beyond' the actual one, but on the differences and inequalities that result from interested action and the necessity of forgiveness that it inevitably invokes. Hegel is often accused of basing his analysis of social life on a 'mutual recognition' that reduces individual difference to a sameness not unlike that of persons; however, the relation of forgiveness is always one of inequality. Judged and judging never coincide. The one who confesses makes himself contingent upon the other. Calculations of virtue and the application of the law may require punishment but, without the supplementary arrival of the word of forgiveness, these also preserve the wrong and extend the injury into a history of revenge, whereas the opportunity to forgive provided by the confession restores the victim to the narrative position and makes the victimizer dependent upon him, waiting for his reply.

A terrible truth of human life is that we must live with those who have wronged us and with those we have wronged. To do so in hard-heartedness and a spirit of revenge both corrupts the single human being and ruins the future, which can only be social. The 'word of reconciliation' in which the confession is given and forgiveness granted overcomes the one-sidedness of the judge as well as the agent. It restores, or rather, realizes for the first time, the genuine interlacing of agents in a world that is *theirs*. It restores to the one who has been wronged the agency that was denied him. It frees him from the deed that made him its object, allowing him to go forward. The deed was not 'imperishable.' He is not doomed to be forever defined by it, but only because the other has confessed and been forgiven. Thus, in the 'reconciling *Yea*' each goes free, but only together.

Through collaborative narration we can go forward into an actual future, a future that is already a social space.

> We complain, we are critical, but we do not build a better world for today and for tomorrow ... Each of us, male and female, as, too, our human activities, needs hope and energy which will create bridges between today and ... between the I and the others. Criticizing, despairing, hating do not create ... but instead exploit energies that destroy them. Projects, hope, love, on the ... , make bonds within and between us possible.
>
> Irigaray (2000, p. 166)

Such projects and hopes require that we are all participating in the same story and that each one has a chance to be the hero of it. The sociality of action implies that, on my own, I am not even the hero of my *own* story. Hard-headedness and hard-heartedness can only bring further conflict and violence. The possibility not only of peaceful coexistence but of productive collaboration depend on collaborative narration, overcoming 'one-sidedness,' and a willingness to suspend the judgments of virtue and reason in order to make way for the arrival of forgiveness. The future requires a collaborative narrative of confession and forgiveness, so that we may live together without destroying one another.

Acknowledgements

I would like to thank Nancy Nyquist Potter for her generous and extremely helpful comments on an earlier draft of this paper. Edward S. Casey, David B. Allison, Anthony J. Steinbock, and Andrew J. Mitchell offered very helpful comments and questions when I presented a version of this paper at the meetings of the Society for Phenomenology and Existential Philosophy in October, 2005 at Salt Lake City, Utah. The panel focused on Hegel's concept of agency, and I benefited by the presentations of my co-panelists, Shannon Hoff and Meghant Sudan.

References

Bush GW (2001). Remarks by President George W Bush at an Anti-Terrorism Event. Washington, DC, Federal News Service, 10 October 2001.

Derrida, J (2002). On forgiveness (trans. M Hughes). In: *On Cosmopolitanism and Forgiveness*. London: Routledge Publishers.

Foucault M (2003). *Society Must Be Defended* (trans. D Macey), pp. 359–60. London: Penguin Books.

Gourevitch P (2000). *we wish to inform you that tomorrow we will be killed with our Families*. New York: Picador.

Hegel GWF (1979). *The Phenomenology of Spirit* (trans. AV Miller). Oxford: Oxford University Press.

Hyppolite J (1974). *Genesis and Structure of Hegel's Phenomenology of Spirit* (trans. S Cherniak and J Heckman). Evanston, IL: Northwestern University Press.

Irigaray L (2000). *Democracy Begins Between Two* (trans. Kirsteen Anderson). London: The Athlone Press.

Kant I (1956). *Groundwork of the Metaphysic of Morals* (trans. HJ Paton). New York: Harper Trochbooks.

Kant I (1987). *Critique of Judgment* (trans. WS Pluhar). Indianapolis, IN: Hackett Publishing Company.

Lacey M (2005). Atrocity victims in Uganda choose to forgive. In: *The New York Times*, 18 April 2005.

Pinkard T (1995). Historicism, social practice, and sustainability: Some themes in Hegelian ethical theory. *Neue Hefte fur Philosophie*, **35:** 56–94.

Rousseau JJ (1994). *Discourse on Inequality* Part II (trans. F Phili). Oxford: Oxford University Press.

Roy A (2002). *The Algebra of Infinite Justice*. London: Flamingo/Harper Collins.

Singer P (2004). *One World*. New Haven: Yale University Press.

Thernstrom M (2002). Charlotte, Grace, Janet, and Caroline come home. In: *The New York Times*, 8 May 2005.

Wiesel E (1982). *Dawn*. New York: Bantam Books.

Woodiwiss A (2005). *Human Rights*. New York: Routledge Publishers.

Chapter 8

Elements of a phenomenology of evil and forgiveness

Gerrit Glas

8.1 Introduction

In this chapter I highlight the topic of trauma, truth, and reconciliation from the perspective of a phenomenology of evil. My basic intuitions are threefold. First, acts of evil have affective, interpersonal, political, and existential components (among others). The power and destructiveness of extreme acts of evil can, nevertheless, not be understood entirely as the sum of what happens in all these spheres. Second, the destructiveness of evil suggests that there is a dynamic at work that manifests itself as denial (in perpetrators) and speechlessness and powerlessness (in victims). Finally, denial and speechlessness have self-perpetuating tendencies that make victims vulnerable to repeating the evil themselves (cf. Card, 2002, p. 214; Card, 2004).

I describe what I mean when I use the term 'dynamic' by exploring acts of evil and their consequences from different angles, mainly psychological and philosophical. I draw on literature on splitting, denial, and shame to gain a better understanding of the denial of perpetrators and the speechlessness of the victims and witnesses of acts of evil. I also compare acts of evil and acts of forgiveness with respect to their underlying existential patterns. My hypothesis will be that such patterns exist and that these patterns oppose one another.

The term phenomenology in the title of this chapter is used in a rather loose way. Phenomenology usually refers to an approach to science and philosophy—developed in the early twentieth century—that aims at describing as accurately as possible how the world appears to us. The word comes from the Greek verb 'phainomenai', which means 'to appear.' This understanding is contrasted with knowledge of essences of things. Some phenomenologists (such as Edmund Husserl, 1922) move in an idealist direction by saying that appearances (phenomena) only exist in one's consciousness and that their reference to a world outside consciousness must be put in brackets. Others (such as Max Scheler, 1916) see these appearances as the result of an interaction between the person and the world. The experience of sadness is then seen as a quality or value that emerges as the result of the interaction between a person and a particular object or event. On this account, my experience of sadness comes neither completely from within (as if sadness were a quality I add to things/events), nor completely from without (as if sadness were a quality of a thing, or event, that has nothing to do with my appreciation of that thing/event). It is an experience that should be attributed to the appreciating and experiencing relation between me and the world (the loss of a loved one; being traumatized). Phenomenologists of the latter type try to unravel the patterns and structures of these interactions.

It is in the latter sense that my approach can be called phenomenological. Phenomenology, here, consists of the careful description and analysis of the interactional dynamic between the person and the world in which he or she lives. However, I am not adopting a strictly phenomenological position, because I do not believe that there is such a thing as pure description. Descriptions are always in some way influenced by one's point of view and certain predilections. Another reason for being reluctant with respect to a straightforward phenomenological position is that I do not concur with the underlying assumptions of some existential phenomenologists, such as the assumption that phenomena such as evil and reconciliation should be approached from the perspective of an already existing and morally neutral 'fundamental ontology' (as suggested by Martin Heidegger, 1927) or be based on an analysis of freedom in which freedom is seen as merely negative (such as in the work of Jean-Paul Sartre, 1943). So, I share the phenomenological approach to a certain extent, but not all of its underlying assumptions.

I begin descriptively, by trying to depict as unbiased as possible how evil appears—how it feels, what it does to people, and how it affects their lives. This chapter is limited to excessive forms of evil and their consequences, because they typically exemplify what I consider to be a relatively neglected aspect of evil—its nontransparency, the speechlessness to which it leads and which is so characteristic for the atmosphere in which evil spreads out, almost like an infectious disease. In the course of this description, we will discover two points. First, we will recognize that, after a while, reporting on evil touches the dynamic of evil itself in the sense that it becomes more and more difficult to just say what evil 'is' and that it is tempting to evade this 'area of speechlessness' by addressing more concrete issues, or by taking an overly neutral and objective stance, or by letting one's attention be diverted to superficial issues.

The other point is that this 'speechlessness' is not only negative but also revealing, in the sense that it brings us to the dynamical core of evil or, at least, close to it. The guiding idea of this chapter is that something exists in the nature of evil itself that resists being spoken about and thought about. It is precisely this resistance that can be analyzed in terms of a dynamic operating in acts of evil and their aftermath. The nontransparency of evil is, then, not just a (static) feature of evil. Nontransparency does not point primarily to our difficulty in describing evil acts and evildoers' motives. Instead, it is a dynamical category: something occurs during the process of experiencing and telling and analyzing that manifests itself in malfunction of one's very capacity to experience, in inability to verbalize, and in the ineffectiveness of the systems with which we categorize our moral world. In other words, it is by concentrating on the nontransparency of evil that we are in a better position to detect the dynamical pattern in the effects and transmission of evil.

In my use of the term 'evil,' I will take Claudia Card's recent definition as the point of reference. She states that 'evils are foreseeable intolerable harms produced by culpable wrongdoing' (Card, 2002, p. 3). This definition combines two points of view: the suffering (harm) and the deed (culpable wrongdoing), and it ties the two together by a relation of dependence or 'causation'. The wrongdoing 'produces' the harm. There are cases in which there is suffering, or harm, without wrongdoing: earthquakes and other forms of natural disaster, for instance; or sufferings produced by (excusable) innocence, coincidence or fortuity. There are also cases in which culpable wrongdoing only leads to moderate harm or suffering. In all these cases there is no evil, according to Card. Evil entails wrongdoing, but it is not identical to wrongdoing. Evil entails harm, but is not identical to harm or suffering. In short, the term 'evil' should be saved for situations in which intolerable harm is caused by culpable wrongdoing.

One important point in this definition is that it does not require intentions or other motivational states in the perpetrator to count a certain act as evil. Intentions do matter, but not for the definition of what it is for an act to be an instantiation of evil. Card accords here to a view held by Neiman, Arendt, and others, which places Auschwitz in the centre of philosophical reflection on moral evil. Auschwitz ruined the assumption that the extent of evil is proportional to the badness of the intention. The morally disturbing effect of mass destruction in the concentration camps was that so much evil could be produced by so little malice and forethought, says Neiman (2002, p. 271). She builds on Hannah Arendt's famous argument on the 'banality of evil,' an idea Arendt originally developed in *Eichman in Jerusalem. A Report on the Banality of Evil* (1965). Eichman did not appear to be the monster that many had thought he was. He did not seem to act on the basis of plainly evil motives; he was simply 'thoughtless' (Arendt, 1965). With Arendt's and Neiman's work, the issue of the relevance of motives and intentions has certainly not been settled. Richard Bernstein, for instance, places a cautionary note by suggesting that there may be different forms of evil. At the end of a thoughtful discussion he says: 'The banality of evil is a phenomenon exemplified by only some of the perpetrators of radical evil—desk murderers like Eichman' (Bernstein, 2002, p. 232).

I nevertheless take Card's definition as a pragmatic starting point. We will proceed, therefore, as if the volitional (or: intentional) aspect—malevolence— is not necessary for an act to be qualified as evil.[1] In the course of this chapter, we will see whether this approach fits the facts or needs refinement. There are, after all, victims for whom it does seem to add to their suffering that the perpetrator deliberately intended their pain and even death. We may expect that descriptions of the harms produced by these intended wrongdoings differ from nonintended (but culpable) wrongdoings, such as acts of recklessness or negligence. This would imply that there are different types of evil—at least at a psychological level. None of the philosophers cited thus far would disagree with this, I think. The question is whether and to what extent such psychological differences matter philosophically. Card's definition is not psychological, but philosophical. It serves as a conceptual umbrella for the more severe cases of culpable wrongdoing, intended or not, that lead to intolerable harm. My pragmatic use of Card's definition of evil entails, nevertheless, that I allow myself to speak of intentions and to refer to acts of malevolence, even if this would not make any difference with respect to what most philosophers consider to be evil.

Philosophy, however, is not the only field that has difficulty in determining the role of intentions in evildoing. Psychiatry and psychology do so too. This is discussed in the next section.

8.2 Two objections against the possible contribution of behavioral sciences to the understanding of evil

Psychiatry and psychology traditionally have been reluctant to define and study acts of evil and malevolence. What is the role of these professions in understanding these acts? Do psychiatry and psychology have the conceptual resources to describe and analyze the nature of evil? Do they have anything to contribute to the debate about moral evil? And, if not, *should* they have anything to contribute? What role do psychiatrists, psychologists, and

---

1 Behind the question whether psychological differences with respect the presence or absence of intention have philosophical significance, lurks the problematic issue of the conceptual status of intentions. We cannot go into this issue deeply, here.

psychotherapists have with respect to the wrongdoings and sufferings of their patients? Do they have any specific responsibility regarding evil and, if so, how is this responsibility accounted for in their professional codes?

Carl Goldberg (1996) argues that there are two assumptions underlying the relative neglect of the topic of evil by behavioral scientists. According to defenders of the *moral* objection, evil is a moral issue better left to theologians and philosophers. Acts of malevolence may be studied in an empirical way, but the nature of evil is such that it resists psychological scrutiny. One can study its superficial layers, such as behavioral and affective expressions of evil or personality dimensions contributing to these expressions but not the moral and existential core of the malevolent person. One can, in other words, study the personality but not the person.

On the other side, there are scientists who deny the existence of malevolence as a moral concept. On this view, malevolence should be discarded and replaced by more neutral behavioral and psychological terms, such as 'behavioral disorder.' Defenders of this view use what Goldberg calls the *psychological* objection. This objection represents a rather crude form of reductionism and scientism. It suggests that there is nothing in the phenomena of evil and acts of malevolence that cannot be expressed and, in the long run, explained by the behavioral sciences.

These objections can be seen as two sides of the same coin. They represent a positivist approach to science that either leads to the separation between moral and other aspects of behavior or to the reduction of moral issues to behavioral or biological facts. Positivism denies that there is a reality beyond what is 'positively' given, that is, beyond what can be described and analyzed in terms of some basic science. All other phenomena are subjective. On this view, morality is either subjective but nonreducible, or subjective and reducible to science.

Both objections are questionable, according to Goldberg, and I think he is right. With respect to the first (moral) objection, it could be argued that it is practically impossible to keep the moral aspects of evil at a distance in clinical practice. Even if we think that the proper object of psychiatry does not entail evil and acts of malevolence, psychiatrists and psychotherapists still have to deal with a reality of which these acts form a part. They treat perpetrators and victims of the acts of perpetrators. I cannot understand how such treatment could take place without the assumption that something terribly wrong has occurred and that this has produced harm for which someone is morally accountable.

One can try to exclude this moral aspect by saying that it is outside the scope of these professions and that practitioners should adopt a professional stance. This professionalism would at least imply neutrality with respect to moral issues. However, the moral aspects of evil cannot be separated from their affective and interpersonal effects on the therapeutic relationship. Attempts to do so may even backfire. An example is the situation in which a patient's explicit questions about the therapists' thoughts about the harm done to her by the wrongdoing of another person remain unanswered on the basis of an overly strict interpretation of professional neutrality. The therapist's unresponsiveness on moral issues may come across to the patient as indifference. This indifference is then interpreted as sign of rejection and lack of attention and can lead to a terrible sense of isolation. It is clear that this outcome is undesirable for many reasons, moral ones included. Efforts to keep psychiatry and psychotherapy free from any moral concern may lead to a backlash in patients, or patients may knock on the clinician's door even more vigorously, not only because they need the emotional and practical support but often, and more importantly, because they want the clinician to take a stance politically and morally. This is one of the reasons why Judith Herman in her classic *Trauma and Recovery* (Herman, 1992) has been so explicit about the fact that personal and political aspects of traumatization cannot be separated.

The second (psychological) objection says that evil and acts of malevolence are reducible to mental disorder. This is, of course, a huge claim that puts a high burden on future scientific research. I am skeptical about this claim. This approach would not solve the problem of how to account for the immorality of evil deeds but would merely transfer it to the domains of psychiatry and psychology. Within this domain, all normative issues with respect to the nature of the ethical would return in disguised form—for instance, in discussions on the boundaries of the concept of disorder. What types of behavior are we going to consider as normal and what types as abnormal? Trying to discard the moral dimension of evil by reducing it to mental disorder will fail, because there is no convincing theory of mental disorder that can avoid the normative, and at least partly moral, questions of what to count as normal or abnormal behavior.

At present, we have many theories about aggression, feelings of inferiority, and shame. But there is a difference between aggression and shame, on the one hand, and sadism and torture, on the other hand. Sadism and torture presuppose a level of deliberateness that is not accounted for in standard theories on (pathological forms of) aggression and shame (however, cf. Baumeister and Vohs, 2004).[2] But even if we could explain the conditions

....

2 Baumeister and Vohs (2004, pp. 96–100) distinguish four roots of evil, violence as: (1) means to an end; (2) in response to threatened egotism; (3) in a misguided effort to do good; and (4) as means of gaining sadistic pleasure.

under which people are inclined intentionally to inflict intolerable harm on others, this explanation still would not answer the normative question of why we consider these deeds and the suffering caused by them to be morally unacceptable. By thinking that we could, we would fall into the trap of the so-called genetic (or: naturalistic) fallacy. Those who make this mistake think that the moral rightness or wrongness of behavior can be accounted for in terms of the causal antecedents of behavior. However, that belief is just as odd as condemning a television program and thinking that its unacceptability can be explained in terms of the electronic processes going on inside the television. Positively stated, behavioral theories describe and explain what occurs when people act, think, and feel. Morality, however, not only concerns what occurs but also who we are and should be. That is, ethics is not primarily about what we do but about who we are and who we take ourselves to be by what we are doing. This point is more fully developed by Paul Ricoeur in his *Oneself as Another* (1990). More generally, this view is true for virtue ethics (and not for Kantian or utilitarian ethics; see Potter, 2002).

8.3 **Evil**

I will now describe three aspects of evil that strike me as important and as related to one another. These aspects do not, of course, exhaust the list of possible features of evil. There are many forms and different degrees of evil. Nevertheless, the aspects of evil described below capture a number of important and related characteristics.

'Evil' is a very general term that lends itself to reification—as if evil were a thing or substance apart from the deeds, suffering, and relationships in which it is embodied. In my usage of the term, however, I am not aiming at qualities of a thing-like entity but at the affective, interpersonal, and existential dynamic in acts of evil and the suffering that is caused by these acts. The aspects of evil I delineate try to give an impression of how acts of evil exert their influence. They aim, in other words, at the dynamic core of evil. I identify the aspects of speechlessness, of splitting and denial, and of shame.

I am very much aware that the few cases I describe below are sketches and far from sufficient to support some of the claims I make with respect to evil's dynamics. These examples should, therefore, be seen as provisional attempts that suggest an approach and should be supplemented with others. At the same time, it should be noted that evil perhaps will always retain its nontransparency (or: incomprehensibility; impenetrability; darkness). All attempts to describe evil are, therefore, somewhat paradoxical and have intrinsic limitations. They will always remain partial and insufficient.

As I stated above, the three aspects described below are attempts to give a more concrete idea of how evil works, first, in the malfunctioning of language (speechlessness), then in the intrapsychic and interpersonal manifestations of splitting and denial, and finally, in the effects of shame. The first point is cardinal: speechlessness is the most concrete manifestation of the dynamic of evil. It also comes closest to what I call the nontransparency of evil. It is in speechlessness that evil's power comes to expression; it is the way evil effaces its own footsteps. Splitting and denial are hardly purely descriptive concepts. These concepts, like the concept of shame, are introduced to understand better why the dynamic of evil is such that it seems to offer resistance to being put into words.

Evil as revealed by speechlessness

One of the intriguing things about the way traumatized people deal with their past is that they may keep silent for a very long time about what has happened to them. Victims of prolonged childhood sexual abuse, women and children who suffer from domestic violence, and people returning from concentration camps are alike in that they often try to forget and to return to normal life. There are many possible explanations for this: fear that perpetrators and others will deny wrongdoing or exact reprisals; avoidance of the stress of remembering; disgust about what happened; or unwillingness to let one's existence continue to be determined by the meaninglessness of what happened. Speechlessness is an aspect of the dynamics of evil that is related to all this, but it highlights a slightly different point: a pervasive sense that what one has lived through is so absolutely different from normal life and represents a reality so totally 'out of joint' that one cannot effectively communicate about it. The victim becomes speechless, because the reality she has gone through is so unreal in the real world that it feels as if words lose their meaning and become futile and powerless. In the presence of normal people with their normal lives and all the tiny occurrences that make human existence human, what happened to her seems unreal, impossible, and of a totally different order. Some people would speak here of the powerlessness of language or the inability to communicate 'the incommunicable' or 'unthinkable.' I would like to suggest that it is not the powerlessness of language, but the dynamic of evil itself that offers resistance to being fully expressed and witnessed.

Nonvictims may experience the same kind of estrangement and powerlessness—but incomparably less intense, of course—when they hear perpetrators report on their crimes. The denial of some perpetrators may have seductive qualities, even sometimes after many years. I give an example that is based on the 8-hour long documentary *Shoah* by Claude Lanzmann (1985a, b). The documentary includes an interview with Walter Stier, former chief of the Sondertransporte (Special Transportations) in Nazi Germany. Challenged by the interviewer, whose biting sarcasm he apparently fails to notice, Stier relates one detail after another of the great logistical and financial problems he faced during wartime and how he successfully overcame them. Every train wagon had to be paid for, and interdepartmental battles made it difficult to build up an efficient transportation system. When one hears Stier speaking, it seems as if time has stopped during the 40 years that passed since then: in his voice, we hear the old excitement. At a certain point in his story he uses a significant phrase—Umsiedlertransporte (removal transports) (Lanzmann, 1985b, p. 168). The term suggests how Stier saw, and still sees, his work during World War II—that is, as a magisterial administrative operation resulting in a 'change of residence' for millions of Jews and others. Of course, he knew about the mass extinction in the gas chambers and about the level of coercion that was needed to organize the transportations. But even 40 years after the events took place, he refuses to use terms that refer to deportation, coercion, and personal responsibility for his enabling of mass extinction. Stier's language suggests that the realities of the Holocaust did not exist.

My point is not to emphasize this denial as such, but to underscore its effectiveness and its seductive qualities. It is the combination of thoughtlessness and ease with which the term 'removal transport' is used that is revealing. By listening to this former Nazi chief, one gets a glimpse of how it once worked and might work again, how lies can support one another and weave together in ideology, how evil deprives persons of their language, and how difficult it is in such a bureaucracy not to let oneself be deprived of verbal means of giving testimony about what is going on—in short: to *not* become speechless.

Nazi bureaucracy's language was permeated with such euphemisms and falsehoods. It is the language itself that is disturbing, but also disturbing is the ease with which it is used after so many years—as if nothing special happened at that moment and as if nothing special has happened since then. Stier's denial is not primarily a negation of something that took place but rather the suggestion that there is nothing to deny. It is instructive to notice the persistence of this (self-) suggestion in former war criminals like Stier. And it is not difficult to imagine how the same mechanisms could work today, both at an individual and a societal level.

The silence of trauma survivors and the denial of perpetrators complement one another. Their behaviors represent two forms of speechlessness. There are many understandable reasons for this speechlessness, as we saw: anxiety, disgust, avoidance of pain, and unwillingness to talk, in the case of victims; self-deception, ideology and lack of judgment, in the case of perpetrators.

Victims sometimes seem to be caught in a self-perpetuating cycle in which all these aspects play a self-destructive role. To speak is the first step in breaking this cycle, whereas speechlessness confirms the victims' expectations that attempts to do so are futile. Therefore, speechlessness is both the expression and the source of a self-destructive dynamic. It is an expression of this dynamic because to speak would mean to resist the dynamic and to take a first step toward a return to the 'normal' world. It is a source of this dynamic because the longer lies are tolerated and remain unaddressed, the more effective the suggestion of their effectiveness may become. Speechlessness, therefore, gives us a clue to understanding the power of the self-enhancing destructiveness of evil.

Perpetrators are caught in a similar way: their speechlessness is the corollary of their lies. They cannot talk about the unsaid, because that would refute their lies. Their lies confirm that what really is occurring has no name and is unspeakable. Lies exert their suggestive influence at least as much by what they conceal as by what they try to lead us to believe. Evil's fertile soil is the lie, but also what comes with the lie: the effective suggestion of the unreality of truth.

To speak in a context in which lies prevail is also, therefore, a moral act. To speak is to witness; it is to give testimony to what has happened based on a conviction that relationships are not meant to be exploited in the way one has experienced. Such testimonies require courage. When traumatization occurs on a larger scale, as in domestic violence or war rape, those who testify also need political support. This is the reason why authors like Herman and Card put so much emphasis on continuity between the personal and the political dimension of traumatization.

Splitting and denial as psychic defenses and as mechanisms consolidating the silence and incapacity to speak

In the previous section, I discussed the importance of lying and the denial that is necessary for lying to become effective. So far, I used the term 'denial' in a specific sense, not just as equivalent to uttering a negation, but in an almost hyperbolic sense as the 'effective suggestion that there is nothing to deny.' In this section, I build on this notion by turning to the intrapsychic dimensions of denial and its underlying mechanisms. Theories about these intrapsychic dimensions are mainly psychoanalytical. Psychoanalysts see splitting as the key mechanism enabling denial. Splitting refers to the processes by which intrapsychic contents are kept apart. So, denial and splitting are closely related concepts; denial is the descriptive term and splitting denotes the explanatory mechanism sustaining denial. I give an example.

Psychiatrist and journalist Robert Lifton is one thinker who attributes a key role to splitting in trying to understand what took place in the minds of physicians who were responsible for the selection and mass execution of people in the concentration camps. In his book *The Nazi Doctors* (1986), Lifton begins with the observation that doctors who supplied the arguments for genocide and who were involved in the execution of it appeared not to be the sadists others assumed them to be. On the contrary, they were often persons who in daily life were reasonable and friendly and respected for their expertise. According to Lifton, genocide and mass murder were not so much the result of individual sadism as of the collective embrace of a medical metaphor. The ulcer of Jewry (and other degenerates) had to be excised from the sick body of humanity.

The adherence to this metaphor, however, came at a price. It could only be sustained by denial, and this in turn by splitting, according to Lifton. The assumption of such splitting processes makes sense of the fact that these physicians maintained their mental stability when confronted with the results of their deeds. In the end, splitting became consolidated in their personalities. Lifton speaks of a split in the personality of some of the most prominent figures. One of them, Joseph Mengele, stroked the heads of children, spoke friendly words to them, and gave them candy. A few hours later, he witnessed their deaths in the gas chamber. The horror of these scenes, Lifton suggests, can only be tolerated by the perpetrator by the artificial separation of different states of mind. It is splitting that can bring about such separation. One state of mind was under the influence of the medical metaphor and all other Nazi propaganda. It denied vital aspects of interpersonal relationships and could only be maintained by splitting off almost all emotions and interpersonal inclinations, like tenderness, compassion, empathy, and the need to attach to others. This splitting is reflected by the emotional numbing and the flattening of affect when these persons were functioning as Nazis. Another state of mind seemed to be operative when these physicians were present in the inner circle of friends and relatives and, perhaps, also in the presence of nameless and unknown children in the camps. In this state of mind, a relatively normal pattern of behavior and feeling emerged—however, at the expense of a proper valuation of what was going on in the world outside.

Lifton does not suggest that physicians like Mengele were suffering from mental disorder. The split in their personality did not conform to what we now call dissociative identity disorder. Even less does he suggest that splitting as a defense mechanism could be the sole explanation of the behavior of these physicians. Lifton is very much aware of the hazards of any attempt to explain the horrors performed by Nazi doctors: explanations would almost inevitably be interpreted or be used as an excuse. But Lifton's primarily descriptive approach gives us the opportunity to suggest another possibility: one might say that splitting is one of the processes that made the genocide psychologically possible. This is what Lifton suggests. However, we also may read this proposition in another direction—that splitting is not only a psychological condition for evil; it is also a *vehicle* for the expression of evil. If this is true, it is by the process of splitting that evil exerts its intoxicating and emotionally and morally numbing power.

I realize that, by these remarks, I leave the realm of psychology proper and enter a domain of existential and, perhaps, metaphysical concerns. However, we are not far from our previous statement about denial as the 'effective suggestion that there is nothing to deny.' All I have done is replace the term 'denial' by 'evil.' Evil consists, then, of the effective suggestion that there is nothing to deny (provided that there is some intolerable harm). This false but effective suggestion is both a condition and a vehicle for evil to break out and to manifest itself in actions. This suggestion is maintained by the process of splitting. Evil's power consists of the efficacy of the suggestion that there is nothing to deny and to feel worried about. This treacherous suggestiveness is a form of (culpable) denial. This denial, in its turn, can be explained by the process of splitting as an inner mechanism of defense.

Moral conflicts cannot emerge in such a context because of the efficacy of the splitting process and the denial to which it leads. Splitting is a condition for the emergence of evil, Lifton hypothesizes. My suggestion is to take the other option just as seriously—the hypothesis that it is evil itself that comes to the surface by the mechanism of splitting and insurmountable denial. I admit that this suggestion is very tentative and may only apply to some perpetrators and to some severely traumatized people with a tendency to overt (self-) destructiveness. It could, however, shed some light on the question of how to understand the destructiveness and power of splitting processes both in traumatized and in traumatizing people.

Evil and shame

I now turn to the topic of shame. Shame can be interpreted as an important psychological source that sustains splitting processes. The prototypical case of shame is a situation in which the person feels exposed and embarrassed by the look of a critical or devaluing other (Lewis, 1995). The typical inclination of the shameful person is to hide and to avoid the look of others. Shame is a complex emotion and there are different types of shame. One can feel ashamed about not meeting the expectations of others with respect to a certain task. Shame may be related to one's body shape or one's way of expressing oneself verbally or emotionally. One may feel shame about who one is and about the fact of one's existence. Shame may be related to actual looks and remarks, but also to what one expects others might think or remark. People who feel ashamed typically show a diminishment of spontaneity and a heightened awareness of interpersonal distance. The most intense experiences of shame are accompanied by a deep sense of isolation and of being pinned down by one's own misery. These intense experiences are sometimes accompanied by feelings of depersonalization. Depersonalization occurs when one looks at oneself through the eyes of the other without the capacity to bridge the gap between the observing ego and the experiencing self. The concept of depersonalization is complex but, in cases of shame, it denotes the incapacity to reconcile the intensely humiliating look of the internalized other with one's basic sense of self. Phrased in these terms, one can understand how early experiences of intense shame may lead to an internalization of the gap (or: split) between the internalized critical other and the experiential self and to the denial of feelings and needs that belong to the experiential self. This internalization, in its turn, is reflected by a predilection for the use of splitting as an inner mechanism of defense. This defense mechanism is activated when the person experiences signals of humiliation or devaluation.

In situations of shame with moderate intensity, we are inclined to respond to our own shame by hiding ourselves and to the humiliation of others with compassion, consolation, and support. Intense shame, however, seems to be related to experiences that cannot be shared with and tolerated by others—at least not in the imagination of the person who feels shame. If one lacks the capacity to bridge the distance between expectation and reality, how could one expect others to do so? I will illustrate this again with a fragment from the documentary Shoah. The fragment shows a person struggling with intense shame (Lanzmann, 1985b, pp. 207–21).

When Jan Karski, the liaison officer between the Polish resistance movement and the Polish government in exile, is asked about his experiences in the Warsaw ghetto, he is initially unable to speak. He struggles with his emotions. He had never spoken of his experiences in the ghetto. The questions burden him too much and he seems to be embarrassed. On his request, the camera is put at a distance and he begins to talk, stammering and with many hesitations. This, together with his diminished spontaneity, is fairly typical for feelings of shame. After a while, he relates how he had been invited by two Jewish resistance fighters to visit the ghetto in order to be a witness later. The stammering of this Polish aristocrat gives us some insight into the reality of the ghetto and how it alienated and depersonalized people, including those who were not victims but only witnesses. Karski speaks of the heaps of corpses along the road, of the animal looks in the eyes of people, and of the stench that hung there. He recalls the almost absurd joy of children who played on the square despite everything that was going on. In trying to find words for these experiences, he reveals a glimpse of a world that is so different from ours that it defies one's imagination. Faced with the horror and absurdity, every word seems to be inadequate, and therefore a distortion, or—worse—even an excuse, an attempt to lessen what really went on and to go back to normality. This is why the philosopher Theodore Adorno wrote that poetry after Auschwitz would be barbarism (quoted in Neiman, 2002, p. 238).

Shame is not simply an affective state in this case; it is not merely the awareness that one does not meet the expectations of others. It is, in its most intense form, an alienating experience of disarray and of loneliness—a loneliness that is effectuated by having been part of a reality that cannot be shared with others. Why not? That is a very difficult question, a question perhaps with more than one answer. Some memories may be too horrible to speak about. Perhaps it is the intensity of one's feelings of helplessness and vulnerability that lead to shame; or, that one's very existence is demeaned; or, the assumption that nobody will ever understand what one has gone through and that others, because of their incapacity to understand, will try to distort or smooth out or normalize what has happened. Returning to these memories may be shameful because one feels exposed again. Shame may become mixed with anxiety in such cases.

Shame, like splitting, is related to denial. The existential experience of the real or imagined incapacity to share one's most troubling experiences is at the basis of denial and splitting, but also of shame. These experiences are warded off by splitting and denial, but may emerge later in situations where one feels exposed and humiliated again, actually or in imagination. Shame, in other words, points at another dimension of the incapacity to share one's most pervading experiences, the dimension of feeling exposed and of having been part of a totally different world, a world that is horrible and disgusting. Even the memory of having been part of this world is humiliating. Parallel to my hypothesis about splitting, I suggest that these experiences of intense shame and their devastating consequences are both a vehicle of evil and at the root of new forms of evil. If this is true, shame is both a result and a cause of evil. It is, like splitting, one of the vehicles by which it spreads out and exerts its influence.

Some authors point to this intermingling of existential, interpersonal and affective aspects of shame. Goldberg (1996), for instance, argues that early experiences of intense shame lie at the root of the development of the malevolent personality and may lead to a recurrent cycle of shame, powerlessness, hatred, violence, and again shame—the 'anger–shame cycle.' This cycle is not just affective; it may influence important interpersonal relationships and, in the end, dominate one's entire existence. Shame is, therefore, also an existential phenomenon. People with such intense shame perceive their existence as totally worthless and as intolerably vulnerable. Their answer to shame is to withdraw and hide and, if this is no longer tolerated, to break out with destructive self-defense.

To summarize, we began with the speechlessness of victims and the denial of those responsible for evil and its workings. We signaled how difficult it is to not let oneself be made speechless in the presence of evil. Speechlessness was a first indicator of the dynamics of evil. In the sections on denial and splitting, we explored this dimension further. Denial and splitting refer to inner psychological processes that help to sustain the 'silence' and incapacity to speak, I suggested. Here I played with the idea of a reversal of perspective in at least some extreme situations—a reversal that suggests that denial and splitting are not only conditions for the occurrence of evil but also expressions of evil, or, better, vehicles for evil to come to expression. This idea was further developed in the section on shame. Shame reveals an interpersonal dynamic that is sustained by splitting processes and that leads to denial, speechlessness, and withdrawal. But perhaps, I suggested, we may again reverse our view by interpreting the interpersonal dynamic of shame as an expression of evil itself, at least in the most severe cases of dominance and humiliation. Purely descriptive, psychodynamic, or interpersonal approaches do not seem adequately to grasp this dynamic aspect, even when analyzed in terms of the so-called shame–anger cycle. We need overarching existential and philosophical concepts to retain a feel for the power and inherent destructiveness of (acts of) evil.

8.4 Forgiveness and reconciliation

I now proceed with an investigation of some of the features of forgiveness and reconciliation. My hypothesis is that the foregoing description of the dynamic of evil may also give a clue to our understanding of forgiveness and reconciliation, and vice versa, especially with respect to their dynamical features. I am interested in the heuristic value of a perspective that considers forgiveness as a way to overcome the dynamics of evil. So, what are the typical features of the dynamic of forgiveness?

There is a large body of extant literature on the concepts of forgiveness and reconciliation (see Murphy and Hampton, 1988; Jones, 1995; Enright and North, 1998; Worthington, 1998b; McCullough et al., 2000; Murphy, 2003). Most authors agree that forgiveness refers to a motivational state or to 'a motivation empowered by basic emotion' (Worthington, 1998a, p. 129). Jeffrie

Murphy considers it as a change of inner feeling that consist of 'the overcoming, on moral grounds, of the vindictive passions' (2003, p. 16) or, more extensively, it is 'the overcoming, on moral grounds, of the intense negative reactive attitudes that are quite naturally occasioned when one has been wronged by another—mainly vindictive passions of resentment, anger, hatred, and the desire for revenge.' (Murphy, 2003, p. 13).

Others add the element of giving: 'Forgiveness exists as a gift that is granted to someone who has harmed one' (Worthington, 1998a, p. 129; cf. also Hampton, in: Murphy and Hampton, 1988, p. 37). North (1998), Enright *et al.* (1998), and Worthington (1998) describe stages in the process of forgiveness. North includes stages the wrongdoer must complete, thereby suggesting that forgiveness cannot entirely be seen as an inner process in the forgiver.

For our discussion, forgiveness is the central concept, but to understand its complex dynamic it may help to turn first to the broader and more diffuse concept of reconciliation. Reconciliation differs from forgiveness. It typically happens within a relationship instead of within a person or regarding one person. It refers to the end point of a process between two (or more) persons as a result of which they are able to live and work together again. Enright *et al.* write: 'Forgiveness is one person's response to injury. Reconciliation involves two people coming together again. The injurer must realize his or her offense, see the damage done, and take steps to rectify the problem.' (1998, p. 49).

Most authors agree that there can be reconciliation without forgiveness, that is, without a change of inner feelings and attitudes toward the wrongdoer or on grounds other than moral ones. Reconciliation is, therefore, not inherently a moral concept, whereas forgiveness by definition is one. Reconciliation may, in other words, be pursued for merely instrumental reasons. Parties of which one has wrongly injured the other may, for instance, agree that to break up would cause more harm than to try to find a way to live or work together. Forgiveness does not seem to be compatible with such an instrumental approach. One may try to give up one's feelings of resentment because it seems wise or in the interest of both parties. These interests may be very practical, for instance, financial or familial. One can even defend these motives on moral grounds other than a duty to forgive or a virtue of forgiveness—for instance by using utilitarian reasoning to the effect that reconciliation will provide the greater benefit for all parties in the long run and does not require a change of the inner feelings and inclinations of the persons that are involved. But most people would not think of these situations as instances of forgiveness. Either resentful feelings are not overcome or the grounds on which the feelings are given up are not appropriate to the feelings. In the first situation, we might speak of pseudo-forgiveness. One example is the victim who says she has overcome her resentful feelings but continually reminds the offender of the injury inflicted on her. In the second situation, the victim has overcome his negative feelings and attitude toward the offender (or at least claims to have done so), but the reason is not rooted in the desire to bring about a change in one's relationship with the offender. So differences exist between reconciliation and forgiveness. Reconciliation allows utilitarian reasoning and absence of change of inner feelings and attitudes towards the wrongdoer. Forgiveness does not. Forgiving on other grounds than the moral impetus to change one's relationship with the offender seems to violate the logic of emotions and attitudes that are involved in the process of forgiving.

There are grey zones, however. In many situations, the moral grounds people have are mixed—mixed with other moral grounds and with instrumental purposes. It seems safe to recognize that cases exist in which both forgiveness and reconciliation occur and cases in which there is reconciliation without forgiveness (restoration of the relationship for instrumental purposes) and forgiveness without reconciliation (forgiveness without the intent of restoration of the relationship).

Let us now turn to a more detailed analysis of different layers or dimensions of reconciliation or reconciliatory behavior. This will also pave the way for a clearer view of forgiveness and its dynamics.

Reconciliation

Rituals of reconciliation are said to exist in animals. They are extensively studied in ape colonies where these rituals function as a form of peace-keeping (de Waal, 1988). Grooming and greeting rituals calm down pent-up emotions that otherwise could lead to intraspecies aggression. These rituals instill a feeling of superiority and of being valued that members higher in the group hierarchy need. Ethology and animal psychology may help to recognize analogous behaviors in humans. I am inclined to emphasize the differences between animal and human reconciliation and to view animal forms of reconciliation as precursors of human forms. When animal precursors are built into human functioning, they gain new significance. These human behaviors can, for instance, now be evaluated in normative terms. Are these behaviors genuine? What do they say about the person and who she wants to be? Are they merely the expression of self-interest or do they serve overarching purposes? Animal psychology can at best only partly account for these normative aspects. It seems realistic, however, to keep in mind that forgiveness and reconciliation are seldom totally pure and unaffected by complicated motives and free of any form of pretending. We may deceive others by pretending to conform to their social and moral order for the sake of our own interests.

Reconciliation-like behaviors in humans may be displayed without and with the explicit intention to reconcile. An example of the latter form of behavior is an employee who, after having been threatened with dismissal, deliberately tries to establish a 'positive' relationship with a supervisor by the display of submissive and pleasing behavior. It is a matter of definition whether or not to count these behaviors as variants of reconciliation.

Reconciliation between humans minimally requires the restoration of an interpersonal relationship, according to Enright *et al.* (1998). For this restoration to occur, it may help to give up feelings of hatred and resentment and the inclination to take revenge. This is the affective and inclinational dimension of reconciliation. It depends on one's definition of reconciliation whether or not to include this dimension as a necessary condition for reconciliation between humans. For now, it is enough to see that reconciliation in humans often involves an affective and inclinational dimension that can be distinguished from the behavioral, cognitive, and moral dimensions.

The same holds basically for change of opinion about the wrongdoer and/or his deeds. It is easier to try to heal a relationship if the wrongdoer can be seen against the background of his biography, education, and social circumstances. However, this does not mean that change of opinion is a prerequisite for reconciliation. This will depend on the persons and the circumstances that are involved. Moreover, understanding the wrongdoer better is not the same as excusing his behavior. One can understand the person of the wrongdoer and his deeds without denying his responsibility. Change of opinion and understanding should, therefore, be distinguished from the moral dimension of reconciliation.

An interesting feature of reconciliation consists of the fact that acts of reconciliation may have moral meaning even if they are not performed on moral grounds. This is so because restoration of interpersonal relationships requires that claims for punishment have been given up and that there is an agreement on compensation. In other cases, punishment has already taken place. Reconciliation is the end point of a process in which parties have negotiated about such claims and have reached some form of agreement. Such agreement forms the basis for restoration of a minimally required amount of trust and may imply punishment or other forms of (lasting) compensation. However, the achievement of such a result implies also that one has given up one's right for further compensation, moral and nonmoral. Moral compensation is the most interesting case for our purposes. It may take different forms: making an apology, showing remorse, feeling repentance, or acting responsibly by solving the problems that led to the infliction of harm. I admit that these latter examples come close to forgiveness. But it is worth at least a thought experiment to imagine situations in which moral compensation is given on nonmoral (for instance, practical and/or utilitarian) grounds. Some of the activities of the Truth and Reconciliation Committee in South Africa could be interpreted in this sense: as events with a moral meaning even in cases in which the reconciliatory acts themselves were not primarily based or performed on moral grounds.

To sum up, reconciliation is an interpersonal process in which two parties come together again on the basis of restoration of the relationship to a level that both desire. There are forms of reconciliation that come close to mere negotiation and—at the other end of the spectrum—forms that include forgiveness. Reconciliation involves affective, interpersonal, cognitive, and moral aspects that play a different role, depending on the context.

Forgiveness

Forgiveness differs from reconciliation (at least) in that it requires moral grounds and the overcoming of vindictive passions (Murphy, 2003). This overcoming of one's passions is an inner process. Let us now make this more precise, by summarizing points of criticism against Murphy's definition that were raised by Jean Hampton (Murphy and Hampton, 1988). Hampton's criticisms will prepare us for a discussion of the dynamics of forgiveness.

Hampton's main concern is that forgiveness involves much more than just a change of one's feeling state. She interprets Murphy's position as arguing for an understanding of forgiveness as primarily a change of feeling on moral grounds. For the present purposes, it is not relevant whether or not this interpretation is right (cf., for instance, Murphy, 2003, for a refinement of his earlier position). Hampton agrees that a change of feelings usually includes change of opinion (judgment). However, this is not enough, in her view. Central to the concept of forgiveness is a change in the relationship to the wrongdoer by which a person is able to absolve the wrongdoer from guilt. Like Worthington (1998a, p. 129), Hampton describes forgiveness as a gift. The gift consists of absolution from guilt. We speak of forgiveness as 'bestowed upon' or 'offered to' the wrongdoer, she says (cf. Hampton, in: Murphy and Hampton, 1988, p. 37; cf. pp. 36–43 and pp. 79–87). The change in the attitude of the forgiver leads to an offer to the wrongdoer that allows the latter to re-enter the community. This is a pretty strong position, so we have to see how Hampton builds up her argument.

Hampton's reasoning about forgiveness is of the same type as our attempt in the previous paragraphs to unwrap the different dimensions of reconciliation. Changes of feelings (on moral grounds) are not enough, she says. Feelings may change because we want them to change (for moral reasons) or because they fade away (with our moral consent). But we may still think about the wrongdoer as an evil person. To forgive involves more than no longer being angry; it is more than suppressing one's feelings or letting them fade away.

Changes in both feeling and judgment will also not suffice to account fully for forgiveness. Change of judgment would involve the acceptance of the moral wrong, according to Hampton. This statement needs explanation. The example Hampton gives is of the instrumental or utilitarian type mentioned above. A stern and rigid father criticizes his daughter-in-law for her sloppy housekeeping; the son advises his wife to give up her resentment (the feeling) and to think well (the judgment) of her father-in-law for the greater good of family peace (utilitarian reason). It is questionable, I think, whether Murphy would count this case as an example of forgiveness in terms of his own definition (overcoming vindictive passions on moral grounds). Even if family peace is considered as a moral ground in this case, and even if the daughter-in-law really would change her feelings and attitudes, Murphy could still maintain that the example does not suffice as an example of forgiveness on his account, because the grounds on which the feelings are given up are not appropriate to the feelings.

Let me explain what I mean here with appropriateness of moral grounds. The issue is intriguing, because it focuses our attention on the nature of the feelings that are overcome and on the quality of the moral grounds for changing one's feelings. For the daughter-in-law, it would, for instance, be inappropriate to give up her anger if it included *moral* indignation. Moral indignation implies that the daughter-in-law's conviction that the father-in-law has done something really morally wrong toward her by blaming her for her inadequate housekeeping. Giving up moral indignation for a reason not related to the indignation implies that she accepts the moral wrong. Asking the daughter-in-law to drop her judgment about the father for the interests of the family and to respond as if no offense had occurred is asking her to drop the moral element of her protest too and to accept a situation that is morally wrong. Such change of opinion under pressure may in the end amount to self-deception. Think, for instance, of a situation in which the daughter-in-law discovers that all family members think her husband is right and in which she finally surrenders her opinion. Would this count as forgiveness? I think that both Murphy and Hampton would answer negatively. Murphy would argue that the grounds are inappropriate to feelings: family peace is, even as moral ground, inappropriate to overcome indignation about what someone else has wrongly and culpably done to us. Hampton would say that changes of judgment under pressure are, in fact, a form of self-deception. Prolonged self-deception undermines one's sense of self-worth and is morally unacceptable as well.

It is in this context that Hampton introduces the concept of condonation, which she defines as '. . . the acceptance, without moral protest (either inward or outward), of an action which ought to warrant such protest, made possible, first, by ridding oneself of the judgment that the action is wrong [. . . .]; and second, by ridding oneself of any attendant feelings which signify one's protest of the action.' (Hampton, in: Murphy and Hampton, 1988, p. 40. The distinction between forgiving and condoning was first introduced by Kolnai, 1973–74).

The latter part of this definition is important. The (moral) protest is already present in feelings: indignation about the father-in-law is a feeling that includes a moral element. The person who is asked to condone is asked to give up such opinions (judgments) and feelings and to accept as moral that which has been experienced as immoral. In short, to condone is to accept the moral wrong, whereas forgiveness does not accept it.

At this point a new problem emerges: if it is true that to forgive differs from to condone and that to forgive is to absolve someone from guilt, how can one remain committed to the idea that the actions of the wrongdoer were wrong and unacceptable? How can one forgive and, by doing so, give up one's moral protest and still think that the actions of the wrongdoer were wrong? Hampton's response to this question is complex and involves a thorough analysis of such emotional states as resentment, indignation, and hatred. I can only summarize her conclusion here. Forgiveness is a process that—after the psychological preparation—involves a change of heart, which change is such that it creates inner room to see the wrongdoer in a different and more acceptable light and to consider him, to some degree, as distinct from his deeds. The victim comes to see the wrongdoer as 'still decent; not rotten as a person, and someone with whom he may be able to renew a relationship' (Hampton, in: Murphy and Hampton, 1988, p. 83). In spite of the fact that the harm cannot be undone and that the moral judgment about what has happened does not change, the person who forgives experiences a change of inner attitude that enables the victim to accept the wrongdoer as 'still decent.'

Repentance and gestures of regret on the part of the wrongdoer may help to bring about this change of inner attitude. But forgiving is not just a reaction to another's repentance, according to Hampton. Acceptance of repentance may still be a proportionate reaction, which is performed because it seems reasonable to do so, or because one thinks one ought to, or because it is what people expect one to do. Such motivations are not inherently moral. They are not distinctive for the concept of forgiveness.

For Hampton the crucial elements of forgiveness are the change of heart and the decision to see the wrongdoer in a different light, namely as still decent. To forgive is to absolve the wrongdoer from guilt and to approve him as a person despite what he has done. This absolution and approval are, in fact, a gift.

Coercive measures to prompt someone to be forgiving change forgiveness into something very different. How could an act that is meant to absolve another from guilt and possible retribution, and that has the potential to liberate the offender from a circle of shame and self-denial, be performed when this liberating act itself is not free? The question is rhetorical: forgiveness is a free act, and it cannot be offered on demand. Coercion and forgiveness exclude one another.

So, those who forgive give up their claims of retribution and compensation but do not condone or excuse the deeds of the wrongdoer. The wrongdoer is still held blameworthy and responsible for the misery he has brought about. These ideas explain why the process of forgiveness is so delicate. It is delicate because the wrongdoer may interpret the attitude of the victim as expressing moral superiority. This perception will keep the wrongdoer from admitting his shortcomings. On the other hand, the victim may give in too soon and on inadequate grounds.

8.5 The dynamics of forgiveness

Section 8.4 provides the necessary preparatory work to suggest in what way the dynamic of evil is counteracted by the process of forgiveness and how this process is related to the points we discussed earlier: speechlessness, splitting and denial, and shame. The hypothesis I investigate in the remainder of this chapter is that, indeed, forgiveness is a process that overcomes the dynamic of evil on these three critical points. First a disclaimer again: I can give here only the skeleton of an approach that would need much more detail to be convincing. What follows is a sketch with many loose ends. I can only hope that the general approach, as well as the loose ends, raise sufficient questions and interest to stimulate thinking on our subject.

Earlier in this chapter, I highlighted the nontransparency of acts of evil and their consequences and connected this nontransparency with features of the dynamic of evil. I interpreted the speechlessness of the victim and the denial of the wrongdoer both (but in a different way) as manifestations of evil (in cases of intolerable harm) and as possible sources of new evil. Later, I suggested that splitting and shame fulfill a similar double role. They can be seen as enhancing and as expressing evil. Neither side of the interpretation was favored above the other. The simultaneity of both aspects suggests they are part of a dynamic process with a cyclic, or spiral, nature. Evil produces speechlessness, denial, shame, and violence, which, in their turn, are at the root of new manifestations of evil.

My attempts to discuss the nontransparency of evil in more detail remain necessarily incomplete and ambiguous: when it is in the nature of evil to deprive us of our language and to shake our moral order to the extent that we feel lost and disoriented, then a certain amount of nontransparency will always remain. I reiterate that speaking has a moral meaning in such circumstances. It means resisting the power of denial and giving witness to the unheard. We have to remember that the dynamic of evil to a large extent consists of the suggestion that there is nothing to deny. In other words, the dynamic itself is 'empty,' like the eye of a hurricane. This emptiness, in other words, reveals both the dynamic power of evil and the speechlessness surrounding acts of evil.

Richard Bernstein, at the end of his book on radical evil, speaks of a 'black hole' in our understanding:

> We seek to comprehend the meaning of evil, its varieties and vicissitudes. We want to know why it is that some individuals choose evil and others resist it. We want to know why some individuals adopt goods maxims and others adopt evil maxims. There is much we can say about someone's background, training, education, character, circumstances, etc. The social disciplines and psychology all contribute to this understanding. But it never adds up to a complete explanation of why individuals make the choices they do. There is always a gap, a 'black hole,' in our accounts.
>
> Bernstein (2002, p. 235)

I have explored this 'black hole' by viewing it as an existential dynamic. Hannah Arendt, while using different terminology, seems to refer to a similar dynamic when she writes about the 'empty space' around friends and loved ones in the year 1933, when the Nazi regime gained power: 'The problem, the personal problem, was not what our enemies did but what our friends did. In the wave of Gleichschaltung (co-ordination), which was relatively voluntary—in any case, not yet under the pressure of terror—it was as if an empty space formed around one.' [*Essays in Understanding, 1930–1954* (ed. J Kohn), pp. 10–11. New York: Harcourt, Brace and Co., 1994; quotation via Bernstein, ibid., p. 22].

This 'empty space' suggests another dimension of evil we have encountered: the erosion of trust and the isolation and unconnectedness to which acts of evil lead.

By invoking forgiveness, I do not mean to say that acts of evil—and especially not the horrible acts of evil we discussed in more detail—should be forgiven. The question of whether and how and when to forgive, is practical, clinical, and theological, but not primarily philosophical. My interest here is conceptual and philosophical—the kind of philosophy that is informed by psychology and psychiatry.

Before finishing my analysis of the dynamics of evil and forgiveness, I want to point out why the contrast between the two is so challenging. I use the concept of forgiveness in its strongest sense, like Hampton, as an inner act that includes the gift of absolving guilt and of approving the person of the wrong-doer; as an act that is more than a change of feeling and judgment; an act that differs from condonation; and is not merely a reaction to the wrongdoer's repentance. Just as the dynamic of evil cannot become completely transparent, the dynamic of forgiveness also retains an element that impresses us as almost unexplainable. I am not saying that acts of forgiveness as such cannot be verbalized or understood, or that the interpersonal and affective dynamic of the process of forgiveness is inexpressible. My point is that, despite all description and conceptual refinement, acts of forgiveness still seem to be groundless to an extent. First, they are groundless in the sense that the forgiver does not have any warrant about the outcome of his offer of absolution to the wrong-doer and, second, they are groundless in the sense that there may be a shortage of grounds to base the gift of forgiveness on. To forgive is to take a risk—a risk that the offer is declined or is interpreted as a sign of weakness, with all the dangers that come with this (humiliation; repetition of abuse; adoption of a submissive attitude).

I take this groundlessness not as a cognitive or evidential error but as a sign that indicates the dynamic of forgiveness. This dynamic is as rich as the dynamics of evil and seems to manifest opposite tendencies compared with the dynamic of evil. What I call 'dynamic' is, again, not distinct from but inter-woven with the affective and interpersonal dimensions of forgiveness. But these affective and interpersonal aspects cannot completely account for the way this dynamic works. The gift of forgiveness is ultimately moral, or even religious. Forgiveness in its most mature forms may have a power that is strong enough to absorb not only the feelings and judgments about someone who behaved immorally toward us but also the dynamic of evil that comes with these feelings and judgments. I am not saying that these feelings and judgments as such are evil, of course. What I suggest is that the dynamic of evil is such that it may make use of these feelings and judgments, for instance, by locking the victim in his world of pain and hatred and by instilling insuper-able feelings of shame in the wrongdoer.

I now return to the three characteristics of the dynamic of evil: speechless-ness; denial and splitting; and shame. Forgiveness is impossible without recog-nition of what has gone wrong (cf. Sharon Lamb, Chapter 10 in this volume shows how difficult this task may be for women). This recognition may take many different forms: remembering, recounting, writing down what has occurred, sharing one's experiences with someone else, or explicit acknowledgment of having suffered from an immoral act. Overcoming speechlessness does not necessarily entail that one speaks. However, some form of internal monologue and of sharing one's thoughts and feelings with someone else seems needed. To recall the hurt is the first step in Worthington's model of forgiveness (Worthington 1998a, p. 113). For the victim, the difficult element in this part of the process is not the speaking itself, but the overcoming of the strong feelings and inclinations that amount to speechlessness, such as the tendency to avoid the anxiety and pain of facing the full burden of what has gone wrong; and the intense feelings of powerlessness, disgust, and shame that may emerge by reliving one's experiences of traumatization. In the offender, similar processes are important; however, here they take the form of giving up one's lies and overcoming denial and, behind this, shame. This is also painful and may go against one's inclinations. In short, to speak and to recognize what has gone wrong is both for the victim and for the wrongdoer a difficult, hazardous, and courageous step in the process of forgiveness. To forgive is to succeed in conquering a dynamic that is still active in oneself.

The same dynamic is possibly also operative in one's dealings with natural evil. In his book on God, medicine, and the problem of suffering, the American theologian Stanley Hauerwas (1990) speaks of 'naming the silences.' The silence he considers is the speechlessness that results from having to deal with incurable cancer or the sudden loss of a child. Such events are not only hard to face and seem to lack meaning: the speechlessness is a kind of paralysis at a more primordial level—a lack of language with respect to the brute facts themselves (instead of to their meaning or interpretation). It is a stammering in the confrontation with the contingency of one's existence.

To forgive is also to give up splitting and denial. One of the interesting questions here is what it means to give up one's defenses. If denial is the result of the workings of a primitive defense mechanism, how is it possible to give it up without giving up oneself? What kind of power is needed to achieve such change and avert self-destruction?

From a clinical point of view, it is sometimes impossible to give up splitting or any other defense mechanism that helps to keep pain and emotional chaos at a distance. Giving up these defense mechanisms may overwhelm the person with undigested traumatic memories, intense negative feelings, and suicidal and other self-destructive thoughts. There is an extensive literature on how to deal with these situations in patients with borderline personality disorder, dissociative identity disorder, and post-traumatic stress disorder, and it is not necessary to discuss this literature here (cf. Herman 1992). For our purposes, it is sufficient to point at a factor that is common to most psychotherapeutic approaches, and that is the development of trust—trust in the patient by the therapist; and trust of the patient in himself, partly as a result of the trust of others (for a philosophical analysis of trust and trustworthiness, cf. Potter, 2002). Trust plays an immensely important role in any therapeutic endeavor. Common to most psychotherapeutic approaches is the powerful assumption of the therapist that the patient will improve, even if there is nothing in the patient's present situation and, even, of the therapeutic encounter that points in that direction and that may guarantee such success. Patients are likely to improve because their being trusted by the therapist helps them to trust themselves.

Forgiveness is not compatible with denial. Giving up denial is essential preparatory work for forgiveness to take place. A special form of denial consists of the use of metaphorical exaggerations and of pseudo-poetic language. Such language transforms horror into something aesthetic. Hannah Arendt (1965) warned against such use of language. The reality of what has occurred is denied once again, which doubles sadness. Arendt is aiming at expressions in which Eichman is called a 'devil' or 'beast' and in which there is an 'Eichman in everyone of us.'

I now investigate the dynamic of the overcoming of denial in nonclinical cases. Here, trust is needed too, both for the wrongdoer and for the forgiver. Trust acquires a more specific meaning here, a meaning that is preparatory for the way we will deal with the next point (shame). The wrongdoer, who gives up his lies and overcomes his denial, is vulnerable to moral criticism and (shame-inducing) rejection. The victim who opens her mind for the horrors of the past makes her self vulnerable for repetition of the dynamics of the interpersonal relationship in which the traumatization occurred or the harm was inflicted. Forgiveness embodies a dynamic of trust that opposes (fear of) moral rejection and repetition of the past.

Trust seems, therefore, similarly 'groundless' as forgiveness. To trust is to place one's fate in the hands of others, at least to a certain extent. Absolute trust is rare, of course. Less absolute forms certainly are not. Think of all those situations in which there is a discrepancy between realistic expectation and the expectations that are based on trust. It seems as if the trusting person acts on a cognitive and moral 'error' because there is insufficient cognitive and moral 'evidence' to warrant the trust of the other.

The same holds for forgiveness. There are many reasons and grounds to forgive (as there are reasons and grounds for trust). But in the end, to forgive is to take a decision that suffers from the same lack of cognitive and moral evidence as in the case of trust. But it is precisely this lack of calculation that indicates where we have to locate the dynamic of forgiveness: in the offer of acceptance in spite of the harm that has been inflicted by the wrongdoer and in spite of the lack of evidence that the offer will be accepted.

Trust seems to be an important intermediate element in the process of forgiving, an element that opposes the existential dynamic that keeps the victim caught in her cycle of pain, avoidance, and denial, and the wrongdoer in his state of guilt. When the wrongdoer trusts the victim with respect to the genuineness of the offer of absolution of guilt, the victim's feelings of self-worth may increase and, with this, her confidence that she can achieve a better life. When the victim offers his or her trust to the wrongdoer, the wrongdoer is asked to view himself as a person that does not coincide with his guilty version. In short, trust may bring about a dynamic that counteracts some of the self-perpetuating moments in the dynamic of evil, most notably the elements of self-closure, denial, and avoidance.

Finally, I focus on how forgiveness counteracts shame. Shame adds a (both real and imagined) interpersonal dimension to the process of forgiveness. The transition to this topic seems natural, because the processes we discussed in the previous paragraphs also include an interpersonal element. By recognizing guilt, the wrongdoer sees himself through the eyes of the victim and may experience his moral inferiority. Guilt is related to acts that caused the harm. Shame goes deeper and is related to one's person or, better, one's core sense of self. In the face of the victim, the evildoer may feel degraded and depraved. The offer of forgiveness confirms his depravity and, at the same time, offers a way out. The wrongdoer teeters between these two. To decline the offer would save his independence: one does not owe anything to anyone. To accept the offer would imply that he acknowledges his immorality and trusts that the forgiver will nevertheless persist in his offer of forgiveness. This is a highly critical moment in the process of forgiveness. It is especially shame that makes it difficult to accept the gift of forgiveness. The power of shame undermines one's belief in the genuineness of the offer and, at the same time, leads to self-absorption and lack of awareness of the real other. Nevertheless, the gift of forgiveness can stop the cycle of shameful and angry disconnectedness and can help the wrongdoer to overcome his isolation and to view his existence as not totally depraved.

To forgive, we saw, is to recognize the extent of the harm. By offering forgiveness, the victim indirectly discloses her pain and vulnerability. For the victim, it is the interpersonal dimension of feeling vulnerable that heightens the shame. Being weak in the presence of strong and dominant others (with sometimes dubious motives) may induce anxiety and shame—anxiety, because of the risk of repetition of trauma; and shame, because of the subtle connotation (and also risk) of humiliation. To feel vulnerable in the real or imagined presence of the evildoer is, therefore, a highly critical moment in the victim's process of forgiving. However, forgiveness is precisely the power that enables the victim to overcome the inclination to hide and to avoid the gaze of others and to make herself invisible. Instead of shrinking back in her private world, the forgiving victim opens her arms and offers her embrace. Forgiveness counteracts evil by this power to open up the victim's closed self and to liberate the wrongdoer from his self-imposed isolation. The power of forgiveness consists precisely in its capacity to break the destructive cycle of shame, anger, and violence and in the healing effects of sharing the person's isolation.

To summarize: it is characteristic for forgiveness to have insufficient grounds; this is not a weakness but indicates forgiveness's power, which manifests itself as courage in the overcoming of speechlessness, as trust in the battle against denial, and as openness and embrace in the context of shame.

8.6 Dealing with evil: beyond philosophy and psychology

Throughout this chapter, I have tried to do justice to the idea that there is a nontransparent element in the phenomenology of evil. This nontransparency was interpreted as an expression of the dynamic of evil. The dynamic of forgiveness runs counter to this dynamic and appears to possess its own nontransparency. Those who forgive hardly ever have sufficient grounds for forgiveness. However, this is not a weakness but indicative of the power of forgiveness to overcome speechlessness, isolation, denial, and shame.

I have built my case from the bottom up. I tried to ascertain the legitimacy of speaking of the dynamic of evil and of forgiveness. Once ascertained, new questions emerge: what 'is' the dynamic of evil and of forgiveness? Where do these dynamics come from? What is their ontological and metaphysical status? What is the place of a religious understanding of evil and forgiveness? And what is the function and value of forgiveness, if evil and its consequences cannot be undone?

This last question is, perhaps, most relevant in our context. As Hampton suggests, it is an issue that leads us to the metaphysical and religious dimensions of evil and forgiveness. How is forgiveness possible, and what could it mean if evil cannot be undone? I close this chapter by sketching two contrasting paradigms with respect to this question, in an attempt to highlight the importance of such paradigms for discussions in the applied sciences and the professions. I first briefly summarize Friedrich Nietzsche's position in *Also sprach Zarathustra* (Nietzsche 1883/1985) and then continue with some remarks on how classical Christianity treats the concepts of evil and forgiveness.

Nietzsche argues that acts of evil cannot be undone and will exist forever. If evil persists and adds up in history, it does not make sense for us human beings to perish under the burden of guilt. We would be better off if we could eradicate the language of guilt and, more radically, if we could deny that such a thing as evil exists. This is indeed what Nietzsche says. The problem of evil is invented by the weak, by people who cannot stand the real world and flee to an idealized version of it. Instead of fleeing, we need a 'will to power' that enables us to embrace our fate. We should eliminate the language of guilt, self-surrender, and love, and replace it by an idiom that takes life as it is and encourages the will to live.

If Nietzsche is right, to restore a relationship with another person who inflicted harm on us, by forgiving that person, is at best a childish form of submission and self-deception. In worse versions, it amounts to 'ressentiment', Nietzsche's favored French term that points at the hidden anger and masochistic destructiveness in the acknowledgment of, and response to, guilt. On Nietzsche's account, we should bear the burden of existence and try to transform it by the will to power. The ultimate consequence of this transformation would be that one has to embrace Auschwitz in order not to fall back into an attitude of weakness and ressentiment. Embracing Auschwitz is impossible, however, according to Neiman (2002, p. 265).

There is no greater contrast than that between Nietzsche's heroic and naturalistic philosophy and the Christian approach to evil and forgiveness. Central to this tradition is not the will to power, but the weakness of human beings with respect to evil. Evil is not directly undone by forgiveness, but 'brought away' and 'covered.' The latter terms are metaphors that refer to the Old Testament ritual of atonement by the sacrifice of two goats of which one was sent away into desert and the other was killed in order to shed its blood in the temple in the face of the Almighty. Jesus' death announced the final overcoming of evil 'in the last days.' So, evil is not undone in the present era, though there is hope that it once will be.

Nietzsche locates the Christian approach to suffering, guilt, and evil at the level of the so-called ethical world view (a term invented by Paul Ricoeur). The ethical world view, according to Nietzsche, connects evil with sin and failure and is, therefore, doomed to circle around in guilt, powerlessness, suppressed anger, and destruction. Thinkers such as Søren Kierkegaard (1844/1980, 1849) and Paul Ricoeur (1955, 1969, 1990) emphasize that the final word about the nature of evil should be spoken at a level beyond the ethical, that is, at a religious level. At this level, suffering and guilt are also inevitable and cannot be undone in the present state of the world, but their burden is taken away by a suffering divine being. The offer of forgiveness is foreshadowed in the self-giving love of the son of God who became 'son of man' and whose suffering on the cross symbolizes his identification with human frailty and sin. The doctrine of incarnation is, first of all, meant to express God's goodness, that is, his will to be part of this world with its suffering, wickedness, and evil. The notion of atonement builds upon this recognition in that atonement is acquired by the acceptance of God's self-giving love.

The Christian tradition suggests that the dynamics of evil and of forgiveness belong to a spiritual reality that can be best approached by faith. To accept the gift of forgiveness is not easy; it is a real 'stumbling block,' because it requires that we give up our presumed moral righteousness. This is painful, humiliating, and shameful. We can overcome this pain, humiliation, and shame by self-surrender and by trust in God's embrace (Volf 1996, pp. 99–166).

So, I end this exposition with the description of two radically divergent paradigms of dealing with evil. Philosophy cannot find in itself the sources that are needed to choose a direction. However, it can bring us to the point where the consequences of our choices become as clear as possible.

References

Arendt H (1965). *Eichmann in Jerusalem. A Report on the Banality of Evil.* Penguin Books (revised and enlarged edition).

Baumeister RF and Vohs KD (2004). Four roots of evil. In: *The Social Psychology of Good and Evil* (ed. AG Miller), pp. 85–101. New York & London: The Guilford Press.

Bernstein RJ (2002). *Radical evil. A Philosophical Interrogation.* Cambridge, UK: Polity Press.

Card C (2002). *The Atrocity Paradigm: A Theory of Evil.* New York/London: Oxford University Press.

Card C (2004). The atrocity paradigm revisited. *Hypatia,* **19**(4): 210–20.

Enright RD and North J (eds) (1998). *Exploring Forgiveness* (with a foreword by Archbishop Desmond Tutu). Madison, WI: The University of Wisconsin Press.

Enright RD, Freedman S, and Rique J (1998).The psychology of interpersonal forgiveness. In: *Exploring Forgiveness* (with a foreword by Archbishop Desmond Tutu) (eds RD Enright and J North), pp. 46–62. Madison, WI: The University of Wisconsin Press.

Goldberg C. (1996). *Speaking with the Devil: A Dialogue with Evil.* New York: Viking Press.

Hauerwas S (1990). *Naming the Silences. God, Medicine, and the Problem of Suffering.* Grand Rapids, MI: Eerdmans Publishing Company.

Heidegger M (1927/1979). *Sein und Zeit.* Tübingen: Niemeyer Verlag.

Herman JL (1992). *Trauma and Recovery.* New York: Basic Books (Harper and Collins).

Husserl E (1992b). *Ideen zu einer Reinen Phänomenologie und Phänomenologischen Philosophie*, I. Halle: Max Niemeyer.

Jones LG (1995). *Embodying Forgiveness. A Theological Analysis.* Grand Rapids, MI: Eerdmans Publishing Company.

Kant, I. (1793/1990). *Die Religion innerhalb der Grenzen der Bloßen Vernunft.* Hamburg: Felix Meiner Verlag.

Kierkegaard S (1844/1980). *The Concept of Anxiety. A Simple Psychologically Orienting Deliberation on the Dogmatic Issue of Heriditary Sin* (trans. Begrebet Angest) (ed. and trans R Thomte in collaboration with AB Anderson). Princeton, NJ: Princeton University Press.

Kierkegaard S (1849). *Sickness unto Death.* London: Penguin Books.

Kolnai A (1973–74). Forgiveness. *Proceedings of the Aristotelian Society*, pp. 91–106.

Lanzmann (1985a). *Shoah. An Oral History of the Holocaust* (documentary movie).

Lanzmann C (1985b). *Shoah* [préface de Simone de Beauvoir]. Paris: Éditions Fayard.

Lewis M (1995). *Shame: The Exposed Self.* New York: The Free Press.

Lifton R (1986). *The Nazi Doctors. Medical Killing and the Psychology of Genocide.* New York: Basic Books.

McCullough ME, Pargament KI, and Thoresen CE (eds) (2000). *Forgiveness. Theory, Research, and Practice.* New York: The Guilford Press.

Miller AG (ed.) (2004). *The Social Psychology of Good and Evil.* New York: The Guilford Press.

Murphy JG (2003). *Getting Even. Forgiveness and its Limits.* Oxford: Oxford University Press.

Murphy JG and Hampton J (1988). *Forgiveness and Mercy.* Cambridge: Cambridge University Press.

Neiman S (2002). *Evil in Modern Thought: An Alternative History of Philosophy.* Princeton, NJ: Princeton University Press.

Nietzsche F (1883/1985). *Also Sprach Zarathustra. Ein Buch für Alle und Keine.* Stuttgart: Alfred Kröner Verlag.

North J (1998). The 'ideal' of forgiveness: A philosopher's exploration. In: *Exploring Forgiveness* (eds RD Enright and J North) (with a foreword by Archbishop Desmond Tutu), pp. 15–34. Madison, WI: The University of Wisconsin Press.

Potter, NN (2002). *How Can I Be Trusted? A Virtue Theory of Trustworthiness.* Lanham: Rowman & Littlefield Publishers.

Ricoeur P (1955). *Philosophie de la volonté. Finitude et culpabilité.* II. La symbolique du mal (Philosophie de l'esprit). Paris: Aubier.

Ricoeur P (1969). *Le conflit des l'interprétations. Essais d'herméneutique.* Paris: Éditions du Seuil.

Ricoeur P (1990). *Soi même Comme un Autre.* Paris: Éditions du Seuil.

Sartre JP (1943). *L'être et le Néant. Essai d'ontologie Phénoménologique.* Paris: Gallimard.

Scheler M (1916). *Der Formalismus in der Ethik und die Materiale Wertethik. Neuer Versuch der Grundlegung eines ethischen Personalismus.* Bern, München: Francke Verlag.

Volf M (1996). *Exclusion and Embrace. A Theological Exploration of Identity, Otherness, and Reconciliation.* Nashville, TN: Abingdon Press.

Waal F de (1988). *Peacemaking Among Primates.* Cambridge: Harvard University Press.

Worthington EL (1998a). The pyramid model of forgiveness: Some interdisciplinary speculations about unforgiveness and the promotion of forgiveness. In: *Dimensions of Forgiveness. Psychological Research and Theological Perspectives* (ed. EL Worthington), pp. 107–38. Philadelphia: Templeton Foundation Press.

Worthington EL (ed.) (1998b). *Dimensions of Forgiveness. Psychological Research and Theological Perspectives*. Philadelphia: Templeton Foundation Press.

Chapter 9

Forgiveness: a critical appraisal

Piet J. Verhagen

The love of God does not find, but creates, that which is pleasing to it. The love of man comes into being through that which is pleasing to it.

Luther[1]

9.1 'Forgiveness, what does it pay?'

Perhaps a question like: 'Forgiveness, what does it pay?' sounds a little crude, when one seriously takes into account the mondial growing attention and interest in forgiveness, in recognition of guilt, and in reconciliation in the domains of religion, society, and politics. The question may sound profane in the ears of religiously committed people and those who are deeply convinced of the spiritual and even revelatory roots of the idea and practice of forgiveness, and of the divine command to forgive even your enemies. In fact, spiritually committed people without any specific church associations or even theistic bonding admit and promote the significance of forgiveness. What evoked this growing interest in forgiveness?

For what possible reason should we speak of a new interest in forgiveness, when we take into account that most religions have advocated forgiveness all along? Since the 1960s, the rise of (post)modern individualism has caused a decline of the Christian churches and a growth not only of nonreligiosity and but also of post-traditional types of religion. Events that might have contributed to the new interest in forgiveness are perhaps legion. Let me recall just two events, other events could be mentioned, that had their impact on a mondial level. The revolution in Iran demonstrated that secularization was not irreversible. Since then, it has become clear that nowadays society at large is characterized by its religious-ideological pluralism, manifested in stressful coexistence and rivalry everywhere in the world. Pluralism relieved

---

[1] 'Amor dei non invenit, sed creat suum diligibile, Amor hominis fit a suo diligibili' (Luther 1518/1957).

secularization as the most appropriate interpretation of the current affairs and religion became a public matter (again) (Schwöbel, 2003). This was illustrated by the second event I would like to recall. During the last jubilee or holy year, 2000, it was the Catholic pope who attracted attention by requesting forgiveness and thereby demonstrating a new attitude on the stage of the world. Until then, it was quite rare to do so in public. Despite this and other worthy examples for asking publicly for forgiveness, we nevertheless see a culmination of vengeful actions between nations, between fundamentalists or otherwise inspired political, religious, and ethnic groups (van Noort, 2003).

Although the feeling of some sort of profanation is understandable where forgiveness is concerned and the question arises as to how profitable it is, this question is in the air. Not only in society and politics but also in mental health, the same interest in forgiveness can be found. Forgiveness, already used in pastoral counseling as a strategy, has become an intervention in marital and family therapy. But as interventions in general became subjected to the current criteria of evidence-based mental health, even forgiveness had to be proven as an effective therapeutic strategy. An intervention should be evidence-based by preference and should be evaluated according to the best evidence available, if it's goal is to attain the status of a meaningful—that is to say, effective—therapeutic intervention. Any intervention or therapeutic approach should be investigated for its efficacy under optimal circumstances and its effectiveness in daily practice. On this line of reasoning, forgiveness should be no exception to the rule. A critical appraisal of any intervention helps to identify whether that intervention does more good than harm for those to whom it is offered. In this way, evidence-based medicine can be a helpful tool in improving quality of care. Professionally speaking, it would be unacceptable to make an exception of forgiveness on opinion or even credulity based arguments under the current emphasis on evidence-based therapy and interventions.

However, the search for the best available evidence, which is the professional translation of the 'what does it pay' question, is not the only matter that concerns me in this chapter. There are other, at least equally important, fundamental questions to ask concerning the constructs used and the underlying models that attempt to explain the process and the meaning of forgiveness.

9.2 **Our relatedness**

Although I will discuss the question of a definition of forgiveness later on in this chapter, I believe it is clear by intuition that forgiveness is embedded in our relatedness. As Martin Buber famously stated, 'In the beginning is the relation' (cited by Jones, 1996, p. 69). That is, human nature is essentially relational. For Buber, the primacy of relationships precedes the primacy of individuality. Embedded in a network of relationships, individuality arises out of relational experiences. This is not just a matter of the very beginning but an ongoing embeddedness that continues to be important our whole lives long. Our identity and our value as persons are determined by fellowship with others. We need to be valued and to be loved. I will follow the line of reasoning by the Dutch philosopher and theologian Vincent Brümmer on love and personal and impersonal relations (Brümmer, 1993). One of his fundamental theses is that most views of love take it to be an attitude rather than a relationship. Brümmer himself develops a relational concept of love. I make use of this model in understanding forgiveness as a relationship rather than an attitude. But first I have to make clear what might be the usefulness of the distinction between attitude and relationship (fellowship) with regard to our personal identity. Once I have clarified this distinction the structure of this chapter will become intelligible.

Every entity shares characteristics with at least some other entities and can therefore be classified as a member of this or that class of entities. But each entity has its own configuration of these characteristics: its own identity. The same goes for human beings. We share the characteristics as members of the same class, yet each individual has its own configuration of these characteristics. In the case of human beings, for example, we share as characteristics ideas and convictions, emotions and needs, wishes and desires. What makes me the person I am is this and not that specific configuration of ideas and convictions, needs and emotions, and so on. The convictions and wishes that have first-person meaning to me, and that give purpose, value, and coherence to my own life and actions, make me the person I am. Brümmer refers to what Harry Frankfurt called ' 'the capacity for reflective self-evaluation that is manifested in the formation of second-order desires', i.e., desires as to which of my first-order desires I consider conducive to my good and therefore authentically want to be the effective motivation of my actions' (Brümmer, 1993, pp. 232–33). In that sense, I take responsibility for the characteristics that I endorse as my own.

It is characteristic of Brümmer's reasoning to state that this authenticity is a *necessary* condition for having my identity as a person, but it is not *sufficient* (emphasis in Brümmer, 1993, p. 234). And here the relational aspect of having a personal identity or being a person comes into the picture. We as humans need others in order to develop as full and authentic human beings. We are inherently social beings. We must be nurtured by others from the beginning. We can only develop and flourish in relationships with partners, friends, mates, children, colleagues, and others. I can only develop as a person to the extent that others endorse my identity and recognize me to be the person I claim to be. We need recognition and validation. My identity as a person is not a matter only in my own hands, nor is it foisted upon me by others. My identity 'is constituted by a consensus in which my claim is endorsed by others' (Brümmer, 1993, p. 234). This idea goes even a step further. It is not only the consensus by recognition of my claim to be the person I am. That recognition is also the source of the intrinsic value I have as a person and that makes me the unique and irreplaceable individual I am. This idea points at the 'human' part of the quotation of Martin Luther at the beginning of this chapter. In my own words: the love, the recognition of humans flows forth and bestows value upon the person who is loved for his or her own unique and authentic characteristics. That love is a value I cannot give myself. And this means also that I, as a person, am not only important to myself but also to someone else, who 'bestows value on me which I could otherwise not have' (Brümmer, 1993, p. 235). To quote Brümmer again: 'Since in this way both our identity and our value as persons is constituted by our relations of fellowship with others, we *need* to partake in such relationships. As persons we therefore *necessarily* long both to love and to be loved' (Brümmer, 1993, p. 235; emphasis in original).

Based on this twofold conception of personal identity, I now proceed with an inquiry of forgiveness and explain the structure of the chapter. We will see that forgiveness shares many characteristics with other attitudinal aspects of human conduct. It has its intentional and evaluative aspects motivated by prejudices, values, and profitableness and, at a more abstract level, by models and definitions. So I briefly discuss the various aspects of forgiveness under these specific headings: prejudices, values, profitableness, and models and definitions. In my view, these are the attitudinal aspects of forgiveness. They tell us something about whether, why, and how forgiveness is a characteristic of me, as the person I am. They can explain whether, why, and how forgiveness as an act of 'reflective self-evaluation' could bring about a change in the 'desires I consider conducive to my good' and, therefore, could bring about a change in the motivation of my actions. These are necessary aspects by which to understand forgiveness in its full meaning. Again, my identity is constituted by a consensus in which my claim is recognized and appreciated by others. I need others to recognize and appreciate me as the person I am and, therefore, to share responsibility with me in realizing the person I am. Evil done to me is a breach in that consensus and shared responsibility. It is from this point that forgiveness is a relationship.

9.3 **Forgiveness: prejudices**

Forgiveness is no longer only a holy matter at the hands of clergy and priests, and no longer a power by which the servant of god can reopen or foreclose the door that would give entrance to ultimate happiness. In our secularized and democratized society, forgiveness has become a moral and therapeutic practice—a matter of restoring effective interpersonal agency against the background of a person's biography of choice (Giddens, 1991; de Lange, 2004). Or should we define forgiveness as a way of dealing with moral failure (Peteet, 2004)? Although undone of its religious and spiritual connotations, forgiveness seems to involve being or longing to be or to become a forgiving person. Why would that be so meaningful? What kind of values can we trace behind this longing? What is effective interpersonal agency within the perspective of forgiveness anyway? Dwelling on prejudices against forgiveness, we can get a glimpse of feasible values that might count in favor of forgiveness.

Contrasted with what people consider to be adequate interpersonal agency is weakness. That is, old objection to forgiveness is that it is a sign of weakness. This weakness could be phrased in several ways. Being forgiving is weak, because forgiving opposes the right to obtain justice, or because forgiving undermines righteousness. Another idea of the way that forgiving could be a sign of weakness is that the forgiving person does not dare to oppose to a religious imperative even though not convinced of its merits. To be sure, weakness as an objection to forgiveness has several facets that need to be considered, such as motivations, needs, morals, and so on. Moreover, the question is not only one of moral strength or weakness, but of interrelated psychological weakness based on a person's psychological make up and his or her moral and religious development. It might be important to evaluate these psychological aspects within a person who has been wronged, because of its possible effects in a therapeutic process aiming at forgiveness. Promoting forgiveness might cause harm instead of benefit. Nevertheless, any construct of forgiveness has to come to terms with this objection of weakness and has to clarify its meaning in connection with justice and righteousness.

The same is true for another prejudice against forgiveness: forgiveness as a misuse of power. I do not mean the misuse of power whereby others impose forgiveness on the forgiving person as a moral or religious obligation—as, for instance, relatives can exert pressure on an abused victim to forgive the victimizer in order to prevent the washing of one's dirty linen in public. What is meant here is the victim as forgiving person who can exert power over the victimizer by repeatedly inducing feelings of guilt, shame, and the like. This power is a kind of strength that, again, might depend on the moral and religious development of a person and might turn out to be a matter of more or less hidden revenge and a destructive attitude. Again, this is an important configuration to evaluate, because it could determine whether forgiveness will do good or will cause harm. The misuse of victim power is a risk factor. How does a construct of forgiveness get rid of this risk of a power play? While I cannot answer this question in the context of this chapter, I point to the two objections to forgiveness, of weakness and misuse of power, to psychological factors, which can be summarized in the question regarding characteristics of mature or immature forgiveness and a psychological healthy development. Just for precaution: I do not mean to suggest that prejudices like these two are always related to psychological immaturity. But in the context of therapy, it is important to evaluate that possibility. Preliminary results of empirical research confirm the intuition that this is an important topic of clinical relevance. Mauger and colleagues (1992) already found in the early nineties that deficits in the ability to forgive others and oneself are related to symptoms of psychopathology.

Enright (1991) considered several prejudices against forgiveness: forgiveness as a reversal of societal justice, forgiveness as a block to personal justice, forgiveness as perpetuating injustice, forgiveness as a logical impossibility, forgiveness as inducing inferiority in the other and in self, forgiveness as lack of respect for others, forgiveness as alienation from our true aggressive nature, forgiveness as producing hypersensitivity to interpersonal hurt. All these 'insinuations' are far from being hypothetical only. On the contrary, many misunderstandings and distortions concerning forgiveness exist despite centuries of catechesis.

I conclude this paragraph by stressing that it is not all difficult to recognize these powerful objections to forgiveness. Confirming my thesis, most of these objections seem to refer to the attitudinal aspects of forgiveness. And these are important enough. But they do not adequately illustrate the importance of the value of the persons involved as persons. Evil is not just done to my emotional needs, moral standards, sensitivity, personal values, and so on. That might be true, but evil done to me goes further than that. I do not want to forgive just because of wrongdoing to my moral standards, view of life, and so on, although that may also be the case. Forgiveness is about 'I and Thou'. I could decide to forgive you despite disagreements over moral standards, or despite personal conflicts, because of an intimate concern about the continuance of our relationship.

9.4 **Forgiveness: values–based**

It is very interesting to discern values involved in thinking about the place of forgiveness in our lives. In what preceded, only nonepistemic values emerged. Nonepistemic values, in contrast to epistemic values, derive from cultural sources (sexual values, racial values, religious values, and so on). Epistemic values are 'truth-seeking values', presumed to promote the truth like the character of science (Ruse, 1999, pp. 30–2). When one looks at the context in which forgiveness (re)appears (see Section 9.1), or the context in which it is studied, it becomes clear that constructs and definitions of forgiveness are partly constituted by social and (sub)cultural needs, and that this blending becomes encoded in the assumptions of research workers. Take, for instance, the cultural context and needs as formulated in a volume such as *Dimensions of Forgiveness* (Worthington, 1998a). The author states that the project is dedicated to the 'scientific foundations of *effective living— how positive mindsets* and *virtues* enhance the *lives of individuals* and, ultimately, the *well-being of society*'. And 'future volumes (. . .) will focus on *optimism* and *hope, wisdom,* and other *life-changing positive states*.' Forgiveness is 'one of the *most life-affirming choices*' we can make (Worthingtona, 1998, pp. ix–x; emphasis added). And what about the next line of thinking: 'We are also cautiously optimistic that this *scientific* understanding might be used to *improve the lot of humanity*' (McCullough *et al.*, 2000a, p. xiv; emphasis added)? These few lines clearly illustrate a set of values and I assume that it fits very well with what has been called the positive psychology movement with its claim to study what is good for humanity. This idea of promoting the good seems to have its roots in eudaimonism. The psychiatrist Cloninger seems to have become one of the new champions of 'The Science of Well-Being' that can be traced back to Plato, Aristotle, and Augustine (Cloninger, 2004). But what is a good life, what is the good than which there is nothing better?

Although as a concept, the content of the good is unclear, practically speaking it is certainly meaningful enough to strive for. It is an element of a view of life. A view of life has a structuring function, insofar as it implies goals to reach for, and it has a regulative function insofar as it provides a life direction, that is, a personal way of living. This is the way in which a concept of the good, valued as part of a view of life—that is, as a comprehensive framework of intentions, norms, values, ideals, and beliefs—is existentially suitable. In this context, the content of the good, or ultimate happiness, could be described as the ideal in achieving, through which one hopes to realize one's individual identity as a person. And, as I stated before, we need our personal ideals to be endorsed and validated by others. So my plea is not against eudaimonism as such, but in favor of intersubjective eudaimonism.

Forgiveness is a more or less dormant element in such a view of life but may awaken with a shock when somebody has been offended. Perhaps it is possible to promote forgiveness without any reference to religious or spiritual concepts, but it is clearly impossible to do so without any reference to a view of life.

In addition to the nonepistemic values, epistemic values are also at stake. One of these epistemic values is the urgency for validity of a concept, i.e., the degree of accordance with our best clinical evidence. Evidence-based medicine is not restricted to the golden standard of the randomized clinical trial or to meta-analysis. The entire method is based on the idea that it is extraordinarily helpful for clinicians and therapists to provide us with the current best evidence in making decisions about the care of individual patients and in a careful use of the patients' preferences in making decisions about their care (Sackett *et al.*, 1996). So when the patient asks for help in becoming a forgiving person, or wants to learn how to grant forgiveness, or how to seek forgiveness, on what grounds is the clinician willing to advise such a patient? According to evidence-based medicine, we do so based on integrating clinical expertise and best external evidence, and with respect for the patients' values. This confronts us not just with the problematic search for evidence. The clinical expertise and attitude in matters of forgiveness is problematic as well.

It is important to be aware of values involved and how diverse they might be and the various ways that values have an impact on experiences and relationships. They inform us about a person's ethos, which is part of our personal identity. Values guide the selection or evaluation of actions, people, and events. In connection with our topic they tell us about the weighted possibility of choosing for or against forgiveness.

9.5 Forgiveness: evidence-based

What kind of evidence can we find in the literature concerning forgiveness besides opinion (or even credulity) based claims? By 'opinion-based' claims, I mean utterances like the one stated by Richards and Bergin that 'despite the relative lack of empirical evidence, we *do believe* that forgiveness is a powerful healing practice, and we *endorse* its careful use in psychotherapy' (Richards and Bergin, 1997, p. 213; emphasis added). I call a statement like this one an 'opinion-based' claim because it lacks an explicit critical appraisal of research.

Worthington conducted two reviews of published empirical research on religious counseling (Worthington, 1986; Worthington et al., 1996). In 1986, he concluded that techniques within religious counseling, and among these techniques regarding forgiveness, have not been well researched. He mentioned just one study as an example. The author worked systematically, which among other things means that he informs his readers about his procedure of the search. As a result, the overall impression is that the research under review revealed a lack of quality.

A decade later, Worthington and his colleagues found that the methodological quality of the research had improved except in outcome studies (Worthington, 1986; Worthington et al., 1996). Nine studies investigating forgiveness are listed this time. The authors made several observations. For instance, research on forgiveness during that period appeared equally in religious and in general psychological journals. Research programs on forgiveness had been developed and were still running. The authors paid attention to their own research program and described two concepts of forgiveness they used in psychoeducational group interventions: forgiveness as helpful in self-enhancement and forgiveness as helpful in restoration of interpersonal functioning. Both interventions generated more forgiveness, but the self-enhancement construct did better than the restoration construct. The authors made an important caveat. Only two studies tested the effectiveness of granting forgiveness in a nonclinical population. Seeking forgiveness was only reported in social psychological literature. In other words, by that time (1996), most evidence was based only on recommendations, case studies, opinions, and, not to forget, credulity.

In 2000, McCullough et al. (2000c) reported in an overview of existing measures of forgiveness that measurements for forgiveness were still improving, but in terms of a (systematic) review, there was not much news to tell. But there are different levels of evidence and there is more to consider when contrasting systematic reviews with credulity based claims. Enright and colleagues published intervention studies using his process model of forgiveness (Enright and Coyle, 1998; the first one of these intervention studies was already accounted for in the second review by Worthington et al., [1996]). That study demonstrated that, in an experimental group of 24 elderly women, higher forgiveness profiles on two forgiveness scales were found. These women suffered from a wide variety of injustices in different relationships. The study also showed a reduction of depression and anxiety. It was that first study (published in 1993, reviewed by Enright and Coyle, 1998, p.147) that showed that forgiveness could be promoted for therapeutic goals. The next three studies were done with different types of offended persons (students, female incest victims, men hurt by the abortion decision of a partner) and different offenses (the students grown up with emotionally absent parents). The studies suggested that forgiveness can be taught and can be favorable for mental health by improvement in variables such as hope and self-esteem and by a decline in anxiety and depression. So one could conclude that the promotion of forgiveness enhances psychological well-being.

Critical questions about this conclusion come from a social psychological perspective (Karremans *et al.*, 2003, 2005; Karremans and Van Lange, 2004). These questions concern the selection of participants and the type of relationships involved. As we saw, participants had experienced rather intense forms of interpersonal offense in close relationships. What does that mean for the claim that forgiving enhances psychological well-being? Is forgiving also associated with well-being among individuals with less intense forms of interpersonal offense, and other types of relationships such as less exclusive ones? (According to Karremans *et al.* (2003), the already mentioned 1993 study (see Enright and Coyle, 1998) did not exclusively include close relationships. In that particular study no significant difference in psychological well-being was found between the experimental and control groups.)

How can we understand in what way, when, and why, forgiving enhances psychological well-being? The hypothesis in these Dutch studies is that forgiving is associated with enhanced levels of psychological well-being when a person experiences a strong commitment to the offender. The association is less pronounced or even absent when a person experiences weak commitment to the offender. In addition, it is suggested that the failure to forgive others to whom we experience strong commitment induces high levels of psychological tension, which in turn may be associated with reduced psychological well-being.

The framework for forgiving in this social psychological model is the interdependence theory. In short, relationships may be challenged by the degree of correspondence of outcomes—that is, the degree to which preferences among individuals correspond versus conflict. This means that, when preferences do not correspond, insufficient appreciation of the partner's needs can easily result in conflict that frequently is accompanied by blaming the other. In light of such an experience, people tend to react in a self-interested manner. At this point, movement away from these given self-interested preferences can only result from a transformation of motivation within that person, in that transformed motives entail broader considerations such as the well-being of the relationship. The relationship-relevant feature that serves as a major factor in the transformation of motivation seems to be commitment, defined as the intention to persist in a relationship, including long-term orientation and feelings of attachment to the partner. Commitment is an important predictor of willingness for accommodation, to make sacrifices, to hold more or less realistic positive beliefs about the relationship, and to shift in thinking from 'I' to 'we'. For this reason, it is likely that not forgiving is in contradiction with strong commitment, creating psychological discomfort.

The findings in this study suggest the following (Karremans *et al.*, 2003). Forgiving does not occur in an interpersonal vacuum. The psychological consequences of forgiving need to be considered in the light of one's commitment to the relationship. The implication for counseling and therapy as to whether or not to recommend interpersonal forgiving is that the question cannot be answered without taking into consideration the nature of the relationship. And there is complementary evidence available, found in the same study, that suggests that the benefits of forgiveness are partner specific, which means that in the context of marital relationships, tendencies toward forgiving one's spouse exhibit a more pronounced association with psychological well-being than tendencies to forgive others in general.

This kind of 'best available evidence' is indeed of interest and great help for the clinician who has to decide about the kind of therapy for this or that patient who asks about the granting or seeking of forgiveness.

9.6 Forgiveness: models or paradigms

In the face of the possible, even idiosyncratic, definitions and constructs of forgiveness we have to consider a full range of models or paradigms (Konstam *et al.*, 2002).

Developmental models

A developmental paradigm focuses on the more or less successful transitions during life span. Based on the Eriksonian paradigm, for example, moral and faith development are of special interest (Fowler, 1981; Imoda, 1998; Kernberg, 2000). But we have to proceed cautiously here. As Lamb (2002) explained, models like the pyramid model developed by Worthington and the process model of Enright are not developmental models in the classic sense. The idea is that forgiveness can be learned. The stages of these forgiveness education models are based on 'philosophers' and clinicians' views of what does and does not constitute forgiveness' (Enright and Coyle, 1998, p. 154). In fact, this approach has very little to do with the traditional developmental stages and possible stage-specific characteristics of forgiveness. Nevertheless, originally Enright started with the presentation of such a traditional moral developmental model that he called a 'social cognitive-developmental stage model' of forgiveness, but later on he turned to a process model (Enright, 1991).

Neuroscientific models

It is interesting to note that a neurobiological paradigm also is being invoked in the understanding of forgiveness. Several lines of approach can be followed, for instance with the help of the popular stress concept and by defining forgiveness as coping with the stressor of victimization (Pargament and Rye, 1998). Forgiveness can be seen as a complex neurocognitive and affective process and, in that sense, neuropsychological functions and neural pathways are involved. In this regard, it is also important to take note of speculations from an evolutionary (Newberg et al., 2000) and an ethological perspective (De Waal, 1997). Several authors attempt to find a connection between their construct of forgiveness and neural pathways (Worthington, 1998b; Newberg et al., 2000). Worthington postulates a connection between the avoidance of forgiveness, classical conditioning, and neural pathways. The idea is that people who are hurt are classically fear conditioned, like the famous rat of Pavlov. Unforgiveness is based on that fear conditioning and avoidance. Newberg et al. (2000) posited their construct in a broader way. For them, forgiveness always concerns an injury that has been inflicted upon a person's self. This is an important aspect that, in general, is hidden behind other factors that might exert great influence on the process, e.g., a person's personality, self-monitoring, and self esteem. This means that a sense of self is always involved in connection with the ability to evaluate behavior as being injurious and the memory of the event. Which brain functions and areas are involved in processes like the formation of memories about emotional experiences? The anatomy of emotion includes several brain regions: the amygdala, the thalamus, and the cortex. These regions interact to create memories about fearful experiences. The intervention strategy to promote forgiveness is said to be based on the idea of extinction of the fear conditioning. Extinction is an active learning process. Such learning is supposed to be situated in the brain between the prefrontal cortex and the amygdala. But as a complex process based on a broad mixture of emotional, cognitive, and developmental ingredients, forgiveness cannot be traced back to a single track in connection with this or that neural substrate. When we take into account this complexity, it is more appropriate to look at the idea of a state of mind. A state of mind can be defined as 'a pattern of recruited systems within the brain responsible for (1) perceptual bias, (2) emotional tone and regulation, (3) memory processes, (4) mental models, and (5) behavioral response patterns' (Siegel, 1999). For example, if an individual had been severely injured, a state of despair or fear may have come upon him or her and become engrained. Perception of the self, the other, and the world around him or her are colored by that fear, resulting in being overcome with shame, denial, and a sense a destruction. Speechlessness may paralyze (Glas, Chapter 8). A model of self may say things like 'I cannot protect myself, I am vulnerable, I am helpless'. Emotions are aroused, alerting for harm. Memories may evoke additional experiences. Denial and splitting may be necessary to struggle to one's feet and to keep oneself upright. The behavioral tendency might be withdrawal. Minor events might activate this state again and again. And so the pattern, including the brain activation, becomes a part of the individual's history.

Cognitive-behavioral and psychodynamic models

The cognitive-behavioral approach focuses on changing one's thinking in order to change one's feelings and behavior. It is quite easy to recognize this way of thinking in the many definitions and step programs to promote forgiveness (Lamb, 2002). Cognitive-behavioral paradigms seem to predominate—although, as we will see, the intrapsychic paradigm has still its own contribution to the description of forgiveness insofar as psychodynamic processes are involved.

A rather typical and worthy example of this line of thinking can be found in the paper written by the psychoanalyst Salmon Akhtar in 2002 (Akhtar, 2002; cf. Kernberg, 2000). The ideas can be illustrated with a few lines from his way of reasoning. Akhtar writes that, in dealing with forgiving, one is immediately faced with the psychology of someone who has something to forgive. And that psychology can be depicted in Kleinian terms, as a move from the paranoid to the depressive position. The move during the therapeutic process toward that depressive position is of special importance for advancing forgiveness. In the depressive position (but not the paranoid position), one can acknowledge that the self is not all good and the other not all bad. A capacity for empathy thus appears on the horizon. And there also emerge feelings of gratitude for what one has received, guilt and sadness for having hurt others, and reparative longings to redress the damage done. Reality testing improves, and the capacity for reciprocal relationships develops. These are all necessary conditions that might bring the possibility of forgiveness closer. According to Akhtar, revenge is taken by the patient in the form of relentless sadistic assaults on the analyst. Reparation is available to the patient in the form of the analyst's lasting empathy that survives these attacks. Reconsideration results from recontextualization and revision of childhood memories. These three factors: revenge, reparation, and reconsideration, are important in allowing the advance from traumatized victimhood to forgiveness. But Akhtar does not mention anything about forgiving and seeking forgiveness other than in the therapeutic relationship, in the transference to the therapist. What about forgiving and seeking forgiveness in real life, and in an effective way between victim and offender? In fact, we would not expect anything a model to offer less; can we hold that Akhtar's theory is what forgiveness is all about? I do not think so. The psychological construct in this or other forms and in these or other words formulated is a necessary but not sufficient condition for forgiveness. What appears to be promoted in therapy is a willingness or preparedness to forgive; forgivingness instead of forgiving. In other words, therapy, like psychoanalytic treatment, works toward expanding capacities for agency—for instance, the capacity to forgive—and toward diminishing constraints of internal forces (Cavell, 2003).

Preparedness for forgiveness can be liberated or promoted in therapy. This is, in fact, not far from what is formulated and aimed at according to cognitive-behavioral approaches. Worthington affirms: 'I am interested in *interventions to promote forgiveness*' (Worthington, 1998b, p. 108; emphasis in original). The unforgiving person, according to his psychological construct, is classically fear conditioned, that is to say fear conditioning is at the root of much unforgiveness. And that fear conditioning motivates avoidance and revenge and makes the individual unfree.

I probably could add other models or paradigms, but it is not my aim to present an exhaustive overview. My position is that forgiveness cannot properly be discussed without the interpersonal or relational paradigm. It is my main focus, but I will come to that in Section 9.8. I conclude this section with a short comment from a more philosophical perspective. It seems to me that one of the reasons for the rediscovery of forgiveness might be the growing sense that the once-prevalent idea about human persons as self-sufficient— the notion of atomism as Taylor (1985) called it—or individualism, as it is usually named, has had its day; we are social beings and not self-sufficient alone. This is important to note: humans are not self-sufficient but social beings. We can only develop our human capacities in relationships with others. In therapy, this idea of self-sufficiency can be traced back to the central notion of 'working through' that enables the evolution from insight to structural change in individual or in group psychotherapy. Whatever you have to work through you, do it in a therapeutic relationship and, in such a way, you eventually will become more autonomous, more self-sufficient. But this could be labeled and valued as a highly atomistic stance. In his discussions of the possibilities and impossibilities of Christian counseling, the philosopher Evans pointed at a similar criticism: contemporary approaches of psychotherapy are far too focused on the well-being and satisfaction of individuals, and far too little focused on our relatedness to others, 'and the framework of obligations these relations create.' On his view, it would be wrong to emphasize that forgiveness is something to be done for your own well-being. Although forgiveness might have that effect, such an emphasis in any motivation program for the promotion of forgiveness would be in the wrong place (Evans, 1996, p. 105).

9.7 Forgiveness: definitions

Given the variety of prejudices, values, models, and paradigms, it is hardly surprising that definitions of forgiveness are quite diverse. In addition, it is quite clear that a lot of work remains to be done on epistemic values such as internal and external consistency, unifying power of the concept, and predictive accuracy. Yet there seems to be a growing consensus; forgiveness is a complex construct that certainly is not unidimensional. It is bidimensional or even multidimensional. I will look now at a few definitions of forgiveness in search of this dimensionality.

At the core of almost all definitions of forgiveness, we will find the idea of a change of attitude, or a transformation of motivation, toward the transgressor. But as Fincham and Beach (2002) explain, in research forgiveness is most often conceptualized as unidimensional. The overcoming of resentment, feelings of revenge and other negative feelings and attitudes are the core of forgiveness; forgiveness is the overcoming of unforgivingness. This dimension of overcoming or counteracting avoidance, or removing internal barriers towards the wrongdoer, is rather typical for the definitions that follow. Fincham and Beach call it the negative dimension. Does it seem reasonable to look for a positive dimension as well? Fincham and Beach call this aspect the dimension of goodwill or an approach toward the offender *as a person* (emphasis my own). This is an important notion for our inquiry. The positive dimension is only a genuine dimension when it is not just a lack of avoidance. In order to be a real dimension, it should have its own determinants and characteristics. I hypothesize that the positive dimension of forgiveness is connected with the value of the (close) relationship and that forgiveness is important in endorsing the meaning of that value, notwithstanding the offense against and breach of the relationship.

Intervention programs to promote forgiveness seem to require a so-called negative, unidimensional definition. For those, forgiveness is '. . . a motivation to reduce avoidance of and withdrawal from a person who has hurt us, as well as the anger, desire for revenge, and urge to retaliate against that person.' (Worthington, 1998b, p. 108).

The second definition is characterized by a bidimensional approach: 'Forgiveness can be conceptualized at two different levels: (1) the inner, intrapsychic dimension involving the victim's emotional state (and the cognitive and behavioral accompaniments), and (2) the interpersonal dimension involving the ongoing relationship within which forgiveness takes place or fails to do so.' (Baumeister *et al.*, 1998, p. 80).

The inner dimension of forgiving is to cease feeling angry or resentful. The social dimension means the return, if possible, toward a meaningful and significant relationship beyond the transgression. Crucial in these approaches is the inner change of the victim, indicated by expressions such as change of heart, change of motivation, change of insight, or even religious conversion.

The same notion of inner change can be recognized when forgiving is defined as a form of (religious) coping: 'Forgiving is transformational in both the ends that are sought [peace of mind and peace with others] and in the means that are used to reach these ends [transformation of motivation].' (Pargament and Rye, 1998, p. 63).

In addition to the two dimensions already mentioned (internal change, interpersonal act), several definitions take into account a more or less explicit moral emphasis: 'In genuine forgiveness, one (. . .) chooses to abandon his or her right to resentment and retaliation, and instead offers mercy to the offender. [Forgiveness] is decidedly moral, concerned with good of human interaction.' (Enright and Coyle, 1998, p. 140), and 'Forgiveness is the recognition of the guilt of the offender and the forswearing of the moral right of revenge or retaliation.' (Glas, Chapter 8).

A last example is the definition proposed by Worthington *et al.* (2000). It is an interesting example for our purposes because of distinctions proposed between forgiveness, interpersonal forgiveness and reconciliation. The authors define: '. . . interpersonal forgiveness [is] a motivation to reduce avoidance of and retaliation (or revenge) against a person who has harmed or offended one, and to increase conciliation between the parties if conciliation is safe, prudent, or possible.' (Worthington *et al.*, 2000, p. 229).

Different from Baumeister *et al.* (1998), these authors use the term 'forgiveness transactions,' distinct from interpersonal forgiveness, to refer to all actions that people need and use to clarify whether granting and seeking forgiveness is at stake. In that sense, forgiveness transactions may or may not lead to a process of reconciliation.

When someone forgives another person because of a violation, it is the forgiver who changes, in his thoughts, feelings, motivations, and so on. But our spokesmen in the above paragraph also put into words the tension presented with such a unidimensional construct. Forgiveness is not just an intrapersonal change; it must be interpersonal as well. Forgiveness is something necessarily in relation not to something but to someone else. Otherwise it is not forgiveness in the complete sense I am looking for. This is why I do not agree with Worthington (1998b), who stated that forgiveness occurs within an individual, and reconciliation within a relationship. The latter is true, the former not. According to my view, intrapersonal change is indeed a necessary condition for forgiveness, but it is not a sufficient condition.

Forgiveness has a dual character; it is both an inner psychic phenomenon and an interpersonal act. The same goes for other psychological phenomena such as trust or empathy. What is the meaning of trust or empathy or forgiveness if there is no important other in whom we trust, or with whom we empathize, or whom we are willing to forgive? Without the other, such trust or empathy or forgiveness would not be real or effective. Even if one were to object by saying self-trust and empathy toward oneself do not require the other, I am not so sure that that would hold true. 'In the beginning is the relation', I quoted before. Self-trust and empathy toward oneself are fostered from the beginning by attachment to the other (Siegel, 1999). Therefore, any construct of forgiveness has to take this dual character of forgiveness into account.

Until this point of inquiry, we did not meet an adequate interpersonal model for forgiveness, although we found some important empirical data that hint in the direction of such a model. It is high time to consider now a relational model for forgiveness.

9.8 A relational model for forgiveness

I take the relational model proposed by Brümmer (Brümmer, 1992, 1993, 2005; Schreurs, 2002) to be very helpful for our purpose. This typology has deep roots in the history of Christian thinking, for instance in the work of Bernard of Clairvaux (1090–1153). Looking at relationships, we are going to separate analytically three basic types of relationships between people although, in reality, human relations are nearly always a mixture of these three basic types. The purpose of my inquiry is not this categorization as such but to find an adequate concept that can help us to understand the bidimensional structure of forgiveness. Once we are able to analyze the structure of a person's relationship with the transgressor, then we can also specify in what way the transgression can be dealt with and the breach in the relationship healed. We can specify the implied challenges and how these challenges may create opportunities either for forgiveness or for creating problems, depending on factors such as personality factors, relational factors, and event factors. If, for instance, a therapist finds that a patient's relationship with another is debilitating or tyrannical and, as such, obstructs that person's mental and spiritual well-being, then the therapist can help such a person discover what this same relationship really looks like and how this relationship could also lead to another, more healthy way of relating. Therefore, I shall try to indicate how we can use this typology of human relationships to connect with forgiveness.

The first type is what Brümmer calls the manipulative relationship. It is an important type of relation in the sense that this relation is asymmetrical; only one partner is the agent, who has almost complete control or power over the other, who has become the object of the agent's manipulative power. Only the agent is personal, the other is object. That is the way in which this relation is an impersonal one. The agent in the manipulative relationship is the one who can start, change, or terminate the relationship. What happens when things go wrong, then—when one or the other is offended? Can we speak in a proper way of forgiveness or seeking forgiveness? That appears to be very difficult, depending on our construct of forgiveness. In a manipulative relationship, the passive partner is an object 'to be managed, cured or trained' by the partner in control (Brümmer, 1993, p. 158). When the passive partner is the offender, it is up to the partner in control to decide how to respond, and by managing or training successfully the breach in the relationship, he will get all the credit. If he does not suceed, he is the one to bear the blame (Brümmer, 1992, p. 439). Only one is responsible, and only he is a candidate for both praise and blame. But with regard to genuine forgiveness—which actually is almost impossible in this kind of relationship—the victim or passive partner is often manipulated or coerced into forgiving, for instance, in the name of paternal authority, or in the name of God. Incest victims in certain religious groups are often forced to forgive, although, and quite rightly, there is, in no way, talk of an inner process of becoming willing to forgive. Or the victim is manipulated with the offender's penitence for God. 'I confessed my sin before God; He forgave me, so now you have to forgive me, would you resist the wisdom of God?' And, as you might expect, the offender is praised for his sincerity or is pitied for the unwillingness of the victim. But what is the meaning of such penitence without seeking forgiveness from the victim? It is difficult to take such penitence to be genuine and sincere, and clearly it cannot be effective as a sincere and convincing expression of guilt and taking responsibility for damaging the relationship.

Treated as an object one could easily take an attitude of passivity. On the other hand, perhaps it is possible, even when one is not in a position to act as a free and responsible person, to choose a certain attitude and develop the inner qualities it requires; that is, to cultivate the inner freedom of being a person.

Without doubt, some people reach an impressive inner strength despite the manipulative relation they have to endure (Schreurs, 2002).

This first type of impersonal relationship corresponds with the relation of slavery, as typified by Bernard of Clairvaux. It is a relation between lord and slave, in which the latter is the property of the former, and servitude is motivated by fear for one's skin (Clairvaux, 1126/1127, republished in Clairvaux, 1995).

But real and effective forgiveness is reserved for personal relationships. In personal relationships, the situation is very different from impersonal relationships in that the people in relation both are free personal agents. Before going on it is important to keep in mind that human relationships are always a mixture of characteristics of the three basic types of relationships. It would be an oversimplification to suggest that we could sustain one of them in its purity. We can be quite inconsistent in our relationships (Brümmer, 1992, p. 436). We can distinguish two types of such personal relationships. The first one is the relation based on agreements of rights and duties. In this type of relation, my partner and the relationship as well have an instrumental value, as means for furthering my own interests. But each partner acknowledges the freedom and responsibility of the other as well as his own dependence on the other for maintaining the relationship. In this situation, an offence is a matter of neglect or refusal to perform one's duties and/or to respect the other's rights. And in such circumstances the offended partner has the right to withhold whatever he or she has promised to deliver. The offended partner has now the right to punish the offending partner for breaking his or her promise. But in fact, there are three ways in which the broken balance of rights and duties in a personal relationship can be restored: you satisfy my rights, I punish you, or I condone what you have done. This second type of relationship corresponds to the relation between a hireling and his boss, according to the terminology of Bernard of Clairvaux. The hireling cares for what is good to him and thinks only of himself, he performs his duties and he wants his rights to be respected.

At this point, we run into a confusion that requires illumination. There are several words in circulation that seem to come close to some an idea of forgiveness, but at the end they do not encompass forgiveness at all. Words like: pardoning, forgetting, denying, and condoning. What is, then, the difference between condoning and forgiving? A willingness to forgive implies that you consider the breach in a relationship a greater evil than the injury that has been done to you and, therefore, are willing to continue identifying with the other person and treating his or her interests as your own in spite of what he or she has done to you. Such forgiveness can only be genuine if there is something to forgive. Unless I really caused you injury by failing to seek your interests as my own, it would make no sense to say that you forgive me. Herein lies the difference between forgiveness and condonation. If you were to condone my action, you would thereby deny that it is an action that caused you real injury, and thus deny that there is anything to forgive. Condoning, as Brümmer suggests, belongs to the repairing of the rights and duties balance and is typical for the contractual relationship. By condoning I say that the failure of the other is of no importance to my interests. An amendation of the contract might be necessary, but that will be all (Brümmer, 1992, p. 440). If, on the other hand, you forgive me for what I have done, you claim that my action did cause you injury, but that you would rather bear the injury than abandon the relationship that I have damaged by my action. Forgiveness entails that you give up your right to pay me back or to punish me, as you would do when our relation was of the 'rights and duties' type. Forgiveness must be bought at a price; it must be paid for with the suffering of him or her who has been wronged. The one who forgives is the primary one who suffers. Forgiveness costs you something whereas condonation is a denial that there are any serious costs involved (Brümmer, 1992, p. 440). The same reasoning goes for the other terms I mentioned, pardoning, excusing, and forgetting. In this verbal usage, the important differences between these words and forgiving might be blurred. But what has been called 'the recall of the hurt' as an essential part of the forgiving process becomes softened or is denied. And, most importantly, in condonation, the price to be paid by the victim is eliminated. Forgiveness occurs when the injured person is able to 'view the wrongdoer with compassion and love while recognizing that he, the wrongdoer, has willfully abandoned his right to them' (Enright and Coyle, 1998, p. 140; McCullough *et al.*, 2000b; Murphy, 2003).

The discussion about words and the constructs behind them brings me to the second type of personal relationships: the relationship of fellowship or mutual love. Bernard of Clairvaux used another metaphor for this type of relationship: the relationship not between the slave and the mercenary, or the between the hireling and his master, but between the son and the father. 'Charity is found only in the son', declares Bernardus. 'Charity converts souls because it makes them act willingly' (Clairvaux, 1995, p. 36). The most characteristic element of this type of relationship is the fact that I identify with the other and treat his or her interests as my own. The value of the other and the value of the relationship are intrinsic for me. Neither the other nor the relationship can be replaced by someone else. In this relation of fellowship the partners appreciate and value each other for no other reason than for the persons they are, without obligations! In that sense relations of fellowship are the ground for the development of highly personal relational qualities as for instance love, trust, security, receptivity (Schreurs, 2002). For these reasons, great differences exist between this type and the 'rights and duties' relationship, even though both are personal and symmetrical. First of all, although not coercive as in the manipulative relationship, the nature of the 'rights and duties' relationship is one of agreements that create obligations. In contrast, in fellowship, it is not the obligation but my freely identifying with the other that binds us, a relation that cannot be enforced. Secondly, fellowship or mutual love is riskier than an agreement. If you refuse my fellowship, you reject *me*. This goes even a step further. Emotions like love, hatred, or grief are highly personal. In other words, my fellowship involves me as a person, because it involves my personally bestowing value on the other. Love, an old and not only Christian claim, not only *recognizes* value in its subject, but also *creates* value in its object! For these important reasons, in fellowship my future actions toward the other do not depend on the other's merits in accordance with rights and duties but, instead, depend on me. And so in becoming unfaithful to the relationship, I also become unfaithful to myself. Fourthly, fellowship is risky because the relationship depends on the partners remaining not only faithful to each other, but also to the identity that they adopt in identifying with each other. The risk is given by the fact that circumstances of our lives could give rise to changes in our identity; partners can grow apart in the course of time. A last characteristic of the relationship of fellowship is that it is a relationship between persons. Brümmer, following P.F. Strawson, makes a distinction between an objective attitude in which we treat things as an object and a personal attitude toward persons, who are the bearers of all those personal characteristics (being free, as moral beings, and who initiate and bear responsibility for their actions) that are the necessary condition for being approached as persons (Brümmer, 1993, p. 158). 'To adopt the objective attitude to another human being is to see him, perhaps, as an object of social policy; as a subject of what, in a wide range of sense, might be called *treatment*; as something . . . to be managed or handled or *cured or trained*' (Brümmer, 2005; emphasis added).

As I said above, forgiveness can only be genuine if there is something to forgive, it can only be freely given, and there is a price to be paid. Inherent in this idea of forgiveness is, of course, a desire for reciprocity, the willingness to identify with me as the offended. Fellowship, in fact, can only be restored effectively if the offender, in his identifying with me the offended, is willing to seek forgiveness. To reiterate what I stated in section two (9.2), real forgiveness is embedded in our relatedness, which relatedness is constitutive for being the person I am. It means that I as the person I am matter regardless of differences of any kind.

9.9 **Conclusions**

In our inquiry after constructs, models and definitions of forgiveness, and evidence for its usefulness and meaningfulness, we found a highly adequate relational model of forgiveness. Its efficacy is that it is free of contradiction and that it is able to unify a mixture of moral, psychological, and social–psychological elements in a coherent way. It most certainly has the potential to offer congruence between theory and practice, through which it is a relevant model. As such, it has a certain simplicity or elegance in that it can shed light on various aspects of granting and seeking forgiveness.

Acknowledgements

First presented as a paper at the Annual Meeting of the Association for the Advancement of Philosophy and Psychiatry (AAPP) 2004, then invited to contribute to this volume, the material grew into a critical, but above all positive, appraisal of forgiveness as potentially a powerful intervention in human relationships. This stimulating enterprise would not have been possible without the necessary and fruitful suggestions and wise comments made by Dr Nancy Potter, editor of this volume, and Dr Agneta Schreurs, outstanding expert in the field of psychotherapy and spirituality.

References

Akhtar S (2002). Forgiveness: origins, dynamics, psychopathology, and technical relevance. *Psychoanalytic Quarterly*, **71**: 175–212.

Baumeister RE, Exline JJ and Sommer KL (1998). The victim role, grudge theory, and two dimensions of forgiveness. In: *Dimensions of Forgiveness, Psychological Research and Theological Perspectives* (ed. EL Worthington), pp. 79–104. Philadelphia, PA: Templeton Foundation Press.

Brümmer V (1992). Atonement and reconciliation. *Religious Studies*, **28**: 435–52.

Brümmer V (1993). *The Model of Love. A Study in Philosophical Theology*. New York: Cambridge University Press.

Brümmer V (2005). *Atonement, Christology and the Trinity: Making Sense of Christian Doctrine*. Aldershot (UK): Ashgate Publishing.

Cavell M (2003). Freedom and forgiveness. *International Journal of Psychoanalysis*, **84**: 515–31.

Clairvaux B (1995). *On Loving God. An Analytical Commentary by Emero Stiegman*. Kalamazoo, MI: Cistercian Publications. (Original work published in 1126–27.)

Cloninger CR (2004). *Feeling Good. The Science of Well-Being*. New York: Oxford University Press.

Enright RD (1991). The Moral Development of Forgiveness. In: *Handbook of Moral Behavior and Development*, Volume 1: *Theory* (eds WM Kurtines and JL Gewirtz), pp. 123–52. Hillsdale, NJ: Lawrence Erlbaum Associates, Publishers.

Enright RD and Coyle CT (1998). Researching the process model of forgiveness within psychological interventions. In: *Dimensions of Forgiveness, Psychological Research and Theological Perspectives* (ed. EL Worthington), pp. 139–61. Philadelphia, PA: Templeton Foundation Press.

Evans CS (1996). Christian Counseling as Aid to Character Formation. In: *Psyche and Faith. Beyond Professionalism* (eds PJ Verhagen and G Glas), pp. 101–17. Zoetermeer: Uitgeverij Boekencentrum.

Fincham FD and Beach SRH (2002). Forgiveness in marriage: Implications for psychological aggression and constructive communication. *Personal Relationships*, **9**: 239–51.

Fowler JW (1981). *Stages of Faith: The Psychology of Human Development and the Quest for Meaning.* San Francisco, CA: Harper and Row Publishers.

Giddens A (1991). *Modernity and Self-Identity. Self and Society in the Late Modern Age.* Stanford, CA: Stanford University Press.

Glas G (2006). Elements of a phenomenology of evil and reconciliation. In: *Trauma, Truth and Reconciliation: Healing Damaged Relationships* (ed. N Potter), pp. 171–202. Oxford: Oxford University Press.

Imoda Fr (1998). *Human Development. Psychology and Mystery.* Leuven: Peeters Publishers.

Jones JW (1996). *Religion and Psychology in Transition. Psychoanalysis, Feminism, and Theology.* New Haven: Yale University Press.

Karremans JC and Van Lange PAM (2004). Back to caring after being hurt: the role of forgiveness. *European Journal of Social Psychology*, **34**: 207–27.

Karremans JC, Van Lange PAM, Ouwerkerk JW, and Kluwer ES (2003). When forgiving enhances psychological well-being: The role of interpersonal commitment. *Journal of Personality and Social Psychology*, **84**: 1011–26.

Karremans JC, Van Lange PAM, and Holland RW (2005). Forgiveness and its associations with prosocial thinking, feeling, and doing beyond the relationship with the offender. *Personality and Social Psychology Bulletin*, **20**: 1–12.

Kernberg OF (2000). Psychoanalytic perspectives on the religious experience. *American Journal of Psychotherapy*, **54**: 452–76.

Konstam V, Marx F, Schurer J, Emerson Lombardo NB, and Harrington AK (2002). Forgiveness in practice: what mental health counselors are telling us. In: *Before Forgiving, Cautionary Views of Forgiveness in Psychotherapy* (eds S Lamb and JG Murphy), pp. 54–71. New York: Oxford University Press.

Lamb S (2002). Introduction: reasons to be cautious about the use of forgiveness in psychotherapy. In: *Before Forgiving. Cautionary Views of Forgiveness in Psychotherapy* (eds S Lamb and JG Murphy), pp. 3–14. New York: Oxford University Press.

Lange F de (2004). Life as a pilgrimage. John Bunyan and the modern life course. In: *Passion of Protestants* (eds PN Holtrop, F deLange, and R Roukema), pp. 95–126. Kampen: Kok Publishing.

Luther M (1518/1957). Disputatio Heidelbergae habita. In: *Luther's Works*, Volume 31, *Career of the Reformer: I* (ed. HJ Grimm), pp. 35–70. Philadelphia, PA: Fortress Press.

Mauger PA, Freeman T, McBride AG, Perry JE, Grove DC and McKinney KE (1992). The measurement of forgiveness: preliminary research. *Journal of Psychology and Christianity*, **11**: 170–80.

McCullough ME, Pargament KI, and Thoresen CE (2000a). *Introduction. Forgiveness, Theory, Research, and Practice* (eds ME McCullough, KI Pargament, and CE Thoresen), pp. xiii–xiv. New York: The Guilford Press.

McCullough ME, Pargament KI, and Thoresen CE (2000b). The psychology of forgiveness: History, conceptual issues, and overview. In: *Forgiveness, Theory, Research, and Practice* (eds ME McCullough, KI Pargament, and CE Thoresen), pp. 1–14. New York: The Guilford Press.

McCullough ME, Hoyt WT, and Rachal KCh (2000c). What we know (and need to know) about assessing forgiveness constructs. In: *Forgiveness, Theory, Research, and Practice* (eds ME McCullough, KI Pargament, and CE Thoresen), pp. 65–88. New York: The Guilford Press.

Murphy JG (2003). *Getting Even. Forgiveness and Its Limits*. Oxford: Oxford University Press.

Newberg AB, d'Aquili AG, Newberg SK, and deMarici V (2000). The neuropsychological correlates of forgiveness. In: *Forgiveness, Theory, Research, and Practice* (eds ME McCullough, KI Pargament, and CE Thoresen), pp. 91–110. New York: The Guilford Press.

Noort van M (2003). Revenge and forgiveness in group psychotherapy. *Group Analysis*, **36**: 477–89.

Pargament KI and Rye MS (1998). Forgiveness as a method of religious coping. In: *Dimensions of Forgiveness, Psychological Research and Theological Perspectives* (ed. EL Worthington), pp. 59–78. Philadelphia, PA: Templeton Foundation Press.

Peteet JR (2004). *Doing the Right Thing. An Approach to Moral Issues in Mental Health Treatment*. Washington, DC: American Psychiatric Publishing.

Richards PS and Bergin AE (1997). *A Spiritual Strategy for Counseling and Psychotherapy*. Washington: American Psychological Association.

Ruse M (1999). *Mystery of Mysteries. Is Evolution a Social Construction?* Cambridge, MA: Harvard University Press.

Sackett DL, Rosenberg WMC, Gray JAM, Haynes RB, and Richardson WS (1996). Evidence based medicine: What it is and what it isn't. Editorials. *British Medical Journal*, **312**: 71–2.

Schreurs A (2002). *Psychotherapy and Spirituality. Integrating the Spiritual Dimension into Therapeutic Practice*. London: Jessica Kingley Publishers.

Schwöbel C (2003). *Christlicher Glaube im Pluralismus*. Tübingen: Mohr Siebeck.

Siegel DJ (1999). *The Developing Mind. How Relationships and the Brain Interact to Shape Who We Are*. New York: The Guilford Press.

Taylor C (1985). *Philosophy and the Human Sciences. Philosophical Papers 2*, pp. 187–210. Cambridge: Cambridge University Press.

Waal F de (1997). *Good natured: The Origins of Wright and Wrong in Humans and other Animals*. Cambridge, MA: Harvard University Press.

Worthington EL (1986). Religious counseling: a review of published empirical research. *Journal of Counseling and Development*, **64**: 421–31.

Worthington EL (ed.) (1998a). *Dimensions of Forgiveness, Psychological Research and Theological Perspectives*, pp. ix–x. Philadelphia, PA: Templeton Foundation Press.

Worthington EL (1998b). The pyramid model of forgiveness: Some interdisciplinary speculations about unforgiveness and the promotion of forgiveness. In: *Dimensions of Forgiveness, Psychological Research and Theological Perspectives* (ed. EL Worthington), pp. 107–37. Philadelphia, PA: Templeton Foundation Press.

Worthington EL, Kurusu TA and McCullough ME (1996). Empirical research on religion and psychotherapeutic processes and outcomes: a 10-year review and research prospectus. *Psychological Bulletin*, **119**: 448–87.

Worthington EL, Sandage SJ, and Berry JW (2000). Group interventions to promote forgiveness. What researchers and clinicians ought to know. In: *Forgiveness, Theory, Research, and Practice* (eds ME McCullough, KI Pargament, and CE Thoresen), pp. 228–53. New York: The Guilford Press.

Chapter 10

Forgiveness therapy in gendered contexts: what happens to the truth?

Sharon Lamb

10.1 Introduction

Writings on forgiveness, reparation, and reconciliation over the last several decades have come from a variety of international sociopolitical sources and are filled with discussions of the necessity for a truthful accounting of the damaging events and the harmful experiences of victims. Within the last 20 years, there has been a concurrent development in psychology in the US, where the idea of forgiveness has been promoted in clinical practice. The clinical literature on forgiveness is unlike the more general literature on forgiveness, truth, and reconciliation in one sense: it appears less interested in truth and accountability and more interested in changing internal feelings about the damaging experiences of patients.

This lack of interest in the truth may be inherent in the practice of psychotherapy which, for decades, has taken a neutral attitude toward events as they 'really happened' and focused on the events as a patient has experienced and remembered them. From the phenomenological, client-centered therapies of the 1950s and 1960s and through the 1990s cognitive therapies, psychotherapists have focused on the patient's interpretations, feelings, and cognitions somewhat independent of the actual events in the person's life. In forgiveness therapy, there is always the perception of a moral wrongdoing that needs to be understood, and those wrongdoings range from ones as seemingly minor as when a loved one has disregarded one's feelings to as significant as sexual abuse by a parent or marital infidelity. From an ethical standpoint, it is important to consider how the truth of what happened is talked about and managed within the psychotherapy. There are several reasons for this, some of which will be developed later in the chapter. But, most generally, when psychotherapists dismiss the need for an exploration of real events in favor of a rendition a client can live with or in favor of a jointly constructed narrative a couple can agree on, they may overlook ways in which the constructed narrative works against the client, and supports a cultural construction of the narrative that is biased, serving the interests of some groups over others. They also may be cutting off a moral accounting of a harm done, an accounting that speaks to larger social issues and about which discussion ought to be promoted for reasons of justice and for greater social good.

While the practice of psychotherapy may promote the suppression of particular truths, there is a second way that the truth may be neglected, distorted, or suppressed other than by individuals within a psychotherapy session, and that is within the broader project of forgiveness psychotherapy. Neither the practice of psychotherapy nor forgiving is a neutral act that has developed outside of social and political contexts. And knowledge is always 'interested,' as Sandra Harding (1991) so aptly claims: there is no knowledge-claim that exists outside of a context of knowers within power structures that permit, distort, and suppress different kinds of information as well as ways of knowing. This chapter examines both the treatment of the truth within psychotherapy sessions about forgiveness as well as within the project of promoting forgiveness in psychotherapy.

My focus is on how forgiveness therapies affect women. This interest arose from my work on issues of blame and responsibility in cases of abuse and victimization and from an observation that those advocating forgiveness therapy, many of whom are white men, use female victims of rape and sexual abuse as examples of those victims who may want unilaterally to forgive a perpetrator who is dead, gone, or unrepentant in order to attain inner relief. In earlier works, I examined the gender issues that went unnoticed in these advocates' discussions of the benefits of forgiveness and argued that women victims have special and gendered concerns that make the advocating of forgiveness problematic (Lamb, 1996, 2002).

In this chapter, I add marital therapy to the discussion of the suppression of truth within psychotherapy practices and, in particular, in relation to forgiveness therapy. The advocates of forgiveness therapy frequently use couples coping with an infidelity as another example of a domain where forgiveness can be psychologically beneficial. At first glance, couples' therapy would seem not to have the same gendered issues found in the victim/perpetrator dyad, where the victim is often female, the perpetrator male, and where acts of rape, sexual abuse, and harassment reflect power differences in a patriarchal society. After all, women in today's society have extramarital affairs almost as often as men do. Yet, as I read the clinical literature on forgiveness therapy with couples who had experienced an infidelity, I notice that every example used is of a man who had had an affair and a woman who needed to forgive him, with little attention paid to the gender imbalance and power hierarchies inherent to traditional heterosexual marriage.

The purpose of this chapter is to analyze the ways in which forgiveness therapy is advocated in two very gendered situations, victimization and marriage, without regard for the history, social lives, and practices that inform the gendered roles in these two areas. I also examine how the moral wrongdoing, or the truth of the moral wrongdoing, is treated within the sessions and within the project of forgiveness therapy, exploring ways in which this practice suppresses particular truths. Keeping in mind that sociopolitical enactments of forgiveness often require a full and truthful accounting of events before forgiveness, I query what exactly is done about the expectation of a full and truthful accounting of the acts and the harm done within the purported healing practices of forgiveness therapy. Does the lack of attention to these issues reflect a motivated ignorance of truths that would be uncomfortable to some parties within a psychotherapy session as well as within our cultural constructions of victimization and marriage?

10.2 Truth in psychotherapy: epistemology

While it might seem obvious that both patient and psychotherapist are involved in uncovering the truth behind a person's injury, this is rarely the case. In psychotherapy, not everyone comes looking for an accurate accounting of what happened to him or her. More frequently, patients want to describe their feelings and reactions to an event that hurt them and to find some relief from the pain of these feelings. In an effort to allow patients to experience and express whatever may come up in a session and to accept rather than deny their responses to life's traumas, psychotherapists are wont to say simply, 'Your feelings are your feelings.' But the truth is already obscured in that an accurate explaining of one's own pain may be impossible and frustrating to a patient trying to depict his or her pain to a therapist. The patient may not be able to find the right words to express the experience. And a patient may need to do therapeutic work reflecting on the wound before he or she has the words to express the pain; for example, it may take many sessions and much work to uncover the ways a particular harm resonates with past harms. It is possible that a person might not ever know the extent of the harm until later in life. A teen who initially may feel that a moral wrongdoing like sexual harassment perpetrated against her is 'no big deal' might later come to believe that this wrongdoing had a greater impact on her development than she had once thought. Patients often do not work consistently toward knowing the full truth of their pain or response to an injury, nor should they in all cases. There also may be times when patients adopt ways of looking at their own harm that go against their own interests.

Furthermore, psychotherapists often do not lead patients into a more accurate and detailed accounting of what happened. Unless the patient comes to therapy with the specific goal of working with the events of what actually happened (e.g., some victims of acquaintance rape pursue the question, Was this really a rape?), psychotherapists may not invest time in leading a client to examine these facts. And even when a patient does want to seek the truth of past events, a therapist may find this search for the truth somewhat irrelevant to the psychotherapeutic work, as in the early days of sexual abuse treatment, when Bass and Davis told readers who might believe they were sexually abused that if a person thinks she was abused, then in all likelihood she was (1994, p. 15) Believing in some cases that the truth is irretrievable, psychotherapists may choose instead to listen to a patient in the present as she is currently feeling and thinking about the harm. Believing that there are no simple truths of the past to be uncovered leads some psychoanalysts and psychoanalytic thinkers to discuss therapy as a process of co-constructing a narrative about a person's life history that makes sense in the present (Spence, 1982). This approach emphasizes that, because we can never discover the truth, and that in fact there isn't one truth, therapist and patient together must find a story of what happened that the patient can live with.

Even if therapists wanted to know the truth, and patients thought it important to get to the truth in order to be healed, the question remains as to whether the truth that is revealed is contaminated in some way. Therapists are trained to be acutely aware of the way the therapeutic process as well as their own interests and psychological issues may influence what can and cannot be said and experienced by a patient in a session. Therapists must constantly be aware of what truths they may be protecting themselves from seeing. Patients also protect themselves from knowing some truths. Psychoanalytic therapy traditionally works through the examination of a patient's defenses or ambivalence towards knowing the truth. The assumption is that the patient wishes that some truths remain undiscovered.

A larger question that is rarely addressed by therapists is whether the truth to be known, uncovered, or shaped in narrative between patient and therapist is also shaped by wider forces. These wider forces could include ideologies of the time and even the very practice of psychotherapy, a practice that developed in the context of particular privileged ideologies that continue to permit some statements of fact and forbid others. These social forces and practices may determine what people can know and how they can know it.

Sandra Harding (1991) claims that knowledge is interested, and so when a harm is done and the injury discussed within a psychotherapy session, we may never get 'just the facts.' There are many reasons why we may not get these facts even if we were to believe that it is possible to get an accurate and object-ive rendering of reality. Lorraine Code, in the book, *What Can She Know?* (1991), explores the possibility that knowing is gendered. She asks the ques-tion, 'what can *she* know?' to emphasize that there are implicit rules and struc-tures governing what *can* be known by a woman and that, at any given time and place, rules and structures prohibit certain acts of knowing depending on one's membership in a group. She argues that statements of facts and events are neither neutral nor objective and that the presentation of them in a neutral way masks that all knowledge is embedded in specific sets of interests. Thinking of experts and academics, she asserts that their interests are interests of a privileged group of primarily white men masking their own interests through the lens of objectivity and neutrality.

So when we extend Code's question to the practice of psychotherapy and ask 'what can she know in therapy?' we see that some aspects of psychotherapy may get in the way of truth-seeking or of a woman understanding or knowing more about the harm that befell her. It may be that, within the framework of psychotherapy, which explores some dimensions of pain and leaves other issues untouched, she can know about her own pain and the truth of this experience, but she may never know much about the political, social, and historical contexts in which those harms took place. The framework of psychotherapy usually does not include an examination of this pain within the broader contexts in which this pain is produced (Code, 1995). A patient and therapist would be likely to understand the harm, for example, of a female victim sexually abused by her father from a so-called objective perspective that depoliticizes abuse and makes it an individual act of harm or immorality or sickness. In so doing, greater social injustices that perpetuate such abuse or play a part in it are ignored and can continue to exist.

It is with these thoughts in mind that I turn to the forgiveness psychother-apy literature to examine this as a subfield within therapy that ignores context and focuses too narrowly on the individual pain and suffering of patients. I then discuss how women are treated in two varieties of forgiveness therapy: therapy with victims of abuse and therapy with married couples. Within these therapies, I argue, subjects are 'abstracted from the particularity of their circumstances' and the links between 'power and knowledge that inform hier-archical social structures' are masked (Code, 1995, p. xii). As Code asks about knowledge, I ask about the truth of a moral wrongdoing: within forgiveness therapies, is there space and climate for a variety of truths to arise, truths that may be uncomfortable to therapist and patient, truths that are rarely aired in public spaces? In 10.4, a section on victims of male violence and 10.5, a section on marital infidelity, I discuss what these truths might be and why they might be suppressed in forgiveness therapy. In forgiveness therapy for both these groups I ask, what sort of climate is created that privileges some communication and suppresses others? But first I provide an overview of forgiveness therapy.

10.3 Forgiveness in psychotherapy

Forgiveness therapy first appeared in Christian counseling journals and single case studies within a therapy setting. Its first serious treatment as a model for psychotherapy appeared within a cognitive-behavioral intervention framework (Fitzgibbons, 1986; Hope, 1987). As cognitive-behavioral therapy grew, so did interest in forgiveness as a component of cognitive-behavioral therapy for those clients who had been harmed. At this time, researchers began to promote the benefits of forgiveness therapy in spite of little research evidence that actual specific benefits existed that were attributable to forgiveness therapy or to the forgiveness component of the therapy (Worthington and DiBlasio, 1990; Hebl and Enright, 1993; Al-Mabuk et al., 1995; Freedman and Enright, 1996). The Templeton Foundation offered rewards for research that explicitly showed the benefits of forgiveness thus, in effect, paying researchers to produce scientific results that this spiritual organization hoped to be true. Forgiveness therapy received additional support from then-APA (American Psychological Association) president, Martin Seligman, the author of Learned Optimism (1991) and Authentic Happiness (2002) among other works, when he announced the Positive Psychology project that he had been working on, a project that urged psychologists to investigate and pursue research that would give us a better understanding of human strengths, including the capacity to forgive (Seligman and Csikszentmihalyi, 2000).

Research in the field of forgiveness therapy is still young, and results about its effectiveness continue to be exaggerated. Take, for example, Belcher, Morano, and DeForge, who claim that 'when individuals are unable to forgive, there are negative psychological and physiological consequences' (2004, p. 73), and who derive this claim from a study of undergraduates whose blood pressure and heart rates went down after they were asked to *imagine* forgiving. There is no research that shows that a temporary drop in blood pressure and heart rate based on imagining something is related to a long-term drop in blood pressure or heart rate. While imagining forgiving someone as a daily practice might indeed bring about such changes, there simply is not research that examines this over time. In another overstatement, Belcher *et al.* claim that 'the inability to seek or provide forgiveness results in a chronic state of anger, which may lead to religious strain, depression, and suicidal ideation and attempts' (2004, p. 73). But there has not been a study of people unable to seek forgiveness. There are studies that show that people who have not forgiven are, in general, more angry (score higher on self-report tests of anger), but the studies do not show a 'chronic state of anger' and, for all we know, they may be justifiably angry.

The use of the phrase 'chronic state of anger' seems an exaggeration. Don't most of us have experiences of hurt in our past, experiences for which we haven't explicitly forgiven the wrongdoer? I have in mind those experiences that are not hard to recall but have become unimportant to us. When we recall these experiences, as when we participate in a psychological study, we may become angry anew. This is different from a chronic state of anger. While some people do become obsessed with thoughts of anger toward their perpetrator and do indeed suffer, others are able to set aside past injuries and go on to live happy lives. The sexual abuse literature shows that around half of those who experienced childhood sexual abuse are symptom-free years later (Rind *et al.*, 1998). Did they all forgive their perpetrators? We don't know, because studies have not been conducted.

Within the pro-forgiveness literature, a few caveats are mentioned with regard to harms, acknowledging that some may be unforgivable. Fitzgibbons (1986) listed these as abandonment, severe continuing alcoholism, rape or incest, long-term victimization, prolonged insensitivity, and intractable selfishness. However, in the 20 years since this article has been written, many of these moral wrongdoings are used as examples for touting the benefits of forgiveness to victims.

It may be important to understand the framework of the psychotherapy sessions before going on to critique the practice (and very few critiques exist about the practice of advocating forgiveness in psychotherapy; Burstow, 1992; Lamb, 2002; Lamb and Murphy, 2002; Furedi, 2004). The programs that have been developed vary in length from one session to as many as 12 steps in a manualized treatment aimed at helping clients to forgive (McCullough *et al.*, 1997; Enright and Fitzgibbons, 2000; Worthington *et al.*, 2005). Forgiving, defined most frequently as a gift of compassion rather than a pardoning or excusing of the act (Enright and Fitzgibbons, 2000), is unequivocably presented as a moral virtue.

The majority of these programs work with individuals in isolation from their perpetrators to help victims forgive a moral wrongdoing independent of whether or not a perpetrator is remorseful. Sometimes the perpetrator is brought into the therapy session or is present because the therapy involves the couple or the family; he or she is asked to listen to and express empathy for what the victim has suffered but not always asked to express remorse. Forgiveness therapy is narrowly focused on the forgiveness itself, not of forgiveness as a response to remorse. (One might wonder why so few therapies teach one how to feel and express remorse and so many to express forgiveness.)

Forgiveness is thus taught and encouraged as a virtue independently of where an examination of what happened might lead. All roads lead to forgiveness. The belief is that forgiveness itself is valuable morally and psychologically whether or not it leads to remorse in the perpetrator, reconciliation with a wrongdoer, or an understanding of what happened.

In unilateral forgiveness, the therapy is meant to help a victim gain control over the way she responds to the moral wrongdoing done to her so that she may eventually be at peace, thinking less about her injuries and more towards the life ahead of her. As Worthington *et al.* write, 'forgiveness can help people psychologically, even if the relationship is not affected (for example, a middle-aged woman might forgive her deceased father for molesting her as a child and thereby eliminate psychological symptoms and achieve a peace she had not previously known)' (2005, pp. 235–6). As with most forms of psychotherapy, the truth of the wrongdoing (whether it happened or not) and the facts (details) of the event seem to matter little unless they matter to the patient herself. Most programs include a phase in which the victim must 'Identify the Hurt' (Coleman, 1998) or 'Name the Injury' (Flanigan, 1992) and this phase is presumed to be a very personal rendition of what exactly about the wrongdoing harmed the person. The therapy focuses on how the patient currently is feeling about and responding to the injury. In many, the expression of anger is permitted and even encouraged in the hope that, if the patient feels her anger is justified, she will more easily give up that anger.

While it is clear how forgiveness therapy may ignore important contextual truths having to do with the wrongdoer, including issues of remorse and possible reparation (indeed, forgiveness therapy is indifferent to the wrongdoer's current state), it is less clear how the accounting of the transgression within the therapy session ignores social, cultural, and historical context. The context of interactions presents options and restraints on the perpetrator as well as the victim. This same cultural context presents a climate for psychotherapy in which some bodies of knowledge and ways of seeing and understanding wrongdoings are supported while others may be suppressed. As Code (1995) explains, this 'rhetorical space' can and does differ for individuals with membership in different groups based on gender, race, class, and ethnicity, all of which groups have different and complicated relationships to structures and practices in society. Women can be pressured during more conservative times or in more conservative political climates, for example, to experience, respond to, and talk about their victimization in ways that deny a history of oppression or their own group memberships, even and especially when such oppression played a part in the wrongdoing. Forgiveness therapy may influence the way patients experience and cope with an injury in a way that minimizes or erases cultural problems that contribute to these harms. It may work to hide particular truths about the moral wrongdoing committed and in this way to support those aspects of a culture that contribute to or even permit such transgressions to take place.

In particular, forgiveness therapies seem to focus on moral wrongdoings that are gendered. Yet the authors who advocate this therapy rarely discuss the history of gendered oppression that may have influenced this kind of transgression or a victim's response to it. Although individual women differ greatly in the degree to which they are affected by gender oppression, there is now no denying that sexual abuse and rape are gendered acts that historically have been supported by the oppression of women as institutionalized in the culture through laws, law enforcement, and male privilege. And although individual women differ greatly in the degree that marriage is an oppressive institution for them, marriage, in a number of ways, has been harmful to women and has reinforced patriarchal, hierarchical relations between husbands and wives. Indeed the norm of marriage in contemporary Western society, provides 'a cover for, if not a license to, the evils of spousal and child abuse' (Card, 2002, p. 140).

Gender and race are two master categories by which US society views the world (Osmond and Thorne, 1993). But gender, in particular, pervades forgiveness therapy in ways that are unnamed or unnoticed by authors and researchers. Although men, too, have been asked to forgive unfaithful wives and have been victims of sexual abuse and rape (for example, in prison or by gang members), the forgiveness literature focuses almost exclusively on women who have been wronged in these ways. (It is almost surprising that with the scandal of priest abuse of boys, few have called on these grown men to learn how to forgive their former priests.) Class, race, and other particularities of their self-concepts and life circumstances make for different kinds of oppressions. Yet I argue in the next section that women belong to a class of women, with a shared history of oppression and, because of that shared history, they may also share in the harm done when forgiveness therapy treats their injuries as separate from this history.

In 10.3, I stated that little research has been done to bolster claims that forgiveness is beneficial. However, several large research enterprises are active today publishing studies that show the benefits of forgiveness. They are headed by Robert Enright at the University of Wisconsin, Frederick DiBlasio at the University of Maryland, Everett L. Worthington at Virginia Commonwealth University, and Michael McCullough, once a student of Worthington's, to name a few. The promotion of forgiveness therapy through these research enterprises follows a pattern in much of psychological research although not more clinical, nonempirical, writing; white males tend to teach in the larger universities where grants are more likely and graduate students are present to take a faculty member's work forward and disseminate the findings as well as the theory, whereas women and minorities tend to be the graduate students and teachers at primarily undergraduate institutions (Curtis, 2005). While not blaming individual researchers for their neglect of gender issues, it seems fair to draw attention to their writing as institutionalized practices that promote those whose views will not disturb the *status quo*.

In the next two sections, I examine the forgiveness research and literature over the past 10 years that have come from these institutions and from followers of the therapies advocated there. I look specifically at two situations that involve women: abuse and marital infidelity. As noted above, neither of these harms exclusively is perpetrated by men toward women. But to ignore the gendered contexts in which they occur leads therapists and clients alike to miss important features of the moral wrongdoing in their quick move to promote forgiveness.

10.4 Victims of abuse and forgiveness: a discussion about gender

Victims of sexual abuse, rape, and battering are overwhelmingly female; perpetrators overwhelmingly male (Finkelhor *et al.*, 1990; Koss *et al.*, 1993; Rennison and Welchans, 2002; Tjaden and Thoennes, 2003). While differing methods of data collection and poor levels of reporting of abuse to the police and social service agencies make it difficult to determine the prevalence of victimization in the US today, researchers agree that 20–25% of women will have experienced some sexual abuse or a rape at some time in their lives and that one-third of women some form of battering at the hands of a partner or husband (Finkelhor *et al.*, 1990; Koss, 1993; Rennison and Welchans, 2002; Tjaden and Thoennes, 2003). Ninety to ninety-five percent of their perpetrators will be male. These statistics are not meant to deny the existence of the rape of men by gang members or in prison or the sexual abuse of boys; the point is that most victimizations are expressions of male power over women. A gendered understanding of these three forms of abuse and victimization is not new. Since the mid-1960s, feminists have pointed out that rape and sexual

abuse are acts of male domination ... women (supported by
public institutions as well as pr... the family and marriage; cf.
Kahn, 1995; Baxandall and Gordon ... and articles from that
period).

The rise in forgiveness therapies ... the end of several decades'
focus in the US on the victim... and so it is no wonder that
forgiveness therapists have taken up the issue of whether or not it is helpful to
encourage victims of abuse (sexual abuse and ... most frequently) to forgive
their perpetrators. This question rarely is examined ... the historical context of
our changing understanding of women and ... tion, and any answer to
this question must first examine the changing perceptions of victims within
US culture.

In the 1960s and 1970s, the uncovering phase of this social problem, victimization of women and children was an issue that played a central role in
women's movements. Women told their stories about abuse in private
consciousness-raising groups and public rallies with an aura of unveiling
truths that had been kept hidden by the culture (Haaken, 1998). There was
anger in their radical writings about male dominance in society when they
pointed their finger at institutions such as the church, the law, the courts, the
family, and marriage as institutions that supported the victimization of
women (Baxandall and Gordon, 2000). The rallying cry was not to forgive and
move on but to change the system so that little girls and adult women had less
to fear and greater freedoms to move about and grow up healthy and unmo-
lested.

Public awareness did change. In fact, the victimization of women and girls
became a national issue with media attention and concomitant changes in the
institutions that respond to (e.g., police) and treat (e.g., psychiatry) victims.
While it was important for institutions such as psychiatry and medicine to
recognize their previous lack of attention to as well as ignorance of trauma in
the lives of girls and women, this new attention was problematic. Rather than
changing the institutions themselves, these issues were made to fit already
existing structures for understanding distress. Victims coming to hospital
treatment centers, for example, were given clinical interviews and checklists to
determine their symptomatology due to the abuse; they were then given diagnoses so that insurance funding could be procured and so that doctors and
researchers could develop treatments specific to syndromes; treatment plans
were devised that followed the general practice guidelines for individuals with
mental disorders. The gendered nature of their injuries no longer was salient
in discussions of trauma. As in most of medicine and psychiatry, the social
causes of symptoms and psychological distress took a backseat to explanations

that focused on genetic predispositions, individual personality traits, and individualized response patterns. In short, trauma was 'medicalized' (Lamb, 1996, 1999; O'Dell, 1997). The medicalization of trauma required specialists and resulted in research aimed at identifying and treating a long list of symptoms documenting the harm of abuse.

The recognition of the problem also went hand in hand with a public representation of victims as overwhelmingly damaged (Lamb, 1996, 1999; O'Dell, 1997). The catch-all diagnosis, post-traumatic stress disorder (PTSD), helped therapists to obtain medical insurance for victims of abuse to pay for their therapy (Lamb, 1999; Becker, 2000), but use of this diagnosis had its drawbacks. The emotional reactions of humiliation, shame, and anger—all of which had been supported and aired in public places (from the consciousness-raising groups to public rallies) where other victims confirmed the rightfulness of such feelings—were of less concern than the PTSD symptoms of numbness, fear, and helplessness. In this way, reactions and feelings were redefined—actually refitted—into PTSD symptomatology.

The prevalence of PTSD as the appropriate diagnosis also shaped the way that victims began to understand their feelings and reactions in response to their abuse. When representations of victims gained preeminence in the media and self-help books, victims turned to these images to understand and name their responses. Diagnoses have the power to reify reactions. That is to say, individuals may respond differently to trauma based on the options for emotion and reaction that are available to them and the labels and meanings in circulation. As soon as trauma is experienced, it is wrapped in cultural meaning and given permitted forms for cultural expression. Anthropologists have long understood the power of labels to define experience. Take, for example, the anthropologist who, when horrified by a rape in the culture she was studying, was told by the victim, 'it's only a penis' (Helliwell, 2000). That culture's understanding of what happened, although both anthropologist and victim agreed that what she experienced was rape, differed immensely in terms of how serious an act the rape was.

In the US during the 1990s, the Victim (with a capital 'V') was represented as the helpless girl and not the angry woman, an image that by then had become associated with feminists. The Victim was good yet still deviant (Haaken, 1998; Lamb, 1999; Becker, 2000) because of her symptomatology. The truths about victimization that were aired publicly were the truths about symptoms and suffering. What truths were suppressed? I suggest that the suppressed truths were those that pictured victims as vengeful, bitter, and angry.

By focusing on the victim and her psychological problems, the truth of what happened—the victimization and the wrongdoer's acts—was less important.

It is unclear whether this focus on the victim is a motivated focus that relieves perpetrators of some responsibility or the result of the mental health professions' preference for treating those harmed rather than those doing the harm. Nevertheless, enter forgiveness.

Forgiveness serves to help victims find some power in their helplessness without turning to vengeance, anger, or even justice. While victimization lowers the status of a person through stigmatization and feelings of helplessness, forgiveness elevates her above her perpetrator and preserves her feminine-appropriate status of 'good woman.' (Frye, 1983; Burstow, 1992; Lamb, 1996, 2002; Haaken, 1998, 2002; Becker, 2000; Jack, 2001; Potter, 2001).

Haaken (2002) writes that forgiveness may undo victimization status. From a psychoanalytic perspective, forgiveness is a method of undoing. Although forgiveness advocates argue otherwise, sometimes in their writing one finds a statement that assumes an unconscious wish to 'undo' a trauma. For example, one author likens forgiveness to acting 'as if the transgression never happened' (Worthington et al., 2005, p. 238). In this way, the truth that an event happened is suppressed or even lost forever.

Clinicians who practice forgiveness therapy claim that forgiveness is a final act in a series of stages. Through these stages, clients are encouraged to express their anger and the therapist lets the client know that the anger is justified (Freedman, 2000). Forgiveness in such circumstances is a gift to an undeserving perpetrator. Even if the perpetrator does not deserve to be forgiven, a victim can ignore that issue and can choose to let go of this anger simply for her own benefit. In an atmosphere or a culture where the angry woman is less acceptable and where compassion, nurturance, and generosity of spirit are viewed as quintessential female traits (Prentice and Carranza, 2002), forgiveness is not such a difficult choice.

There are several reasons why advocating forgiveness to women who have been abused is problematic. The first is that, historically, women have been excluded from positions of power with regard to justice. The second is that women have been encouraged to choose self-enhancement over social change even in areas of abuse and victimization (Becker, 2004). And the third is that, in the years following the uncovering of the problems of rape, sexual abuse, and domestic violence, women have been given less 'rhetorical space' (to borrow Code's phrase) for the expression of anger. All of these reasons are developed below. Each reason speaks to the context of women's oppression through victimization and the rewards given to women who conform to stereotypical gender norms.

With regard to the first problem of asking women to forgive—that women historically have been excluded from positions of power with regard to justice—forgiveness therapists have an answer, although they do not address the issue of gender. They simply have claimed that, while forgiving her perpetrator, a victim still can seek justice in the courts. In this case, forgiveness means letting go of a grudge and extending benevolence but does not mean giving up one's right to seek justice or even to see that a wrongdoer is properly punished.

A closer look at this reply shows that, although in principle, women can seek justice while forgiving, it is really institutions such as the courts, the police, and the penal system who are given the main task of holding the perpetrator responsible and making him pay his debt. They do the grudge-holding. Such a feat is called 'splitting off' in the psychoanalytic literature, which phrase refers to the inability of a person to integrate all feelings within the self and so she splits off feelings by compartmentalizing them out of awareness or assigning them through projection to other people (Klein and Riviere, 1964). In the case of a victim who is asked to forgive, more than feelings are split off. The entire role of 'vengeful victim' is assigned to the institutions, leaving the victim only the nicer, more palatable role of the forgiving victim.

If the victim really were encouraged to forgive and still hold a perpetrator accountable, we would see within the explanations of therapy ways in which therapy can help a person to hold on to and express both acts simultaneously. Instead, when a female victim forgives, thus taking on the more nurturing role, the role of judge and jury is handed over to other people, other institutions.

Why would a woman prefer this more nurturing role or give up her right to hold her perpetrator accountable? I return to the point that women have been excluded from places of power within the judicial system. Politicians, lawyers, judges, and police, the ones who uphold justice in society, have been overwhelmingly male until recently. Through such exclusion, women may grow to believe not only that a place for them doesn't exist, but also that they don't have the qualities demanded for such positions of judgment and responsibility. Potter (2001) writes that we need to understand how structural power relations have socialized us to view virtues and vices differently for different groups. Thus women may come to believe that it is more virtuous to forgive while men hold others accountable, even though, as Regehr and Gutheil (2002) suggest, having justice served may be every bit as 'releasing' as finding forgiveness in oneself.

The second reason why asking women to forgive is problematic concerns the fact that, historically, women have been persuaded to seek self-improvement over social change. Dana Becker writes of this trend, arguing that women have been encouraged through practices developed at the Stone Center as well as following Carol Gilligan's work 'to believe that by taking care of their psycho-logical 'selves' they are becoming ever more powerful' (Becker, 2004, p. xii). Becker writes of the psychotherapy movement's disruption of more political goals of feminism through the 'repackaging of the psychological as power' (p. 1). What she calls 'the colonization of the interior world of the psyche' (p. 1) through endless self-help advice has served to refocus women away from more activist projects and into what Lynne Segal calls 'more manageable [feminist] protests' (1999, p. 46). Asking women to give up vindictive feelings and the expression of them may be similar to asking women to remain nurturant and warm (traditionally feminine qualities.) But assuming these qualities at the cost of development of one's self and self-interest has been a long-standing problem for women, one described well by Dana Jack in her research on depression (Jack, 2001), Lyn Mikel Brown in her exploration of the politics of anger among middle school girls (Brown, 1998), and Carol Gilligan in her discussion of women's feelings of being unwomanly when considering abortions (1982).

Anger is one emotion that the self-help industry seems to have colonized— anger that otherwise might have promoted more social activism and assisted women in struggles for real power, not just self-empowerment. Murphy first remarked that women have been taught to forgive and forget instead of to resent and resist (1982). Forgiveness advocates do report a lessening of anger in their subjects. But they assume that giving up one's anger is almost always a good thing psychologically.

Marilyn Frye writes that anger, both felt and expressed, presupposes 'what kind of being one is and what sort of relations are possible between oneself and another' (1983, p. 89). She argues that a woman's anger is accepted only when it is expressed on behalf of others and not herself: 'Hence it is safer to get angry about nuclear power, than about one's own rape; the former is more likely to be intelligible, to get uptake' (Frye, 1983, p. 92). Potter (2000) explains this use of J. L. Austin's (1962) term 'uptake' to be a response that goes beyond attending, empathizing, and respecting what another says; it is to take in someone's communication in a way that gives it depth, importance, and fullness of meaning. Both Frye and Potter note that men (and many women) have been socialized to dismiss women's anger. The effect of such socialization is that women's anger is not given uptake. Psychologists Carol Tavris (1982) and Dana Jack (2001) argue that an angry woman is punished for her anger more frequently than that of an angry man and that women see being angry as inconsistent with being a woman. Expressing the more traditional role of woman as nurturer may result in feelings of acceptance by a society that rewards nurturing and compassion in women.

Murphy's (2003) question, 'What kind of victim should I try to be, a vindictive or a forgiving victim,' can be reframed for women: 'What kind of a woman should I be, angry and vindictive or compassionate and giving?' Or, better yet, 'What kind of woman *can* I be?' Why must victims be persuaded to give up their anger in exchange for psychological health? What makes anger so unhealthy for women? Do any spaces exist—or can we imagine any—in which the voicing of anger can bring about greater health for women and for men?

It is suspicious that the writings on forgiveness therapy for women who have suffered abuse convey such a negative view towards the vindictive emotions (cf. Murphy, 2003, chapter 2) and betray a perhaps unconscious wish to make women conform to gender norms of niceness and nurturance. And it is suspicious that the psychology literature expounds on the practice of forgiveness whereas it is extremely difficult to find even one cognitive-behavioral program that helps wrongdoers move toward remorse. This contrast speaks to the shift of focus from the wrongdoing to the victim's psychology. [Madanes' (1990) work with sex offenders in family therapy is one exception wherein she instructs offenders to make self-humiliating pleas for forgiveness with no demand or expectation that the victim, often a child, forgive.] It is also suspicious when gender issues are ignored in research that implies there are no differences in the benefits of forgiveness for men versus women, as if such research could answer such a serious question as 'What are the problems for women in forgiving?' Finally, it is suspicious when the bulk of the literature on forgiveness examines gendered issues such as abuse and victimization, post-abortion suffering, and marital infidelity without examining the gender issues involved.

10.5 Marital infidelity and forgiveness: a discussion about gender

Forgiveness in marriage is another area in which gender matters. Roles within marriage are delineated historically and linguistically (wife/husband rather than partner) and, over the past 30 years, there has been a number of analyses of the institution of marriage and the power hierarchy within (Perelberg and Miller, 1990; Kahn, 1995; Baxandall and Gordon, 2000; Card, 2002). However, although advocating forgiveness in marriage is commonplace in the literature, there is no corresponding discussion of gender and power.

Advocating forgiveness in marriage is very different than advocating for forgiveness in the case of a past abuse or victimization where the perpetrators are often missing, jailed, or dead. In cases of abuse, forgiveness therapists advocate a unilateral forgiveness whose purpose is to ease the distress of the angry and unhappy victim rather than to reconcile the pair. The kind of forgiveness usually associated with a marital infidelity is that which not only will ease the distress of the wounded party but that has the potential to repair the relationship. While it is possible to practice forgiveness therapy with members of a couple who do not intend to see each other again or who need to work out an amicable relationship for the sake of children in a divorce (Gordon and Baucom, 1998), it is probably unusual for a couple divorcing to seek couples therapy. The examples of forgiveness therapy used in the literature tend to be of heterosexual couples attempting to heal their marriage. If the goal of this type of therapy is to repair the relationship, too vigorous a pursuit of the truth may be antithetical to the preservation of a relationship. I will address this idea after presenting a brief history of feminist family therapy and the work done by several theorists on blame and responsibility within family therapy sessions.

Feminist family therapy has been in existence since Rachel Hare-Mustin's seminal article in 1978, 'A Feminist Approach to Family Therapy' and the founding of the journal, *Feminist Family Therapy* in 1988 (Silverstein, 2004). Following feminist critiques of the family as a system that institutionalizes gender bias, feminist family therapists challenged traditional conceptions of how to conduct therapy with couples and families. At the time, family therapists tended to see problems in families as caused by overinvolved ('enmeshed') mothers and disengaged fathers, blaming women for not 'allowing' fathers to become more involved with their children (cf. Minuchin and Fishman, 1981). Feminist family therapy theorists, when they began critiquing family systems theory, were interested in the ways in which theorists diffused the blame, making the whole family or both members of the couple responsible for the wrongdoing of one member. Feminist family therapy theorists uncovered the misogyny in this conceptualization; they argued that wives were being blamed for patriarchal gender roles that both partners were fulfilling (Hare-Mustin, 1978, 1989; Leupnitz, 1988) and that mothers were being blamed for the way fathers were treating their children (Minuchin and Fishman, 1981). Bograd (1984) and Goldner *et al.* (1990) challenged the treatment of husbands who batter their wives as a mutual problem between the couple and, along with other feminist therapists and researchers, pointed out that husbands and wives operate from different power positions in the family (Hare-Mustin, 1978; Goldner, 1988). Virginia Goldner (1988) argued that, although husband and wife may be in a reciprocal relationship where each influences the reaction of the other, this does not mean that each person has equal influence. Hare-Mustin (1991) and Margolin *et al.* (1983) argued that equal does not mean equitable, in the sense that each person in a couple participates equally as in two halves of a whole, yet one half has more power. Haavind (1984) added that both men and women were equally invested in preserving inequalities in the marriage, working to conceal rather than reveal gender subordination so that inequalities appear as equalities, particularly through a discourse of intimacy between equals.' Generally, feminist family systems theorists showed how the oppression of woman is enacted and perpetuated within the family and how therapists could avoid supporting this oppression in their practice (Goodrich, 1991, 2004).

They also showed how the oppression of women within the family intersects with other oppressions. Feminist family therapy theorists dramatically changed the way family and couples therapy was carried out by bringing up issues of sexuality as well as ethnicity and race (Krestan and Bepko, 1980; Goodrich, 2004). By the 1990s interlocking oppressions became a topic for theorizing within the field of family therapy (Silverstein, 2004).

Given this history of changes to the field of family and couples therapy, one wonders why there is little or no discussion about issues of gender, race, or ethnicity in the forgiveness literature that focuses on marital counseling. If, as forgiveness advocates suggest, forgiveness is a virtue and universally so (Enright *et al.*, 1998), in that it can be applied to any situation by any person, then surely it would help their advocates' goals to include a variety of situations and couples. But readers undoubtedly find that case examples are of traditional couples—white and middle-class with white Protestant names such as Julie and Bill—dealing with marital infidelity (Worthington and DiBlasio, 1990; Coleman, 1998; Freedman, 2000; Brown, 2001; Hill, 2001; Barnett and Youngberg, 2004). Taken as a whole, what do these examples tell us about the project of forgiveness therapy for marriages? And what's missing from the analysis that might give therapists pause before advocating forgiveness within a marriage? An analysis of gender; an analysis of power.

Couples and family therapists take the dyad or the group, respectively, as their unit of analysis. Rather than asking why Jerome did such-and-such, these therapists typically ask what was going on in the system that enabled Jerome to do such-and-such, and what benefit he and DeShawn derived from it. That is to say, individual problems are viewed as group problems and, in some cases, responsibility is shared. Thus, in working with a couple in which one partner has committed adultery, it is not uncommon for the therapist to try to uncover hidden aspects of the relationship that allowed for or even promoted the infidelity. This is tricky, because the act of exploring the environment in which adultery took place can release the wrongdoer from responsibility for the act and diffuse the blame so that both partners in a couple take responsibility for one person's wrongdoing.

This problem occurs in the writing on forgiveness where the couple in an example is asked to discuss their mutual misdeeds, and sometimes the wounded partner is asked to consider her own accountability for her husband's misdeed. This would seem to be a search for a deeper truth about the adultery. Did she make herself unavailable to him? How did they each contribute to problems in their marriage? In one session described, both partners are asked to come up with 'transgressions' for which to forgive each other and to practice listening empathically to these 'transgressions' (Worthington et al., 2005). Brown, not a forgiveness advocate *per se* but a therapist who writes on infidelity, says forgiveness for two married adults involves 'each of them owning their own responsibility for having let their marriage deteriorate to the point of crisis' (Brown, 2001, p. 254). Worthington and DiBlasio (1990) describe their form of couples' therapy as encouraging 'additional introspection and accountability that brought insight to each partner about his or her contributions to the fractured relationship' (p. 222). While it is true that an affair may reflect the deterioration of a marriage, it is also possible that focusing on mutual responsibility for marital problems derails the discussion from the wrongdoer's responsibility for the way he (or she) chose to respond to that deterioration. This way of approaching infidelity presents mutual responsibility as the deeper truth and decenters the particular responsibility of the wrongdoer. All responses to a bad marital situation are not morally equal but, in much of the literature, one partner's choice to ignore the problems in a marriage is viewed as equally problematic as another's choice to seek sex elsewhere. Because family systems theorists see the system as responsible, mutual responsibility is often presented as the deeper truth.

The practice of couples' therapy may indeed be quite different than writing about it. In my interest in what truths are permitted and what rhetorical space is available to discuss and explore these truths, I go on to look at the writing about therapeutic technique. Writers about models of psychotherapy are the 'experts' who lay out the space in which a problem is discussed. In doing so, they define the parameters of the problem. Before examining what they take as the truths of the situation, I present an analysis of who is included in their examples.

Forgiveness experts write primarily and at greatest length about *women's* need to forgive their husband's infidelities. This focus (and concomitant lack of focus on women's infidelities) may reflect the bias of the authors who are mostly male and who may in some ways hope, if only unconsciously, to soften women's responses to male failings. By writing on this particular problem, they unwittingly reinforce cultural stereotypes of men as wanderers and as more sexual than women, and women as patient responders who are less sexual in their needs and demands. While this bias in the writing may reflect the authors' client load—that is, perhaps men who need to forgive their wives rarely come to therapy—I suspect a deeper bias. Women traditionally have borne the responsibility of maintaining relationships and are perhaps more economically dependent and so may feel more pressure to forgive, whereas men more frequently have the economic opportunity to address a problem by leaving the marriage. By focusing on women's need to forgive men, like evolutionary theorists who argue that it is man's instinct to have sex with many women (Buss *et al.*, 1992), these forgiveness authorities may be apologists for men's bad behavior. Because of this bias in their use of examples, the writing about forgiveness therapy thus suggests particular truths about harm done that excludes other truths, certain acts one ought to be forgiving about that excludes other acts.

I now go on to explore what happens to truth-telling in therapy sessions advocating forgiveness. Within a step or phase program employed in marital therapy for forgiveness about infidelity, truth-telling becomes more about telling the truth of one's harm and having the husband who committed adultery listen with empathy. Gordon and Baucom (1998) write that 'the injured partners have such a strong need to insure that participating partners understand the impact of their actions' and that 'Feeling "heard" can bring about a reduction in the injured partner's immediate anger because it signals the participating partner's willingness to engage in the process and to acknowledge the effects of his or her actions' (p. 433). A factual detailed accounting of the act from the wrongdoer's perspective seems cruel, and truth-telling as such has the potential to require the injured party to relive the event or to know more than she would like to know.

And yet, given that committing adultery often involves lying and distorting the truth, a truthful accounting of the wrongdoer's lies might be important in bringing about forgiveness. Telling the truth *that* one did what one was suspected to have done could be a necessary act before the process of forgiveness takes place. It is interesting to note, however, that advocates of forgiveness for sexual abuse claim that the therapy is *just* as effective for those who want to forgive a perpetrator who has not admitted and has not shown remorse. The advocates for forgiveness in *couples'* therapy never say that it is fine for a wife to forgive a husband for an affair that he has not admitted to but that she knows he has committed. However, by emphasizing the full accounting of the harm caused rather than a full accounting of the moral wrongs committed, they shift the focus from the act of wrongdoing to the feelings of the injured party about the person who did the moral wrong.

This is similar to other kinds of therapeutic forgiveness work. There is often an exercise in empathy whereby the victim is asked to look at the person who hurt her in a different light. In the case of abuse, it involves making the sex offender a human being and no longer a one-dimensional monster and, in the case of marital infidelity, it involves understanding the husband as a person with complexity and not as someone who set out to do her wrong. Enright *et al.* (1991) calls this exercise 'recontextualizing the offender.' Hargrave (2001) refers to it as transforming a wrongdoer from a devil to a person. Gordon and Baucom (1998) write that the wounded individual should develop a deeper understanding of the partner's weakness even though a new view of the partner should be realistic.

It is true that wrongdoers are human beings with complex motives and feelings as well as with histories and traumas that influence their decisions and judgments. And seeing people in their particularity seems to be a good thing because it reflects a humanistic understanding of people and because presumably we all would like to be seen multidimensionally. But this particularity, in forgiveness therapy, is always reduced to an individual's history and rarely understood in terms of the particularity of a person's group membership, in this case, gender.

For example, take the case of Joe whose father recently died and who, after 20 years of a good marriage, had an affair with a younger woman. That his father recently died is introduced in the article as a piece of information about an individual that particularizes this man's wrongdoing and lends some understanding, if not excuse. (This example is based on a case cited in Hill, 2001.) The author lays out Joe's grief as a primary cause for his wrongdoing, particularly because he had 20 years of a good marriage prior to the point where he had an affair. But in addition to seeing Joe as a man grieving, we can look at him through a more gendered lens and consider his acts as representative of his gender and his gendered role in his marriage. For example, the death of his father may have raised issues with Joe about his own vitality as a man. His choice of a younger partner is a gendered choice in that young women are status symbols for older men, helping them to defend against aging, get admiration from other men, and feel more masculine. His wife, though, had fewer options to get a younger man in bed. And in having the affair, Joe contributes to his wife's oppression as a woman who lives in a society that devalues women the older they get and overvalues women for looks and their potential to enhance men's status. In having the affair, Joe enacts societal oppression of women and reinstates his power in the relationship, his greater privilege and opportunity to move on, and his greater power in the world by virtue of his being a man. This gendered analysis does not erase the more individual history of his father's death and his prior relationship with his father. Instead, it contextualizes it within a culture in which this relationship takes place. Widening the focus to the gendered society in which the marriage takes place yields a different way of looking at infidelity.

Lynn Parker (2004) directs therapists as to how to think about how power is distributed and expressed in any relationship. Distribution of power and privilege is at the heart of many couples' relationship problems, Parker argues, whether or not a woman feels disempowered or a man feels privileged. She asks the following questions of clients: Who tends to be the decision makers? Who accommodates more? Is there one partner who does the greater share of housework, child care, elder care, relationship care? Whose moods dominate? Does one person in a relationship have the power to threaten the other? Do both people in a relationship have the financial ability to leave the relationship? Can each person support him or herself and the children if needed? Does one partner use physical or verbal force or violence as a means of intimidation or control?

Following suit, I raise the question of whether it is different when a wife has an affair from when a husband has an affair. Within a feminist family therapy framework, it is—and the differences are linked to power imbalances between men and women in society. The choice to have an affair is not only about intimacy and sexual pleasure but also about gendered issues such as attraction, feeling like a 'man' or a 'woman,' and feelings of desert such as 'I deserve to have a good sex life' or 'I deserve to have a woman take care of me during this time.' Such feelings of desert arise from stereotyped notions of what a person might expect given one's gender and place in society. Expectations of public condemnation for a marital affair are also influenced by one's gender and place in society. Given different stereotypes about women's and men's sexual appetites, public condemnation of an affair will differ for men and women. While a man may even get approval for being a 'player' by some colleagues at work, women will be condemned more heartily by men and women alike for having an affair. There is particular condemnation for women with children.

Within this context, an act of forgiving will often corroborate or reinforce more general stereotypes about men and women such as the following: 'He can't help what he did because men have less self-control;' 'If I didn't give him sex, he deserved to get it elsewhere;' 'It's a woman's role to make her husband feel like a man;' and 'A woman should keep herself attractive for her husband.' These are the kinds of reasons for an infidelity that women are asked to consider when forgiveness therapists request that women look at their contribution to the marital infidelity, making the responsibility for the marital infidelity mutual. Given what we know of power differences in marriage, forgiving may be so gender-loaded an act that advocating it for a woman could be tantamount to telling her to go back to her role as good wife and mother.

I take issue not with helping a wife or husband to forgive her or his remorseful spouse but in advocating a position that reinforces women's unequal position within the family. Women are the ones with primary responsibility for making relationships work, often the ones with less means to be able to leave the relationship, and also the ones whose anger is more likely to be seen as disruptive to the relationship. While couples are mutually responsible for their marriage in a proactive way, when looking back on the dissolution of a marriage, they may not have equally committed bad acts or made equally bad decisions in coping with the problems of their marriage. Forgiveness therapists, in their discussion of mutual responsibility, cover over the truth of the infidelity and the truth of the wider cultural context in which marriage occurs. When there are differential rewards and punishments for men and women who adhere to or defy stereotypes and who have different responsibilities and power within their relationship, the advocating of forgiveness becomes problematic.

10.6 Truths be told

There are two ways in which the truth of what wrongdoings occurred and why becomes unclear in the advocating of forgiveness therapy. Both have to do with the creation of a rhetorical space in which only some truths can be aired. The first is in the presentation of forgiveness therapy through experts who publish. I have tried to show that both in cases of abuse and victimization as well as marital therapy, writers and researchers present versions of a moral wrongdoing that hide the gendered nature of the acts in a way that protects males and places equal if not more burden on females to forgive and, in the case of infidelity, to share responsibility for the wrongdoing. Couples therapists no doubt would argue that they would take the same frame of reference for a woman who was not faithful to her husband, but the fact of the matter is that forgiveness therapists do not often write about this type of case.

The second obscuring of the truth happens within the therapy session itself. There the 'truth' is represented as the truth of the harm that was done to the person and the truth that the perpetrator is a complex human being, but not the truth regarding the actual events of the wrongdoing. The truth that gets obscured is that even in all his particularity, a wrongdoer may still be a person with privileges, entitlements, and power that are exercised through his transgression.

With truth obscured and diffused, it then becomes easier for forgiveness therapists to advocate more speed in the process. As with all forgiveness therapy, there seems to be an assumption that a specific time period exists in which wounds should heal and that, if they do not, the wounded party has a problem that therapy can address. Rather than requiring an extended period of good deeds, trustworthy behavior, and renewed commitment from a partner who has committed adultery—a more action-oriented form of therapy that surely would have some effect on a wounded spouse—forgiveness couples therapists attempt to help the process move along. As in all forgiveness therapies, noted earlier, the therapy lessens the moral burden of reparation that belongs to the wrongdoer and redistributes it within the couple. Forgiveness therapists may have good intentions, believing that the victim has suffered enough from her abuse and that there is no need to prolong her suffering in her inability to forgive. Coleman (1998) warns against therapists bringing up forgiveness too early because it places primary burden on the victim; the victim is doubly burdened by the betrayal she must cope with as well as the struggle to find forgiveness. But Freedman (2000) takes a more hurried stance; in discussing a case of infidelity in a marriage between Max and Molly, she says that it had been 'one month' since Max's confession, and Molly couldn't get the picture of him and the other woman out of her head. One month? The implication is that forgiveness ought to be considered one month after an infidelity; how soon after a rape should a victim begin the process of forgiving?

Couples may find that there is no way to forgive and not reinforce the stereotypes or uneven power relations they seek to avoid. The same may be true for victims of abuse. If gender matters in acts of abuse, and if it impacts a marriage, then gender surely influences forgiveness. If an accounting of the truth of what happened and the suffering incurred is an essential task before forgiveness, then whether therapists are working with victims of abuse or with couples dealing with an infidelity, truths about power and gender must be addressed. And so, like most of us who at some time in our lives have struggled to live in the gendered and hierarchical composition of the family, victims of abuse and couples coping with a marital infidelity must live embracing the ambivalence of histories that cannot be changed as well as the hope for a difference in the future.

References

Al-Mabuk RH, Enright RD, and Cardis PA (1995). Forgiveness education with parentally love-deprived late adolescents. *Journal of Moral Education*, **24**: 427–43.

Austin JL (1962). *How to Do Things With Words*. London: Oxford University Press.

Barnett JK and Youngberg C (2004). Forgiveness as a ritual in couples therapy. *The Family Journal: Counseling and Therapy for Couples and Families*, **12**: 14–20.

Bass E and Davis L (1988). *The Courage to Heal: A Guide for Women Survivors of Child Sexual Abuse*. New York: Harper and Row Publishers.

Baxandall R and Gordon L (eds) (2000). *Dear Sisters: Dispatches from the Women's Liberation Movement*. New York: Basic Books.

Becker D (2000). *Through the Looking Glass: Women and Borderline Personality Disorder*. Boulder, CO: Westview Press.

Becker D (2004). *The Myth of Empowerment*. New York: New York University Press.

Belcher JR, Morano C, and DeForge BR (2004). Treating resistant couples: the use of forgiveness in conservative Christian and Jewish traditions. *Family Therapy*, **31**: 71–85.

Bograd M (1984). Family systems approaches to wife battering: a feminist critique. *American Journal of Orthopsychiatry*, **54**: 558–68.

Brown EM (2001). *Patterns of Infidelity and their Treatment*. Philadelphia, PA: Brunner-Routledge Publishers.

Brown LM (1998). *Raising Their Voices: The Politics of Girls' Anger*. Cambridge, MA: Harvard University Press.

Burstow B (1992). *Radical Feminist Therapy: Working in the Context of Violence*. Newbury Park, CA: Sage Publications.

Buss DM, Larsen RJ, Semmelroth J, and Westen D (1992). Sex differences in jealousy: evolution, physiology, and psychology. *Psychological Science*, **3**: 251–5.

Card C (2002). *The Atrocity Paradigm: A Theory of Evil*. New York: Oxford University Press.

Code L (1991). *What Can She Know? Feminist Theory and the Construction of Knowledge*. Ithaca, NY: Cornell University Press.

Code L (1995). *Rhetorical Spaces: Essays on Gendered Locations*. New York: Routledge Publishers.

Coleman PW (1998). The process of forgiveness in marriage and the family. In: *Exploring Forgiveness* (eds RD Enright and J North), pp. 75–94. Madison, WI: University of Wisconsin Press.

Curtis JW (2005). Inequities persist for women and non-tenure track faculty: the economic report on the status of the profession 2004–05. *Academe*, **91**: 20–30.

Enright RD and Fitzgibbons RP (2000). *Helping Clients Forgive: An Empirical Guide for Resolving Anger and Restoring Hope*. Washington DC: American Psychological Association.

Enright RD and the Human Development Study Group (1991). The moral development of forgiveness. In: *Moral Behavior and Development 1* (eds W Kurtines and J Kurtines), pp. 123–52. Hillsdale, NJ: Erlbaum Press.

Enright RD, Freedman S, and Rique J (1998). The psychology of interpersonal forgiveness. In: *Exploring Forgiveness* (eds RD Enright and J North), pp. 46–62. Madison, WI: University of Wisconsin Press.

Finkelhor D, Hotaling G, Lewis IA, and Smith C (1990). Sexual abuse in a national survey of adult men and women: Prevalence, characteristics, risk factors. *Child Abuse & Neglect*, **14**: 19–28.

Fitzgibbons RP (1986). The cognitive and emotive uses of forgiveness in the treatment of anger. *Psychotherapy*, **23**: 629–33.

Flanigan B (1992). *Forgiving the Unforgivable: Overcoming the Bitter Legacy of Intimate Wounds*. New York: Macmillan Publishers.

Freedman S (2000). Creating an expanded view: How therapists can help their clients forgive. *Journal of Family Psychotherapy*, **11**: 87–92.

Freedman SR and Enright RD (1996). Forgiveness as an intervention goal with incest survivors. *Journal of Consulting and Clinical Psychology*, **64**: 983–92.

Frye M (1983). A note on anger. In: *The Politics of Reality: Essays in Feminist Theory*, pp. 84–94. Freedom, CA: The Crossing Press.

Furedi F (2004). *Therapy Culture: Cultivating Vulnerability in an Uncertain Age*. London: Routledge Publishers.

Gilligan C (1982). *In a Different Voice*. Cambridge, MA: Harvard.

Goldner V (1988). Generation and gender: normative and covert hierarchies. *Family Process*, **27**: 17–32.

Goldner V, Penn P, Sheinberg M, and Walker G (1990). Love and violence: gender paradoxes in volatile attachments. *Family Process*, **29**: 343–64.

Goodrich TJ (ed.) (1991). *Women and Power: Perspectives for Family Therapy*. New York: WW Norton & Company.

Goodrich TJ (2004). A feminist family therapist's work is never done. In: *Feminist Family Therapy: Empowerment in Social Context* (eds LB Silverstein and TJ Goodrich), pp. 3–16. Washington DC: American Psychological Association.

Gordon KC and Baucom DH (1998). Understanding betrayals in marriage: a synthesized model of forgiveness. *Family Process*, **37**: 425–449.

Haaken J (1998). *Pillar of Salt: Gender, Memory, and the Perils of Looking Back*. Camden, NJ: Rutgers University Press.

Haaken J (2002). The good, the bad, and the ugly: psychoanalytic and cultural perspectives on forgiveness. In: *Before Forgiving: Cautionary Views of Forgiveness in Psychotherapy* (eds S Lamb and J Murphy), pp. 172–91. New York: Oxford University Press.

Haavind H (1984). Love and power in marriage. In: *Patriarchy in a Welfare Society* (ed. H. Holter), pp. 136–67. New York: Columbia University Press.

Harding S (1991). *Whose Science, Whose Knowledge: Thinking from Women's Lives*. Ithaca, New York: Cornell University Press.

Hare-Mustin R (1978). A feminist approach to family therapy. *Family Process*, **17**: 181–94.

Hare-Mustin R (1989). The problem of gender in family therapy theory. In: *Women in Families: A Framework for Family Therapy*. (eds M McGoldrick, CM Anderson, and F Walsh), pp. 61–77. New York: WW Norton & Company.

Hare-Mustin R (1991). Sex, lies, and headaches: the problem is power. In: *Women and Power: Perspectives for Therapy* (ed. TJ Goodrich), pp. 63–85. New York: WW Norton & Company.

Hargrave T (2001). *Forgiving the Devil: Coming to Terms with Damaged Relationships*. Phoenix, AZ: Seig, Tucker, & Theisen.

Hebl JH and Enright RD (1993). Forgiveness as a psychotherapy goal with elderly females. *Psychotherapy*, **30**: 658–67.

Helliwell C (2000). 'It's only a penis': rape, feminism, and difference. *Signs: Journal of Women in Culture and Society*, **25**: 789–816.

Hill EW (2001). Understanding forgiveness as discovery: implications for marital and family therapy. *Contemporary Family Therapy*, **23**: 369–83.

Hope D (1987). The healing paradox of forgiveness. *Psychotherapy*, **24**: 240–4.

Jack D (2001). *Behind the Mask: Women and Anger*. Cambridge, MA: Harvard University Press.

Kahn K (ed.) (1995). Front Line Feminism. In: *1975–1995: Essays from Sojourner's First 20 Years*. San Francisco, CA: Aunt Lute Books.

Klein M and Riviere J (1964). *Love, Hate, and Reparation*. New York: WW Norton & Company.

Koss MP (1993). Rape: scope, impact, interventions and public policy responses. *American Psychologist*, **48**: 1062–9.

Koss M, Goodman L, Fitzgerald L, Keita G, and Russo NF (1993). Male violence against women: current research and future directions. *American Psychologist*, **48**: 1054–8.

Krestan JA and Bepko CS (1980). The problem of fusion in the lesbian relationship. *Family Process*, **19**: 277–89.

Lamb S (1996) *The Trouble with Blame: Victims, Perpetrators, and Responsibility*. Cambridge, MA: Harvard University Press.

Lamb S (1999). Constructing the victim: popular images and lasting labels. In: *New Versions of Victims: Feminists Struggle with the Concept* (ed. S Lamb), pp. 108–38. New York: New York University Press.

Lamb S (2002). Women, abuse and forgiveness: a special case. In: *Before Forgiving: Cautionary Views of Forgiveness in Psychotherapy* (eds S Lamb and J Murphy), pp. 155–71. New York: Oxford University Press.

Lamb S and Murphy J (eds) (2002). *Before Forgiving: Cautionary Views of Forgiveness in Psychotherapy*. New York: Oxford University Press.

Leupnitz D (1988). *The Family Interpreted: Psychoanalysis, Feminism, and Family Therapy*. New York: Basic Books.

Madanes C (1990). *Sex, Love, and Violence: Strategies for Transformation*. New York: WW Norton & Company.

Margolin G, Talovic S, Fernandez V, and Onorato R (1983). Sex role considerations and behavioral marital therapy: equal does not mean identical. *Journal of Marital and Family Therapy*, **9**: 131–46.

McCullough ME, Worthington EL, and Rachal KC (1997). Interpersonal forgiving in close relationships. *Journal of Personality and Social Psychology*, **73**: 321–36.

Minuchin S and Fishman HC (1981). *Family Therapy Techniques*. Cambridge, MA: Harvard University Press.

Murphy J (1982). Forgiveness and resentment. *Midwest Studies in Philosophy*, **8**: 503–16.

Murphy J (2003) *Getting Even: Forgiveness and its Limits*. New York: Oxford University Press.

O'Dell L (1997). IV. Child sexual abuse and the academic construction of symptomatologies. *Feminism & Psychology*, **7**: 334–9.

Osmond MW and Thorne B (1993). Feminist theories: the social construction of gender in families and society. In: *Sourcebook of Family Theories and Methods: A Contextual Approach* (eds PG Boss and WF Doherty), pp. 591–625. New York: Plenum Press.

Parker L (2004). Bringing power from the margins to the center. In: *Feminist Family Therapy: Empowerment in Social Context* (eds LB Silverstein and TJ Goodrich), pp. 225–338. Washington, DC: American Psychological Association.

Perelberg RJ and Miller AC (eds) (1990). *Gender and Power in Families*. New York: Routledge Publishers.

Potter N (2000). Giving uptake. *Social Theory and Practice*, **26**: 479–508.

Potter N (2001). Is refusing to forgive a vice? In: *Feminists Doing Ethics* (eds P DesAutels and WJ Lanham) MD: Rowman & Littlefield Publishing Group.

Prentice DA and Carranza E (2002). What women and men should be, shouldn't be, are allowed to be, and don't have to be: the contents of prescriptive gender stereotypes. *Psychology of Women Quarterly*, **26**: 269–81.

Regehr C and Gutheil T (2002). Apology, justice, and trauma recovery. *Journal of the American Academy of Psychiatry and Law*, **30**: 425–30.

Rennison CM and Welchans S (2002). Intimate partner violence. Special Report. Washington DC: US Department of Justice, Office of Justice Programs, Bureau of Justice Statistics.

Rind B, Tromovitch P, and Bauserman R (1998). A meta-analytic examination of assumed properties of child sexual abuse using college samples. *Psychological Bulletin*, **124**: 22–53.

Segal L (1999). *Why Feminism? Gender, Psychology, Politics*. New York: Columbia University Press.

Seligman M (1991). *Learned Optimism*. New York: Alfred A. Knopf.

Seligman M (2002). *Authentic Happiness: Using the New Positive Psychology to Realize your Potential for Lasting Fulfillment*. New York: Free Press.

Seligman M and Csikszentmihalyi M (2000). Positive psychology: an introduction. *American Psychologist*, **55**: 5–14.

Silverstein LB (2004). Classic texts and early critiques. In: *Feminist Family Therapy: Empowerment in Social Context* (eds LB Silverstein and TJ Goodrich), pp. 17–36. Washington, DC: American Psychological Association.

Spence D (1982). *Narrative Truth and Historical Truth: Meaning and Interpretation in Psychoanalysis*. New York: WW Norton & Company.

Tavris C (1982). *Anger: The Misunderstood Emotion*. New York: Simon and Schuster.

Tjaden P and Thoennes N (2000). Extent, nature, and consequences of intimate partner violence: Findings from the National Violence Against Women Survey. Available from http://www.ncjrs.org/pdffiles1/nij/181867.pdf [Accessed 11 Sept 2003].

Worthington EL and DiBlasio FA (1990). Promoting mutual forgiveness within the fractured relationship. *Psychotherapy*, **27**: 219–23.

Worthington EL, Mazzeo SE, and Canter DE (2005). Forgiveness promoting approach: Helping clients reach forgiveness through using a longer model that teaches reconciliation. In: *Spiritually Oriented Psychotherapy* (eds L Sperry and EP Shafranske), pp. 235–57. Washington, DC: American Psychological Association.

Chapter 11

Telling the truth about mental illness: the role of narrative

Christian Perring

11.1 Introduction

A typical scenario in therapeutic truth-telling is one where a victim or survivor tells the truth about a painful episode to expose the treatment he or she suffered at the hands of another. The harm may involve physical beating, sexual assault, emotional attack, emotional neglect, discrimination, or lack of recognition of a person's value. Telling the truth about these events may be painful and, in some cases, reliving the trauma can itself be a traumatic experience, especially in a hostile context such as testifying in a courtroom. Despite the emotional pain that can accompany truth-telling, it is a fundamental assumption of our therapeutic age that telling the truth is an essential ingredient in the healing process. There are psychological and sociological questions about when such truth-telling is helpful and what makes it a valuable process, and the investigation of that process is naturally the province of psychologists and sociologists. These questions are answered with models for how and when truth can be therapeutic. Most of us are familiar with the Freudian model of the repression of traumatic experience and the neurotic symptoms caused by subterranean memories that are so unpleasant that they have been repressed. When these memories are brought to consciousness with appropriate affect, the neurotic symptoms should disappear, according to this theory. Freud himself initially believed he had discovered cases of the abuse of young people (what is often problematically referred to as the 'seduction hypothesis') but then, at least according to most histories of psychoanalysis, abandoned this belief in favor of the view that these events were imagined rather than actual. However, his method of treatment of the resulting neurosis remained basically the same, i.e., a cure by talking and discovering the truth of the past. For example, in *Studies on Hysteria*, Freud describes the case of Katharina, whose father made sexual advances towards her when she was in her early teens. At the age of 18, she developed anxiety attacks. She saw Freud, who uncovered the truth of what her father did. While he does not report a cure, he does say he hoped 'she derived some benefit from our conversation' (Breuer and Freud 1895, p. 133). In Freud's *Five Lectures on Psychoanalysis*, Freud describes the talking cure as a process of sweeping the mind clean through remembering with accompanying expression of affect the occasions in which hysterical symptoms first occurred (Freud, 1977, p. 13).

Modern psychological theories may place more emphasis on the shame felt by victims of abuse, the internalization of the degrading opinion of the oppressor or abuser, and the irrational guilt often experienced. Telling the truth about events and going public with them may empower the survivor with the understanding that there is no need to feel shame. A central example of a modern approach that emphasizes truth and accurate perception of the world is cognitive therapy, associated with the work of Aaron Beck. The methods of cognitive therapy are to identify cognitive errors and distortions and then to correct them (Wright *et al.*, 2003). As I say, these are familiar models well established in both psychiatric and popular consciousness and there is no need to expound on them further here.

My aim in this chapter is to explore how a narrative approach might provide a useful alternative tool for understanding how truth-telling can help people fight both political oppression and stigmatizing ways of representing themselves. I will draw attention to some ways in which telling one's story is not simply a matter of laying out the facts but rather involves choosing a narrative to describe one's life. There are many aspects to this contrast, and I will focus on cases where the language and categories we use to describe ourselves are indeterminate or in flux. I will not attempt to provide a precise definition of narrative (a task that I take to be extremely difficult if not impossible) and my claims do not require a precise definition. We are familiar with paradigm cases of people telling the story of their lives, or portions of their lives, and these stories generally involve explaining what happened to them, who they interacted with, what they did, how they felt, and what they thought. These narratives are often structured chronologically and aim to make clear why events unfolded as they did and why the narrator's life turned out as it did. Thus a central aim for most narratives is to provide understanding of a life, so that it makes sense. This notion of 'making sense of a life' may be hard to analyze, but I trust that it at least has some strong intuitive appeal. One aspect of this work that I take to be interesting and important is that it suggests how the concept of narrative can show some links between personal autonomy and social liberation. I will be particularly interested in cases where telling the truth about oneself is an act that contributes to political self-liberation.

Telling one's story may be therapeutic not just as a way of revealing previously hidden truths, but also as a way of fighting prejudices and correcting mistaken conceptions of what kind of person one is. Furthermore, telling one's story may sometimes be a way of creating an identity for oneself. A central question is to what extent individuals or groups of oppressed people have the power to counter or neutralize stigmatizing mainstream narratives, demeaning names, and distorted images. I will use the case of transsexuals as an example and I will conclude with a discussion of the ways in which people with mental illnesses have tried to develop stories and language with which to describe their lives that fight demeaning stereotypes.

11.2 Theoretical perspectives on narratives and counter narratives

In this section, I outline ways in which a number of theorists from different disciplines have argued for the importance of a concept of narrative, and I especially focus on those who have introduced the concept of a counter narrative as a way to combat the constraining effects of dominant narratives.

Within the medical humanities, there has been a surge of interest in narrative, and these theoretical and professional focuses on narrative tie in well with movements in popular culture (Charon and Montello, 2002). Within academic philosophy, two of the most important authors on narrative are Alasdair MacIntyre and Paul Ricoeur. In *After Virtue* (MacIntyre, 1981), MacIntyre argues that our ideas of living morally are essentially tied to the notion of narrative. Rejecting utilitarian and deontological accounts of ethics, MacIntyre argues that in order to assess the value of actions, we need to understand them in the context of a person's life. Ricoeur (1992) emphasizes how narrative constructs the character of a person, and he calls this the 'narrative identity.' These pioneers in the field have had an important influence on current philosophical discussion. In this chapter I especially draw on the ideas of a philosopher who has recently worked on narrative, Hilde Lindemann Nelson.

A narrative describes a person's life or a portion of a person's life. A useful starting point is Nelson's emphasis of four general elements of narrative that are particularly important for her purposes (Nelson, 2001, p. 11). First, a story is depictive, representing human experience. Second, it is selective in what parts of experience it represents. Third, it is interpretive, offering a certain construal of the experience. Finally, it is connective, creating relationships among its elements and to other stories.

We can tell stories of nonhuman animals, other biological organisms, and inanimate objects, but it is plausible that narratives primarily apply to people and only secondarily to other kinds of beings. They are generally told, explicitly or implicitly, from one or more points of view, with some authority as to how events were experienced and what the narrator thought and felt during the events. (There may be some stories that are narrated in the third person, an all-knowing observer who makes no explicit self-disclosures, but this too is a point of view.) Paradigms of narratives are well-structured, typically with a beginning, middle, and end, although narratives can also be radically incomplete. Stories necessarily do more than simply list events though, because, inevitably, they have to focus on some events more than others and omit some events altogether. Thus they prioritize some aspects of what happened over others. Two stories about the same time of a person's life may be consistent with each other yet give very different descriptions of what happened by their different focuses.

11.3 Narrative and political liberation

Narrative plays a role in political struggles in rather obvious ways. In contemporary culture, we place great value in people speaking in their own voices and telling their own stories rather than having their stories told for them. This is especially true for women and minorities who have lived in oppressive societies that devalued their points of view. Feminist theory and women's movements have argued that scholars and researchers must pay attention to the realities of women's experiences that have been previously neglected, leading to a bias in our understanding of women's lives (Longino, 1990). Furthermore, the very ability to tell one's own story is a mark of autonomy, so in respecting the equal right of women to control their own lives, society must honor their ability to say what their lives are like and to tell the truth about what they experience. The same holds for any oppressed group that is striving for equality. This is one of the senses in which telling one's personal story is a potentially political action that helps to give an oppressed group a voice in society.

However, common experience has often shown that liberation is not guaranteed or even promoted simply by a person being allowed to tell the story of her life. People may use words, phrases, and forms of stories that work against their own liberation. Ways of telling stories carry values with them, and if a person adopts a mode of story-telling with values that demean her or endorse her oppression, then telling her own story may be self-defeating. Oppressed people find it difficult to speak with their own voices distinct from that of their oppressors, or to identify their own point of view as distinct from what they are told to adopt. For example, in patriarchal countries, women often agree with men that they are not capable of thinking rationally and should not be entitled to be part of government. Women have endorsed the view that they are too emotional and irrational to make important decisions that affect the rest of society. To put the point in a very simple way, oppressed people may have been coercively socialized into adopting the language and values of their oppressors. To make the point more complexly and more directly related to narrative, oppressed people may not have language or ways of telling their stories readily available to them that allow them to distance themselves from their oppressors' point of view. We can express this by saying that there are 'dominant narratives.' This means primarily that within a particular culture on a given topic, people have only limited ways of describing their lives, and those ways pervade the culture. There is also a secondary connotation that the main narrative forms that are employed tend to sustain the domination of weaker groups by stronger groups.

We can link these observations about the political role of narrative to theories about the psychology of narrative. We can note that some of the most noted psychoanalytic theorists have tended to neglect the political dimensions of narrative. For example, Donald Spence and Roy Schafer have emphasized the importance of clients in psychotherapy becoming narrators of their own lives (Spence, 1982; Schafer, 1992). While these approaches draw on Freud's psychodynamic theories, they do so with a reformulated metapsychology, replacing quasi-mechanistic models of the interactions between the different parts of the mind with narrative models. Strict Freudians take the terms of Freud's metapsychology very seriously: they believe in the existence of psychic energy and mechanisms of defense quite literally. However, one of the many reactions against strict Freudianism, partially under the influence of thinkers such as Jean-Paul Sartre and Gilbert Ryle, was to reconceive these theories about the mind, not as literal truths but as metaphors, and to refigure theories of human psychology not in terms of entities within the space of the mind, but rather in terms of what the *person* talks about and what actions he performs. Yet while thinkers such as Spence and Schafer challenged the ontology of Freud's metapsychology, they tended not to argue against the claims about the psychosexual development of children such as Freud's theory of the Oedipus complex. Furthermore, they did not explore narrative in political terms, and they placed little or no emphasis on working against dominant narratives.

A far more political approach to linking personal change to social change stems from a number of leftist thinkers in Britain whose work has come to be identified as 'critical psychology.' One notable work in this group is *Changing the Subject: Psychology, Social Regulation and Subjectivity* (Henriques *et al.*, 1984). This group of authors draws on psychoanalytic theory, the work of Foucault, Althusser, Adorno, Lacan, and a number of feminist theorists, and their project scrutinizes how psychology perpetuates differences in race, class, gender, and sexuality. For example, Wendy Hollway examines the interactions between heterosexual couples and how couples describe those interactions in interviews. One of her central theoretical concepts is 'discourse,' which is broader than narrative. Although Hollway does not give an explicit definition of 'discourse,' she appears to mean the set of concepts, assumptions, and even theories that guide one's actions. Given that neither narrative nor discourse is precisely defined, it is not possible to set out the precise relation between them. However, we can at least tentatively equate a person's narrative to be her discourse about herself. Hollway identifies three relevant discourses in the interviews she conducted, and she calls these 'the male sexual drive discourse,' 'the have/hold discourse,' and 'the permissive discourse' (Henriques, 1984, p. 231). She characterizes them with broad strokes, and I can only summarize them here. The first is the 'male sexual drive discourse,' a theoretical assumption that men have a biological need to have sex with women, in the sense that their actions are biologically determined. The second is the 'have/hold discourse,' which is identified with Christian ideals that women should want to have a family and children, through monogamous relationships with men. Finally, the third is the 'permissive discourse,' which is most easily identified with the ideas of the 1960s that people should be not be confined by the restrictions of society but instead should recognize that sexual pleasure is a good and, so, any sexual activities that result in pleasure are good.

Without following these ideas in more detail, we can consider Hollway's assumption that discourses largely determine the relations between people, or as she puts it, make available positions for the subject to take up (Henriques, 1984, p. 236). So gendered discourses, rather than biology, are what determine the social relations between men and women. Nevertheless, there is some room for maneuver with respect to discourse, and some people choose alternative liberating discourses. It is through such choices that personal, social, and political change becomes possible. The central theoretical aim of Hollway's paper is to examine in more detail how such changes occur. Her conclusion is worth quoting at length:

> The circle of reproduction of gender difference involves two people whose historical positioning, and the investments and powers this has inserted into subjectivity, complement each other. When there remain contradictions in each person's wants of the other, there is ground for an interruption of its reproduction. These contradictions

are the products of social changes. It is through the kinds of social changes that I outlined at the beginning of this chapter that alternative discourses—for example feminist ones—can be produced and used by women in the struggle to redefine our positions in gender-differentiated practices, thus challenging sexist discourses still further. Changes don't automatically eradicate what went before—neither in structure nor in the way that practices, powers and meanings have been produced historically. Consciousness-changing is not accomplished by new discourses replacing old ones. It is accomplished as a result of the contradictions in our positionings, desires and practices—and thus in our subjectivities—which result from the coexistence of the old and the new. Every relation and every practice to some extent articulates such contradictions and therefore is a site of potential change as much as it is a site of reproduction.

Henriques et al. (1984, pp. 259–60)

Her interviews with subjects in 1980s Britain suggest that they adopt all three discourses mentioned previously, to some degree, and that the tensions or contradictions between these different discourses are what lead the interviewees to search for new ways of thinking about their roles in relationship to other people. For all the indeterminacy of the meaning of the term 'discourse' and the controversy over the relative weight of biology and culture in determining how people behave, I believe that Hollway's passage presents a plausible and exciting approach for how people are able to change their relationships to others. It is largely an empirical question how such changes become possible, and it is certainly difficult empirically to show the truth of a theory such as Hollway's either as a general claim or as applied to particular people, but nevertheless, it can provide a starting point for conceiving the role of narrative as a therapeutic agent and as a cause of social change.

A more recent collection of articles from critical psychology focuses on the concept of counter story. In *Under the Covers: Theorizing the Politics of Counter Stories* (2001), editors Michelle Fine and Anita Harris collect work by a variety of scholars on how people resist dominant narratives by telling their own stories. The collection includes analyses of how some women with breast cancer resist the imperative to think positively, several pieces on how indigenous peoples resist the depiction of their lives as inferior, irrational, and emotional compared with colonizing whites, and a provocative piece positing the lyrics in some rap music as a counter story to the depiction of young black males as aggressive, criminal, and irresponsible. In their introduction to the collection, Harris, Sarah Carney, and Fine evade providing a definition of counter story with the observation that narratives are constantly changing. Their main point is that counter stories are forms of political agitation even though they have not previously been much recognized as such. Rather than provide a grand theory of counter narrative, the work the editors have gathered together serves to enrich our understanding of what can count as a counter narrative and the way the conflict between dominant narrative and counter narrative tends to play out. (For another recent collection on the notion of counter narrative, see *Considering Counter-Narratives: Narrating, Resisting, Making Sense* (2004), edited by Michael Bamberg and Molly Andrews.)

11.4 **Nelson and narrative repair**

One of the most interesting recent philosophical explorations of therapeutic storytelling is Hilde Lindemann Nelson's *Damaged Identities: Narrative Repair* (2001). Nelson uses the concept of narrative to shift attention from the personal level to the level of social justice. She argues that personal identities are complicated narrative constructions that can be damaged by unjust social relations. In particular, she argues that 'the master narratives used by a dominant group to justify the oppression of a less powerful group distort and falsify the group's identity by depicting the group . . . as morally subnormal' (Nelson, 2001, p. 106). Many familiar examples exist, such as the depiction of slaves in slave-owning America, the depiction of women in patriarchal societies, or the depiction of homosexuals in homophobic cultures.

Nelson further argues that in order to resist such a construction, the oppressed group needs to do more than simply disagree with the master narratives. Instead, it needs to create its own counterstories that not only tell the truth about the lives of those in the group but also offer alternative ways of conceiving how to live. Counterstories in this way repair damaged identities, according to Nelson.

One example Nelson discusses is that of transsexuals. Nelson defines a transsexual as a person whose gender identity is opposite to that normally associated with his or her bodily sex (Nelson, 2001, p. 125). Transsexuals thus experience a mismatch between their identities and their bodies and are diagnosed with gender dysphoria. Standard treatments involve extensive counseling, hormones, and surgery. Nelson argues that the master narrative that dominates the way that both professionals and most nonprofessionals describe transsexuals has the implication that 'a preoperative male-to-female transsexual living as a man isn't really a man in any ordinary sense of the term and certainly doesn't identity with that gender, but he passes for a man. If, postoperatively, she starts living as a woman, then in one sense she becomes a woman.' However, in another sense, her genesis as a woman is so unusual that she isn't really a woman either, and so she can only pass for a woman. So, according to what Nelson calls with irony the Clinically Correct story, she fails to be either male or female authentically. This makes it a morally degrading narrative, because with this use of categories, transsexuals are not only abnormal, but their humanity is intrinsically deficient, because they fail to count as either really male or female, when on the binary conception of gender, humans must be either one or the other. Nelson argues that this master narrative, 'itself a tissue of incompatible stories and fragments of stories,' (2001, p. 126) is imposed by a dominant group, the medical community, and has come to be accepted by a large number of transsexuals. She points out that transsexuals themselves were avid readers of Harry Benjamin's definitive 1966 book *The Transsexual Phenomenon* and adjusted their descriptions of themselves to doctors so as to conform to the book as a way of maximizing their chance of being recommended for surgery. Nelson argues that the best known personal memoirs of transsexuals conform to the Clinically Correct story.

Some astute writers on the topic have argued that one of the central flaws in the discourse of transsexualism is the assumption of a gender binary of either male or female, and Nelson agrees with this criticism. The gender binary is not common to all cultures; indeed, even Western cultures sometimes have ways of talking about gender that introduce subtleties in the categorization of gender (cf. Nanda, 1999). However, Nelson points out that 'what is socially constructed is often dreadfully hard to deconstruct' (Nelson, 2001, p. 129). It can be easier to get gender reassignment surgery than to reshape our cultural understanding of gender. For such a shift in cultural understanding to take place, she further argues, it is not enough to have theoretical insight. In order to avoid the oppression caused by our categories of gender, people must have stories available to them that offer alternative ways of being gendered. They need both first- and third-person stories that are not morally degrading and, furthermore, 'that don't leave the entire burden of deconstructing the gender binary to transsexuals, and that allow the more interesting differences among transgendered people to emerge' (Nelson, 2001, p. 134). In particular, she suggests that we need stories that 'leave ordinary norms for 'man' and 'woman' in place but rehabilitate the concept of passing.' It would also be possible to expand the concepts of man and woman to include those transgendered people who have adopted those identities. Finally, it would be possible to allow people to *refuse* to be either men or women (Nelson, 2001, p. 135).

Nelson rejects the reduction of the social category of gender to the biological category of sex, and she does not believe that we can solve the oppression of transsexuals simply by using more biologically accurate descriptions. As social beings, we inevitably use some concepts of gender that are related to, but not reducible to, the biology of sex differences. While Nelson's discussion does not make sharp distinctions between concepts of gender, narratives of gender, and theories of gender, her fundamental point is clear: we need to expand the ways we categorize people so that they have a way to describe themselves, and that we have a way of describing them, that enables them to live nondemeaning lives.

Assessing Nelson's ideas gives us a method of understanding the role of truth in liberating and healing oppressed groups. What is especially stimulating about her approach is its synthesis of the psychological and social. While Nelson's approach is still profoundly psychological, it moves the repair of damaged identity from an individual process to a group one. The onus to create an alternative narrative is the responsibility of larger groups, transsexuals as a group, the medical and psychiatric professions, and society as a whole. The process requires the creation of new narrative forms that individuals are then able to employ to narrate their own stories in ways that enhance their autonomy and resist the master narratives that reduce their humanity.

11.5 Counter stories in psychiatry

For the remainder of this chapter, my aim is to apply Nelson's approach to more central cases of purported human rights abuses in which psychiatry plays a role.

First, I will discuss the problems of master narratives and stigmatization in psychiatry and the effects of these on identity. What are the master narratives of psychiatry? My interest here is on the narratives available for people who are diagnosed with mental disorders, rather than the narratives available to psychiatrists, psychologists, and other mental health professionals. The central narrative available is the medical one. It goes like this. The mentally ill patient has a mental disorder that needs to be treated through the methods of psychiatry and clinical psychology. These include psychopharmacology, talk therapy, and social support. While serious mental illness is rarely if ever cured, it can often be treated successfully if the patient complies with the treatment. Compliance generally requires accepting one's diagnosis and following the doctor's orders. When possible, the mental patient should accept the help of friends and family. With perseverance and some luck, the patient can come to live a worthwhile life and triumph over the mental illness. These broad features are present in many memoirs by both clinicians and people who have lived with mental illness, with many individual variations. The medical narrative is often hopeful and helpful.

Nevertheless, being labeled as a mental patient generally brings a great deal of shame and stigma in our culture. This has deep historical roots, as the figure of the mad person has long been portrayed as provoking and even deserving fear, derision, rejection, and horror. We should be clear that the medical narrative does not, in itself, imply stigma, and indeed psychiatry has often fought to oppose and end the stigma of mental illness. Nevertheless, because stigma still exists, and medicine and psychiatry are the main ways that people become labeled as having mental illnesses, they inevitably work in tandem with stigmatizing forces.

In contemporary Western society, the stigma associated with mental illness is less prominent than it has been in the past, and there have been many attempts to fight stigmatizing representations of the mentally ill. Arguably, current portrayals of mental illness are still stigmatizing, but in more subtle ways than in the past. What is beyond argument is that the lingering effects of stigma are still present, and people place themselves at social risk by admitting that they have serious mental disorders.

Now, I want to clarify what a counter story might look like in this realm and how it might help to fight stigma. Creating a narrative involves choosing which experiences, events, emotions, and thoughts to report. Creating a counter story involves selecting these things in ways that will fight stigma. I will not be able to cover all these elements, but I will focus on a few.

In exploring the concept of a counter story, it is important to see its relation to other ways of depicting people and efforts to help oppressed groups through language. Recent decades have brought greater sensitivity to the power of derogatory language and the need to avoid it (Wahl, 1995). There are countless derogatory ways of referring to those with mental disorders and, indeed, ways that appear neutral or even positive can quickly be turned around. The most obvious example from recent years comes from education, where the label of 'special education student' has largely failed to confer a status of 'special' on students in special education programs and has done little to fight the stigma associated with words such as 'idiot,' 'retarded person,' 'moron,' or 'cognitively deficient person.' Further, some have criticized the practice of using mental illnesses to refer to or identify patients, as when a clinician says 'I have a schizophrenic and a borderline to see this afternoon.' The 'people first' movement has recommended referring to those with mental illnesses as persons or people 'with schizophrenia' or 'with borderline personality disorder,' for example, so as to emphasize that the sufferers are people first and that their illnesses do not constitute their identity. It is difficult to find where the notion of 'people first' language originated, but it has now become widespread, at least in some areas of education and service provision (Titchkosky, 2001).

A different form of resistance to derogatory language has been to try to reclaim offensive words. In recent decades, some feminists have attempted to reclaim words such as 'hag,' 'bitch,' 'slut,' and 'witch,' and to use them openly and proudly, so that they cannot be used against women. Some disability activists have reclaimed the term 'cripple' for themselves, and have even built on it, creating new words such as 'supercrip.' Similarly, there have been attempts by people with mental illnesses and their allies to reclaim words such as 'mad,' 'crazy,' and 'schizo' and to valorize them so they do not carry the same negative charge.

It is debatable to what extent attempts to fight stigmatizing language have been successful. It seems clear that the old terms of abuse for those with mental illness have not been neutralized, but still carry great power to offend. Nevertheless, the focus on language may have been somewhat helpful in sensitizing the general population as to the destructive power of derogatory language (Corrigan, 2005). Yet it is reasonably clear that simply changing our ways of referring to emotionally troubled and cognitively challenged people will not by itself do much to help them. The negative terms that are used to identify those with mental illness and disability are symptoms of deep underlying prejudices and, while there has been much more sensitivity to language in recent decades, especially in education, with the replacement of labels such as 'retarded' with more positive ones such as 'special needs,' there is little evidence that this has done anything to remove the underlying stigma. Similar remarks apply to images and the iconography that tend to be used in picturing the mentally ill, from the old depictions of Bedlam to depictions of homicidal maniacs in horror movie posters (Gilman, 1982; Wahl, 1995). Portrayals of mental illness in the mass media have improved in recent decades, but self-consciously positive images designed to destigmatize have modest success at best.

Counter stories must be more than a matter of finding new words to describe people. We have no guarantee that creating counter stories will be any more successful in liberating people than creating new phrases to refer to people, but it is at least a different sort of project, albeit overlapping. Counter stories of people with mental disorders will be distinctive in the forms of language they use, but they will also be distinctive in terms of their plots, perspectives, and styles. Similarly, creating a counter story is a different project from proposing a different model or theory of mental illness. One of the main claims made for seeing mental illness as a disorder of the brain is that it is destigmatizing (Andreasen, 1984). The suggestion is based on the idea that older models of mental illness conceived of it as a flaw in personality or a sign of bad parenting by the mentally ill person's family. To see mental illness as a brain disorder is supposedly to eliminate the possibility of those judgments. On this view, the brain-based model shows that suffering from a mental illness is just a matter of biological bad luck and is no reflection on the sufferer or his or her family. While it is certainly true that which model of mental illness one adopts will affect how one tells one's story of one's experience of illness, it is important to be clear that a counter story, or the form of a counter story, is more than a theory. Plots, perspectives, and styles are not determined solely by one's theory of mental illness.

11.6 The consumer/survivor movement

I will now focus on a provocative example of possible counter stories of people with mental illness, namely, the growth of the psychiatric consumer/survivor (C/S) movement. While this movement does not refer to a precisely defined group of people, but rather to a collection of loosely associated different groups, it does have some identifying value. The name of the movement is somewhat self-explanatory: consumers are users of psychiatric services, but the concept is narrower than the label 'users of mental health services.' The 'consumer' concept is an alternative to the label of 'patient,' which many since Carl Rogers have found objectifying and have seen as a failure to recognize the agency of the person with the medical or psychological problem. The term 'survivor' is more complex, being ambiguous as to whether the survival is of mental illness (similar to the use of the term 'cancer survivor') or the psychiatric treatment for the illness (similar to the use of the term 'rape survivor' or 'war survivor'.) The C/S movement is distinct from the Recovery Movement, which tends to be allied with 12-step programs that adopt a medical model of addiction. The Recovery Movement more generally seems to be sympathetic to a medical understanding of most forms of addiction and self-destructive behavior. By way of contrast, the C/S movement tends to be rather hostile towards a medical approach to people's emotional distress. This feature of the C/S movement also distinguishes it from that of National Alliance of the Mentally Ill (NAMI) in the US. NAMI quite explicitly adopts a medical model of mental illness, is run largely by family members with mentally ill relatives, and is partially funded by the pharmaceutical industry, while the C/S movement is largely run by users and ex-users of psychiatric treatment. The C/S movement has no central organization or funding, although the advent of the Internet has enabled it to achieve more publicity for itself.

In the UK, the C/S movement has recently been associated with a 'Mad Pride' movement; the book *Mad Pride: A Celebration of Mad Culture* (Curtis, 2000). In Canada, there has been work on the promotion of businesses run by mental health consumers with some signs of success, and there is even collaboration and a sense of community among some psychiatric survivors, at least in Ontario. In the US, the C/S movement has been less visible, but it seems to exist not just online, but to some extent in and around the community mental health movement and in rehabilitation services. There is a strong alliance between the C/S movement and the disability rights movement, and this provides a particularly interesting parallel. Disability rights activists do not deny that people with disabilities have physical and mental differences from the norm; rather what they tend to resist is the medicalization of those differences and the stigmatization that is often associated with such medicalization. Members of the C/S movement may identify specific episodes in their lives when they have received electroshock treatment, were heavily medicated against their will, or have been involuntarily restrained, as violations of their human rights and thus experience telling the truth about their medical treatment as a way of coping with the trauma caused by the medical establishment. Within the psychiatric/consumer movement, people may simultaneously fight for their right to receive new medications and proper psychiatric treatment while at the same time criticize the psychiatric and medical establishment, the stigmatizing treatment they have received, and the labels that have been attached to them. Some in the movement would even identify themselves as victims of psychiatric torture, where torture is understood as intentionally malicious medically unnecessary treatment (cf. the website titled 'The Government Psychiatric Torture Site', http://www.mk-resistance.com/. Last accessed May 17, 2005). The movement would place itself alongside other political liberation movements such as the civil rights movement, the women's movement, the disability rights movement, and the opponents of apartheid in South Africa. Thus they identify psychiatry, possibly paradoxically, as both an oppressive force in their lives and also as a means by which they can get some help to achieve greater autonomy. This tension of attitudes might be seen as a mark of the vulnerable position that people in the C/S movement find themselves in. (One might view this in the manner of Hollway as a contradiction between different discourses, and thus a potential site for change, rather than a self-defeating inconsistency.)

Defenders of psychiatry may well accept that psychiatry has been involved in human rights abuses and would agree that this is unacceptable. Some historical incidents of major ethical misconduct have been well documented, such as human rights abuse in the Nazi era, Japan, and the Soviet Union

(Bloch and Chodoff, 1991). Contemporary cases of psychiatric misconduct are more disputed, but one need only look to the recent past in the USA for clear cases, such as the use of lobotomy in the mid-twentieth century (Valenstein, 1986). Psychiatrists are likely to make distinctions between proper and improper psychiatric treatment and to call for the condemnation of immoral psychiatrists who violate patients' rights. Nevertheless, they will defend the standard and excellent practice of psychiatry. In contrast, what is striking about the C/S movement is that it tends not to make such distinctions between good and bad psychiatry, or the good practice of psychiatry and the stigmatizing attitude society as a whole toward mental illness, but rather to retain a stance of hostility and suspicion to the whole establishment. The C/S movement fights stigmatization, labeling, and forms of treatment that it considers disabling or damaging, and fights for the recognition of people who are labeled as mentally ill as fully human with full moral status. We can see within this range of activities the attempt to generate counterstories that fight stigmatizing narratives and the expansion of the dominant understanding of what it is to be mentally ill. These activists are trying to perform a narrative repair, to hark back to Nelson's terminology. In particular, the collaboration between people within the C/S movement to tell new stories about their lives and the writing of memoirs and recollections by people within the movement does this very explicitly. In recent years, there have been many published narratives of mental illness, in memoirs, news stories, novels, and films (cf. Vonnegut, 1976; Sheehan, 1983; Greenberg, 1984; Sacks, 1985; Sechehaye, 1985; Styron, 1992; Jamison, 1995; Kaysen, 1994; Schiller, 1996; Neugeboren, 1998; Lindner, 1999; Slater, 1999; Millett, 2000). (See also the *Metapsychology Online* website for an exhaustive set of reviews of narratives of mental disorder.)

A central problem for the C/S movement as a way of developing an alternative understanding of mental illness is that its credibility as truth-telling is questioned by much of the rest of society. When people with mental illnesses protest against abuses of their rights and systematic discrimination, they are often dismissed as unreliable witnesses precisely because they have been diagnosed with major mental illnesses and they are not considered to be psychiatric experts. A practice of 'truth-telling' may simply increase the chances of their being dismissed as mad and in need of treatment. A second primary problem for the C/S movement and those who fight for the rights of the mentally ill is that we have good reason to believe that society today doesn't much care about their rights even when abuses have been well documented. In recent years, at least in the USA and the UK, there has been much preoccupation with the 'problem of the dangerous mentally ill' with legislation aimed to protect society from this group. When there are exposés of terrible conditions in housing for the mentally ill, as exposed by Clifford Levy in his Pulitzer Prize winning series 'Broken Homes' in New York in the *New York Times* in 2002 (April 28–30, 2002), there were no repercussions for the politicians or those in control of mental health policy in the state. It is hard to think of a case of revelation of the abuse of the rights of the mentally ill that led to sweeping reforms in the last 30 years, and it seems highly unlikely that this is because all the rights of the mentally ill are now respected.

Serious mental illness remains one of the most stigmatized conditions in modern society, and one doesn't need to be a believer in antipsychiatry or radical psychiatry to see the truth of this claim. A practice of 'truth-telling' can and often does lead to the 'truth-teller' being seen as a difficult patient, a trouble-maker, or a paranoid person, and can even lead to diagnoses of further mental illness. My aim here is not to cast aspersions on the integrity of the psychiatric profession nor to deny that there are in fact difficult patients, trouble-makers, or paranoid people, although I should say that, considering the history of the treatment of the mad (Grob, 1994), I would recommend looking at current practices with a critical stance sensitive to concerns about human rights abuses. Instead, my main point in using the example of the C/S movement is to point out that this movement has the goal of providing a group identity for at least a portion of the mentally ill as sufferers of discrimination, abuse, and stigma. This has a strong political element to it.

We can bring now bring in Nelson's account of counter stories as a way to repair damaged identities. According to Nelson's view, what the C/S movement would need for full success is the creation of new narrative forms that help achieve the aims of the movement. It is not enough for healing that people tell the truth about what happened to them as former patients or as victims of stigmatization. They need to find ways of telling their stories that show them as people who understand the ways that society is intolerant and even abusive of people with their characteristics, so they can develop positive, nonstigmatized ways to tell their stories and live their lives.

11.7 **Stories of mental illness**

Nelson's examples of members of disempowered groups coming to be more empowered through counter narrative emphasizes the *process* of telling stories to each other; through such a process, people can achieve more solidarity as a group and become more confident in their individual judgments. The process enabled them to shirk off the prejudices of others and to speak up for themselves. Nelson's account of transsexuals had a different emphasis: she showed a need for a wider conceptual scheme that does not force people to describe themselves in confining ways when their bodies do not match their self-conceptions. Our present binary ideals of true man and true woman leave no room for other alternatives.

Both uses of counter storytelling should be available to those with mental illness. People with mental illnesses should be able to come together and trust their own judgments as opposed to the demeaning judgments of those in power. They should also be able to find a new set of concepts to describe themselves so as to escape the dilemmas that come with our current vocabulary of madness. However, there is another feature of telling one's own story that enables one to resist demeaning stereotypes and images that expands on Nelson's account. This feature is the richness and complexity that inevitably comes with telling a detailed story of a life, and it is worth emphasizing because it shows how counter stories are different from new theories or alternative concepts.

There are many ways to tell the story of an experience of mental illness, and there are many memoirs, novels and films that contain narratives of mental illness exploring those different ways. Some stories are richer than others, and a few are so one-dimensional that they are no more than case illustrations of particular theories. However, my claim here, which is akin to Hollway's discussion of the inevitability of contradictory discourses in our everyday practices around gender, is that the details of a life when adequately described will humanize the subject of the story and contain points of potential resistance to demeaning master narratives. Thus, every detailed story of a person's experience over a sustained period of time is a potential counter story.

11.8 Conclusions

It is clear that to tell one's story typically is to go beyond stating value-neutral facts about oneself. It is at the least an opportunity to reflect on and assess one's life and to try to make sense of how one came to live the life one has had. Telling one's story is personal (while at the same time political), not so much in being biased but rather in being full of meaning, as a sequence of emotionally significant events. It is hard to imagine a narrative that does not come heavily laden with implicit or explicit value judgments and, should one attempt to construct a value-neutral narrative, this very effort would give the narrative an unusual significance, with an implicit and presumably unexplained valuing of neutrality. Nearly all narratives are full of moral and aesthetic valuations. This is another way in which telling the truth about oneself cannot be captured in a narrowly construed theory of basic facts.

Telling the truth about oneself can be helpful in ways that are not standardly captured in psychological theory, and it is crucial to pay attention to conceptions of narratives and counter narratives in order to see ways we have of describing ourselves and thus gaining control over our lives. Sharing one's story can fight demeaning and confining master narratives and stereotypes and exploring different narrative forms can open up new ways of being that were not previously available with older conceptual schemes. My hope is that through a careful examination of the narrative forms employed, we can come to understand better how these stories inform and mold both public and professional conceptions of the nature of mental illness.

I began by arguing that people can heal themselves by telling the truth about themselves and then focused on nonoppressive forms of narratives. The connection between these ideas should be clear: in revealing truths about oneself, one has to use language and narrative forms to tell one's story. Counter stories are a way to resist the stereotypes, demeaning categories, and oppressive labels that are used in dominant narratives. Stories of transsexuals are particularly illuminating because they help us to see how the subjects to whom these labels apply may themselves embrace problematic concepts and theories in their self-descriptions. While we don't have a ready-made set of alternative narratives to replace the old ones with, it is fairly easy to at least imagine the possibility that we could improve on the narratives we have and enable people to describe themselves in less confining ways. I believe that the same holds true for the people we describe as mentally ill. The stigma associated with madness and being emotionally distressed is still powerful and, while it is conceivable that moving toward a medical model of mental illness will help to reduce that stigma, it is far from clear that it will completely remove all stigma, and it is debatable whether or not it helps at all. People in Western societies do seem increasingly prepared to be open about their experiences of mental illness, thus revealing previously hidden truths. Yet we should still pay careful attention to how people express these important aspects of themselves, and look for ways in which they can tell their stories that resist the powerful forces of stigma.

Acknowledgments

Thanks to Daniel Calcutt, Hilde Lindemann Nelson and especially to Nancy Potter for comments on earlier drafts of this chapter.

References

Andreasen N (1984). *The Broken Brain: The Biological Revolution in Psychiatry.* New York: Harper & Row.

Andrews M (2004). Memories of mother: counter-narratives of early maternal influence. In: *Considering Counter-Narratives: Narrating, Resisting, Making Sense* (eds M Bamberg and M Andrews), pp. 7–26. Amsterdam: John Benjamins Publishing.

Bloch S and Chodoff P (eds) (1991). *Psychiatric Ethics*. Second Edition. Oxford: Oxford University Press.

Charon R and Montello M (eds) (2002). *Stories Matter: The Role of Narrative in Medical Ethics*. New York: Routledge Publishers.

Corrigan P (ed.) (2005). *On the Stigma of Mental Illness: Practical Strategies for Research and Social Change*. Washington, DC: American Psychological Association.

Curtis T (ed.) (2000). *Mad Pride: A Celebration of Mad Culture*. London: Spare Change Books.

Fine M and Harris A (eds) (2001). *Under the Covers: Theorizing the Politics of Counter Stories. The International Journal of Critical Psychology*, **4**. London: Lawrence and Wishart.

Freud S (1977). *Five Lectures on Psycho-Analysis* (ed. and trans. James Strachey). New York: WW Norton & Company.

Gilman SL (1982). *Seeing the Insane*. New York: Wiley Publishers.

Greenberg, J (1984). *I Never Promised You a Rose Garden*. New York: New American Library.

Grob G (1994). *The Mad Among Us: A History of the Care of America's Mentally Ill*. New York: Free Press.

Henriques J, Hollway W, Urwin C, Venn C, and Walkerdine V (1984). *Changing the Subject: Psychology, Social Regulation and Subjectivity*. London: Methuen Publishing.

Jamison KR (1995). *An Unquiet Mind: A Memoir of Moods and Madness*. New York: Random House.

Kaysen S (1994). *Girl, Interrupted*. New York: Vintage Books.

Levy C (2002). April 28–30. *Broken Homes*, a series. *New York Times*. http://www.pulitzer.org/year/2003/investigative-reporting/works/index.html.

Lindner RM (1999). *The Fifty Minute Hour: A Collection of True Psychoanalytic Tales*. New York: Other Press.

Longino H (1990). *Science as Social Knowledge: Values and Objectivity in Scientific Inquiry*. Princeton, NJ: Princeton University Press.

MacIntyre A (1981). *After Virtue: A Study in Moral Theory*. New York: Oxford University Press.

Millett K (2000). *The Loony-Bin Trip*. Chicago, IL: University of Illinois Press.

Nanda S (1999). *Neither Man nor Woman: The Hijras of India*. Belmont, CA: Wadsworth Publishing Company.

Nelson HL (2001). *Damaged Identities: Narrative Repair*. Ithaca, NY: Cornell University Press.

Neugeboren J (1998). *Imagining Robert: My Brother, Madness and Survival: A Memoir*. New York: Henry Holt.

Ricoeur P (1992). *Oneself as Another*. (trans. Kathleen Blamey). Chicago, IL: University of Chicago Press.

Sacks OW (1985). *The Man Who Mistook His Wife for a Hat: And Other Clinical Tales*. New York: Summit Books.

Schafer R (1992). *Retelling a Life: Narration and Dialogue in Psychoanalysis*. New York: Basic Books.

Schiller L (1996). *The Quiet Room: A Journey Out of the Torment of Madness*. New York: Warner Books.

Sechehaye M (1985). *Autobiography of a Schizophrenic Girl*. New York: New American Library.

Sheehan S (1983). *Is There No Place on Earth for Me?* New York: Random House.

Slater L (1999). *Prozac Diary*. New York: Penguin Group USA.

Spence DP (1982). *Narrative Truth and Historical Truth: Meaning and Interpretation in Psychoanalysis*. New York: WW Norton & Company.

Styron W (1992). *Darkness Visible: A Memoir of Madness*. New York: Vintage.

Thornton T (2004). Reductionism/antireductionism. In: *The Philosophy of Psychiatry: A Companion* (ed. J Radden) New York: Oxford University Press.

Titchkosky T (2001). Disability: A rose by any other name? 'People-First' language in Canadian society. *Canadian Review of Sociology and Anthropology*, **38**(2): 125–40.

Valenstein ES (1986). *Great and Desperate Cures: The Rise and Decline of Psychosurgery and Other Radical Treatments for Mental Illness*. New York: Basic Books.

Vonnegut M (1976). *Eden Express*. New York: Bantam.

Wahl OF (1995). *Media Madness: Public Images of Mental Illness*. New Brunswick, NJ: Rutgers University Press.

Weitz D (2004). Insulin shock: a survivor's account of psychiatric torture. *Journal of Critical Psychology, Counseling and Psychotherapy*, **4**(3), 187–94.

Wright JH, Beck AT, and Thase ME (2003). Cognitive therapy. In: *The American Psychiatric Publishing Textbook of Clinical Psychiatry*, Fourth Edition (eds RE Hales and SC Yudofsky) Washington, DC: American Psychiatric Publishing.

Chapter 12

Healing relational trauma through relational means: aboriginal approaches

Lewis Mehl-Madrona

12.1 Introduction

The effects of trauma within intimate relationships can be devastating for people, families, and communities. Consistent with modern psychiatry and psychology's focus upon the individual, an illness has emerged in the twentieth century to encompass the after-effects of trauma—post-traumatic stress disorder. Also consistent with modern psychological culture, when an illness appears, a treatment industry arises to cure it. As a result of these developments, theories multiply about post-traumatic stress and how to treat it. This chapter will focus on trauma within intimate and family relationships and how it can be addressed within a relational context. Other chapters have addressed trauma in interpersonal relationships and upon communities (war, genocide, ethnic cleansing), but this chapter is distinct in that it rejects Eurocentric assumptions about trauma and healing.

European concepts of trauma and recovery focus on fixing people who are damaged and punishing people who do the damaging. Aboriginal concepts tend more toward restoration and healing and concepts of reconciliation, consistent with recent social movements (Lamb and Murphy, 2002). Forgiveness, for example, is becoming more prominent, as evidenced by its place in the 2005 Works of Love conference sponsored by Case Western University. Aboriginal culture strongly encourages forgiveness, reconciliation, and restorative justice over concepts of punishment and retribution but how these attitudes are brought about is different from European-American approaches.

Therefore, we will consider how forgiveness works between intimate and formerly intimate partners when trauma has occurred from the context of aboriginal communities.

12.2 Forgiveness, accountability, and healing

Anger and resentment diminishes the quality of intimate relationships and are known to produce free fatty acids that accelerate arteriosclerosis and end-organ damage from hypertension. Because of this, anger and hostility are associated with earlier coronary events (myocardinal infarctions) and strokes. Anger and resentment fuel violence; overcoming resentment heals and restores the physical body. Resentments, bitterness, vengeance, and helps fuel wars, domestic violence, familial vendettas, and other acts of violence. As Potter notes, distress from trauma can be aggravated by holding on to rage or other negative emotions (Potter, Introduction).

Wrongdoers also benefit from forgiveness. Being forgiven signifies, to the wrongdoer, that he or she is not reducible to his or her bad actions (cf. Glas, Chapter 8, this volume). This point emphasizes an important counterpart to healing as a victim/survivor of trauma, and that is the possibility of healing as the wrongdoer. So when we consider questions of accountability for psychological harm, we need to think both individually and sociopolitically about who comprises this group in its various contexts.

As Perring argues in Chapter 11, a story-telling approach to healing has advantages. As a person of Cherokee heritage, I find telling stories to be central to traditional healing, and I draw upon this tradition in the chapter. So I ask: What stories must be told and how do we negotiate the stories of the recipients of violence and those who inflict it? What are the underlying relationships in which connections are forged and what are these relationships? What is healing?

To address these questions, let us use an aboriginal approach. I will tell three stories. These stories represent common scenarios that I encounter in my work with relational trauma. They will help us to consider the questions posed. They are not isolated stories. Each story recurs many times. Despite the uniqueness of each story, each has a representative quality as well, and we can learn from the situations they represent.

12.3 Carol's story and how community story-telling facilitated healing[1]

The trauma

Carol was a 38-year-old Dakota woman who lived in a remote, rural community. Carol's community had largely been converted to Catholicism, of a

---

[1] The identities of all persons involved in each of the three stories have been disguised to preserve confidentiality.

fundamentalist type. Carol presented with acute anxiety. She feared she had committed a mortal sin, as she had just asked her husband to leave. Various family members and acquaintances (as well as the priest) were reminding her that marriage was for life, for better or for worse, and could not be put aside no matter what the husband had done.

Carol had been drinking heavily and had decided that either she was going to die or her husband had to leave. She had not revealed to him a previous relationship with his brother during a time when he had been away from the community, living in the major city of the Province. During that time he had been drinking heavily and seemed unlikely to stop or to return to the community. His brother, who was not a drinker, had begun to help Carol to maintain her house and to care for her children. They became progressively more intimate until they were sleeping together. Just as her husband was returning, Carol became pregnant with the child of her husband's brother. She gave birth to a girl some months later. On the one hand, Carol worried about her sin of adultery. On the other hand, she believed that her husband's brother was a good man, perhaps the only man who had ever loved her with respect and dignity. She longed to be with him, but feared committing a sin by divorcing her husband.

Earlier in their marriage, Carol had learned that her husband had molested their daughter. This had included actual intercourse, which happened when he was drunk—but he was drunk most of the time. She had pressed charges as social workers had urged her to do. Then the pressures of her parents, the priest, and the community fell hard upon her. She was told repeatedly that spouses did not testify against each other. She was told repeatedly not to threaten her marriage. She was urged to retract the charges, to say that she made them up. Carol collapsed under this pressure and recanted. Mysteriously, other witnesses and evidence disappeared. No one was willing to discuss what had happened and the charges were eventually dismissed. Carol began drinking heavily during this time. Her husband eventually left again and Carol stopped drinking.

Carol described a history of violence throughout their marriage. Her husband hit her when drunk. She had suffered some broken ribs on two occasions. Once he had broken her wrist. She described frequent episodes of being forced to have sex with him when he was drunk. She did not like having sex with a drunk or being forced into it. On more than one occasion, she had sustained vaginal trauma from this sex. It even occurred at knife point or with a gun to her head.

Carol decided to make her husband leave when she caught him looking at her second daughter (the child from her husband's brother) in a way that she thought was suspicious. She couldn't bear the thought of another daughter being molested. Then he had left and she felt so relieved until the community began working on her.

What are we to do?

Healing steps taken

The husband had been charged on multiple occasions, but nothing had changed. Retributive justice systems had been tried in this context and had not worked. In part, this was because violence had become, to some extent, normalized. This type of violence was not unusual in the community. Sexual molestation was common but not discussed. Men often took sex when drunk. Furthermore, community-interpreted Catholic values demanded that the women tolerate this behavior as part of their marriage vows.

I was on shaky ground. My values were different from those of the community. I didn't know to what extent I could challenge those values, especially with the priest on the side of marriage at all costs.

As Carol's psychiatrist, I had to respond. I told Carol that I couldn't comment on the local interpretation of Roman Catholicism, but I could say that I had friends who were Catholic priests, though admittedly in major urban areas. I told her that my friends would certainly say that Carol also had a duty to protect herself and her daughters and that some behavior actually broke the marriage vows. I know priests who would say that your husband broke the bonds of marriage by his behavior, I said. My friends would say that you were being courageous in protecting your daughter and asking him to leave. Carol agreed that she had friends who told her this as well. I complimented her on her ability to survive her life. I told her that many women in her situation would have just given up to drugs or alcohol or depression. She smiled at that. I guess I'm a survivor, she said. The more I drew attention to her courage and her ability to survive, the more she relaxed. I suggested that she surround herself with friends who supported her decision and that she ask them to buffer her contact with the community members who thought she was sinning. I suggested that her friends could engage those people in discussion about what constituted sin in marriage so that she wouldn't have to argue with others about her behavior.

That was an acceptable beginning. But in aboriginal communities, people who leave the community often return; few stay away for good. Over time, I suspected that Carol's husband would be back and that he would ask her to take him back. Family members would put enormous pressure on her to do so. This likelihood necessitated a community meeting. I asked Carol to bring family members and friends to our next appointment. When she didn't appear to the next appointment, I called her. She was sitting at home with some of her family who were telling her not to come to the appointment. I asked if the community mental health worker and I could come over to her house. She agreed.

Carol lived in a ramshackle prefabricated house that looked like a trailer without wheels. She was embarrassed by her small space. Her mother and father were there. So was her husband's brother, though no one was supposed to know that she and he had been involved. I wondered if that was really a secret or just a pretended secret but knew better than to ask. We began a curious discussion about how family members felt about Carol's decision to ask her husband to leave. Slowly, the strict Catholic values of her parents emerged along with the more liberal perspectives of her husband's brother. Children were playing videogames at the end of the room. I tried hard not to push my values, but to be curious and ask questions. At the end of an hour, the mental health worker and I had to return to the office, so we asked if we could visit again. When the family agreed, we scheduled another meeting and invited them to bring more people, both in favor and against what Carol had done.

For our next meeting, Carol invited friends who supported her. Her parents asked the priest to come. We continued to dialogue about right and wrong. At the following meeting, her parents brought her husband. He wanted to return to Carol's home. Carol refused. We continued to encourage the community members to stay in dialogue. Carol raised issues of his violence upon her. I wondered what the community perspective would be. Everyone agreed that violence was wrong, but the conservative opinion was that he was still her husband and should be allowed back. The liberal opinion was that Carol could refuse to take him back. The meeting ended with Carol remaining insistent that he not return. Arrangements were made for him to spend time with the children at the homes of other relatives.

We continued meeting and Carol continued to refuse to let her husband return. Eventually he went back to the city. A total of 10 meetings were held. Discussions seemed productive. The question of sexual abuse had emerged, though no one had really been able to address it, as the topic was too charged. Some sisters told me privately that they would make sure that the husband was never alone with his daughters. This seemed like the best we could expect.

Over the course of the next year, I met with Carol and her family three more times. At the end of the year, she divorced her husband, over the objections of her parents and the priest as well as some of the more conservative members of her community. Her husband's brother eventually moved into her house and they were living together 2 years later.

How did story-telling help Carol and others?

Could legal involvement have helped this situation? Apparently not. Police reports had generated no change in behavior. In the past, community and family pressure had prevented Carol from speaking up. The question is why this approach worked even to the extent it did. Was it because we were trusted members of the community who Carol and others felt safe enough to invite into their anger and pain? It doesn't seem so: the community mental health worker was part of the community, but I was not. I usually visited only every other week. They may have looked up to me as a person with authority, but I am not sure what kind of authority they perceived. My view is that the sustained dialogue was important and useful in that it was relational—it brought together people in conflict and provided a space for them to speak their mind and to listen to others who disagreed. They continued to disagree but, over time, they learned to understand each other better. Dialogue made that possible—dialogue in which people talk in order to listen. In traditional Hawai'ian medicine, this approach to relational healing is called Ho-opono-oho. Regardless of its name, the idea of creating dialogues of accountability for healing and reconciliation through the world's indigenous cultures.

Reconciliation of a sort occurred, not in the form of the couple getting back together, but in the form of peaceful resolution. Previously, Carol had managed her anger by drinking. Telling her story at our meetings presented the opportunity for a different way of coping with her anger. Carol was able to express her anger at what she considered abuse and at her parents for not protecting her or agreeing with her. Her parents were able to express their values. Other community members expressed themselves. Would her husband have been allowed back into the house and the relationship without our support and without the meetings? I suspected so. I suspected that our fostering of dialogue was helpful in achieving the ending that occurred. Carol did get to tell her story, and she said things to her husband she had never been able to say before. She was able to receive support from friends, if not her family. She didn't go back to heavy drinking.

12.4 Alfred and Trina, stuck in a repetitive story

An arrest and blame

Alfred's story was different. Violence occurred in his home as well. Alfred's wife, Trina, tended to hit him. Alfred broke things in response.

Alfred was Cree and Trina was Metis. Alfred worked out of town and came home on weekends. Trina was chronically ill with systemic lupus erythematosus, an autoimmune disease. She had terrible joint involvement and was on high doses of narcotics for her pain. Trina had been arrested for domestic violence several times. Neighbors would call the police and, though Alfred generally covered for her, on several occasions she had freely admitted she had hit him 'because he deserved it.' Once, that admission earned a trip to jail, which she blamed on Alfred. The family came to me because therapy was mandated by the court. Though they were supposed to go to a court-ordered provider, Alfred had manipulated the system to get them to approve me, as he had heard that I was interested in aboriginal healing and mental health.

I didn't know if it would do any good, but I asked them to sign an agreement that I would not be brought into court to testify under any circumstance. This was to avoid their temptation to turn me into a judge and to argue in an adversarial way in front of me about who was right and who was wrong. I did not want to hear evidence. I did want to hear everyone's stories, but in a manner of moving those stories toward a place of mutual understanding in which change could occur. I did not want to be in a position of reporting to a higher authority except to acknowledge that they had appeared for their mandated therapy. I did not want my records to become another piece of evidence. When that is at issue, the sessions become a means to get the records to speak in one or the other party's favor.

Court and the law usually interfere with dialogue. They create too powerful an audience. People fall into the trap of wanting to prove to the judge which story is correct, of wanting the judge to determine which partner is right. This one-up, one-down approach mitigates against the parties having conversations in which new understandings occur. The adversarial approach of our British-based legal system only serves to create adversaries. An aboriginal relational approach to healing begins with the foundation that all stories are equally correct. There are no privileged truths and there is no need to establish which story is true. This is not to say that limits are not drawn. Continued violence is wrong. But violence can stop without declaring a moral winner. The capacity for reconciliation is limited when the focus is on who should be punished.

One of the best, recent films to compare and contrast aboriginal justice with British-based justice recently appeared on Aboriginal People's Television Network, entitled Trial and Fortitude Bay. The movie was about an accidental "rape". A young man thought his former girlfriend wanted to have sex with him. She didn't, but it took more time to convince him than it should have. He got the message when she bit him. Over the six months he waited for trial, the community worked things out. He brought food to the girl's family in restitution. He went back to the traditional ways of hunting in order to do that and accepted mentoring by an elder who was judged the best hunter in the village. He gave up drinking, smoking up, and incessant television. The community forgave him and re-incorporated him. The movie shows the mockery that the British-based legal system made of a healing that had already taken place.

Trina was angry about her arrest. If only Alfred hadn't called the police. Alfred insisted that he hadn't called the police, that it had been a neighbor. Trina insisted that it had to have been Alfred. He responded that he didn't want the police involved in their lives; it was too embarrassing. Then Trina was shouting back at him, why did he call them? They were caught in a vicious cycle, a rut of communication. Trina was sure that Alfred had told the police she had been hitting him. Alfred said that the police told him that Trina had admitted hitting him and 'that was all she wrote,' by which he meant that no further statements from him were necessary: she had incriminated herself. Alfred, however, could not convince Trina to accept this point of view.

Just what was their pattern? I asked. Alfred's version was that Trina boxed him in a room and would go on for hours about whatever was bothering her, whatever real or imagined insults he had done to her. Trina's version was that Alfred was never home and that he didn't love her and wouldn't talk to her. Alfred countered that he came home just about every weekend for a long weekend and that Trina could move to where he worked if she wanted to be with him more. Trina countered that she had offered to move to where he worked and he had refused to allow her. The cycle went on and on.

Clearly Trina was hitting him. She believed she had the right since she was the woman and Alfred deserved to be hit. Her logic was that women had the right to slap around men because women were smaller and could not do any real damage like men could do. Also, she justified slapping and hitting as righteous responses to rage for a woman, as women needed to get men's attention. Besides, she argued, she wasn't hurting him. He could do a lot more damage to her. Alfred insisted he never hit her. Trina countered that he had hit her once when they were scuffling over his computer. Alfred countered that he hadn't meant to hit her; he was just trying to grab it from her because she was threatening to smash it on the ground. 'That computer means more to you than me,' Trina countered.

As best as I could tell, Alfred was not hitting Trina. He did, however, admit to smashing things and throwing cups across the room, even through a window. He insisted that was the only way to get Trina to stop haranguing him. He said she could continue her diatribe against him for hours. Alfred admitted in a private moment with me that spending too much time with Trina made him crazy, no matter how much he loved her.

Violence, fear, and the ineffectiveness of the law

Here was another situation in which the retributive judicial system was clearly making matters worse. Trina was not impressed or subdued by their power. Instead, she used her experiences with the legal system as further fuel against Alfred. Nor could Alfred use the legal system in any effective way. Their older children had made it clear they would retaliate in any number of ways against him if he ever called the police on their mother. Alfred was terrified of the police—not because of them, but because of what other family members might do to him if they believed that he had called the police. He said he would run out of the house to hide if he thought the police were coming. He was terrified that they would take him off to jail as the perpetrator since the men always went to jail, he said. He was worried about losing his job if he had a criminal record. He worked as a commercial truck driver for a company that had a strict policy against hiring anyone with a criminal record. Background checks were frequently updated.

Trina didn't seem to care. She wanted justice. She wanted Alfred to be punished for his wrongdoings, including having an affair when he was living in another city. Alfred admitted the affair but countered that he had thought that he and Trina were breaking up and had even filed divorce papers. Trina countered that she had seduced him back and that he had only filed divorce papers so that he could get laid.

The consequences of failing to listen to another's anger and suffering

Where could we go with all this? The next logical step was to see the children. They came and talked to me but then refused to return because of their embarrassment about talking and their wish for privacy. They thought our meeting was stupid and that the family's business should never be heard outside the family. They would have no further part in such nonsense. The dialogue continued about how Alfred should be punished. Trina claimed that he was mentally ill with a panic disorder. Alfred admitted being afraid of Trina. He talked about being beaten as a child and waiting for his step-father to come whip him at night. He explained that Trina's waking him up in the middle of the night to be angry or to hit him reminded him of those experiences. He said he sometimes had nightmares and woke up in a cold sweat. Trina proudly agreed with this. He has panic disorder, she announced. He needs treatment.

Over eight sessions, we made little progress. The dialogue was stuck. Other family members would not come. While I did get permission to invite some of them (and others were forbidden to come by Trina), none accepted my invitation. I suspected a behind-the-scenes process in which family members were told not to come, either by the children or other adults. Perhaps the issue was shame. Perhaps they were ashamed of a more public discussion about Trina and Alfred, even though the privacy rules would be followed. Additionally, many of the key family members who might have had some leverage were far away in Eastern Canada. This prevented them from coming even if they wished. I had suggested that Trina and Alfred go east for a family mediation, but that also fell upon deaf ears.

Trina continued hitting Alfred. He announced that he was going to learn to stop breaking things and that he was going to take her hits 'like a man.' Alfred had a traditional sense of values that conflicted with his clear desire to get out of the marriage; he was also afraid to leave. Once, while waiting for Trina to return from the wash room, he said to me that he didn't know which would be worse—his life as it was or his life as Trina would make it if they broke up.

Epilogue

I saw Alfred 2 years later. Nothing had changed. He was alternately living out of his truck or at friends' houses or was returning to the family for a few evenings before things exploded and he moved out again. Trina remained addicted to narcotic prescription drugs for her pain and her lupus was getting worse. I couldn't help but wonder if her anger and her need to inflict that anger on Alfred had some relationship to the 'fire in her joints,' which is a metaphorical way of describing lupus arthritis. Perhaps her brain was also inflamed. I worried with Alfred that one day they might kill each other by accident. He worried, too. Trina had recently chased him around the house with a knife in each hand. He had been terrified and had slept outside despite the cold. Everyone was stuck in their story. Trina attributed her lack of friends to her illness. She had no way to meet people. She was isolated inside the house. Her pain kept her prisoner.

Alfred and Trina's story illustrates some further points about relational healing. Unlike our first story, the emphasis on being right did not shift. Family members did not come to provide fresh perspectives and leverage. No real listening occurred. Their relative isolation worked against a truly relational approach. The dysfunction in their relationship could not be healed through a lattice of functional relationships around them. They had no accountability to relational communities. They had no shared traditional stories for how to treat each other. Trina's illness also prevented dialogue—right or not, she could withdraw from discussions when her illness flared or when she was in pain. She also appeared (to me) to be using her pain medications to modulate her feelings, which also restricts dialogue. Drugs and alcohol prevent genuine listening.

I have often thought about what could have been done differently. I think that if Alfred had taken a stand and pursued separation or divorce, that step might have forced a dialogue if separation or divorce was not what either party truly wanted. In this case, involvement of the legal system could have restored a dialogical process, as the couple was unable to move out of the competition for moral superiority and victimhood. A pending divorce action could have potentially 'upped the ante' to force negotiation or, at least, resolution of some type. The avoidance of that community of accountability (family court) served to maintain the dysfunctional interactions. I have also wondered if the outcome would have been different had I been more effective or forceful in enrolling family members or the children to contribute to the discussions. Maybe I should have seen the children first without Trina and Alfred.

Regardless, the keys to successful use of relational healing, which the next story will illustrate, seem to be embeddedness in family relationships that matter (accountability), the existence of important relationships within a community that matters, the openness of involved parties to moving beyond the competition for moral superiority toward a solution focus, the presence of traditional and family stories supportive to dialogue and to listening and conflict resolution, and avoidance of misuse of alcohol and drugs during the conversations.

12.5 Robert's story and aboriginal relational healing

Robert, Betty, and the Elder

Here is a final story to consider. Robert had been an alcoholic. He had beaten his wife, Betty, so severely that she had been hospitalized. He had gone to prison for that act, but he was now released. He had gotten off alcohol while in prison and had not resumed drinking. He wanted to get back together with his wife.

Betty said she loved Robert but didn't want to go to the hospital again. She said she had received enough scars from him. She sent him to see me because she didn't know what else to do. I listened to Robert tell his story and then his version of Betty's story. I sent a letter back to Betty telling her what I had learned about Robert's version of her story about him and his story about her. I suggested we all meet.

Two weeks later they came. Robert was begging to come back to the family. Betty stood her ground.

They were Dene and, as they were inclined to be traditional, I asked them if an Elder could join us for the next appointment. From failures such as my second story, I have learned that Elders command more respect from traditionally oriented people than I could ever deserve. Their support lends needed weight toward relational resolution. In the first story, I involved the priest as the closest acceptable spiritual leader, along with the positing of my priestly friends as 'imaginary' members of the dialogue since, as I claimed, they would have taken an opposite position from the local parish priest. The lack of support of that 'elder' may have contributed to our inability to move toward reconciliation and healing, and led to the outcome of divorce. Paradoxically, the priest may have precipitated what he hoped to avoid by his own biases. A more neutral, 'not knowing' approach on his part could have fostered reconciliation. (I elaborate on the concept of 'not knowing' in Section 12.6, 'Listening attitudes'.) No mutually agreeable Elders could be identified for the second couple. This third couple were surprised at my request to include an Elder, but quickly agreed. It matched their cultural views.

For this situation, I knew just the Elder to suggest. He met with us 2 weeks later. He was also employed by the Drug and Alcohol Treatment Program, so he had expertise that I thought might be helpful in assisting Robert in continuing his abstinence from alcohol. I will never forget what transpired next. The Elder requested an evening meeting with both of their families. At this meeting, he proposed a preparatory sweat lodge ceremony. I asked to join them and, to my gratitude, was permitted. Two weeks later, on a Sunday afternoon, we had the sweat. Both Robert and Betty attended, along with several of their relatives. After the sweat, we ate food in the kitchen and eventually the time for the meeting came. It lasted all evening. The Elder told stories about the role of men and women in traditional society. He told how the first man and the first woman were created. He told stories that explained how the men recognized that they couldn't get by without the women and vice versa. This story-telling lasted long into the night. Then he proposed another meeting.

De-colonization and the law

I couldn't make all their meetings, but I attended enough to watch a fascinating process unfold of what I would call de-colonization. The Elder was gradually removing the veneers of hardness and toughness that had been required for Robert's survival in and before Prison. He was gradually introducing an entirely different view of what it meant to be a man. He was imparting what could be called local knowledge about male and female relationships. He was imparting his understanding of the traditions about how men and women treat each other and about the process of intimate relating. He did this in a way that engaged Robert to believe in the stories out of cultural pride. Through the telling of traditional stories, the Elder was able to persuade the man that being aboriginal required behavior consistent with the traditions. We do not hurt the women, he said. Warriors do not hurt the women or the children. It is not right.

Later, like Elders from other cultures have explained to me, this Elder said to me that the white culture was wrong. 'You do not stop a man from being violent by tearing him down, humiliating him, punishing him, and putting him in jail,' he said. 'This makes him more violent. The values he learns to survive in jail are the opposite of the traditional values. In jail they teach them how to solve problems with violence and by being tough. They beat all the feelings out of them. I know this from looking in the eyes of the young men as they return from jail. Often there is no one there. Their spirit has left them. You stop violence,' he continued, 'by building people up. You stop violence by respecting people and by teaching them the traditional values. We were not a violent people,' he said. 'We did not abuse our wives and children. At least, not before the fur traders came. We hunted. Sometimes we fought, but as warriors. I am building him up,' he said. 'I am returning him to the old ways. I am giving him a sense of personal power. I am reconnecting him to his people—to the ancestors and the spirits, to Creator. This is how you stop violence.'

'Once he is a traditional man again, then his wife can love him. She cannot love a jailbird or an alcoholic. Those are not our ways.'

Reconciliation and healing

The man did change. He stayed with the Elder. He went to the ceremonies. His wife softened her heart and invited him back into the family. He came as a traditional man, just as the Elder had said, and not as a jailbird or a drunk. This interaction inspired me. It led me to always consult the Elders as soon as possible in these situations. I recognized that they had tools for reconciliation. It was what might be called unconscious local knowledge. Many could not articulate their approach; they could only perform it in collaboration with others.

Why was this story so much more successful than my previous efforts alone? All the parties were embedded in a community in which the Elder commanded respect. His words were considered teachings to be followed and not questioned. Traditional stories exist that explain acceptable social and moral behavior within the culture for how men treat women and children and the duties of women and children toward men. A cultural basis exists for reciprocal relationships of accountability to each other. The Elder possessed unconscious local knowledge regarding how to facilitate Robert's taking a different position toward violence and women without losing face. Regardless of how well he could articulate this knowledge, the Elder was able to increase self-esteem instead of decrease it as courts and prisons do.

12.6 Drawing implications from the stories of others

The truth and nothing but the truth?

What did these stories tell me? First, I have come to believe that a commitment to 'truth-telling' doesn't itself bring about reconciliation and healing, as Alison Mitchell's analysis shows (Mitchell, Chapter 5, this volume). Everyone has a story—even violent people. They have a story that explains their behavior. Theory does not explain their behavior. Concepts do not explain their behavior. Psychodynamic constructs do not explain their behavior. As Gergen and Kaye (1992) argue, the theories we use to support our actions (psychoanalytic theory, Biblical theory, Hegelian ethics, feminism, etc.), whether these theories give rise to punishment and retribution or forgiveness and reconciliation, are merely ideas with historically created reality, 'furnishing no more accurate picture of reality than fiction' (p. 173). People's behavior makes sense within the context of their life story, the one they are living that lives through them. Change the story and you change the man, as one Elder told me. The facts are less important. What happened, happened, as one Elder shrugged; now we must go on.

As Mitchell notes, the intuitive realist position of looking for truths that correspond to historic matters of fact (which is what plagued the couple in my second story) rarely works. Practically speaking, this is a poor approach. Nothing changes, as we saw in the second story. Facts matter less than stories. Change the story, the future changes. Obsessively collect facts, and the past becomes the future. What we expect determines our future, not what happened in the past. If we expect the past to continue because of its facticity, it will. If we expect transformation, it can happen. Fact-finding is less important than genuine dialogue. Social networks of accountability are necessary to foster genuine dialogue. European and American culture presents values of talking in order to get a point across. Aboriginal cultures present values of talking in order to listen. Men must be accountable to women, and vice versa. Power disparities interfere with real conversations. These disparities exist for women, ethnic minorities, immigrants, prisoners, and other marginalized members of society. Our role as professionals is to find ways to correct power imbalances. Reconciliation is only effective in an atmosphere of social justice, in which involved parties have equal power. Power imbalances end conversations and lead to monologues, lectures, and diatribes, not dialogue.

Listening attitudes

The best attitude to adopt when telling stories about trauma is what Anderson (1997) calls a 'not knowing' curiosity. In another article, Anderson and Swim (1994) wrote: 'By not-knowing we mean a general attitude or stance that does not have access to privileged information, can never fully understand another person, and always needs to learn more about what has been said or not said… The best language for moving toward understanding those with whom we work is the storyteller's own language.' (p. 27).

Through language and collaborative partnerships, healing can occur. All shareholders in the trauma co-produce the eventual result. An attitude of not-knowing, along with what Anderson calls a *not yet said* stance, is best for healing trauma within relationships in that these attitudes allow all involved shareholders in a trauma to become conversational partners in resolving a painful situation. Through the ensuing dialogue, through hearing all the stories, new meaning co-evolves that is representative of the existent relationships and the inseparable generation of new understandings.

Shotter describes this process:

> [C]hanges in ways of talking can bring to prominence previously unnoticed features of our relations to each other and to our surrounding circumstances, and in this way, lead to the institution of new 'forms of life' (to use Wittgenstein's term), new ways in which people routinely related themselves to one another and thus treat each other as being . . . In other words it is in the momentary relational encounters occurring between people in their dialogic exchanges that everything of importance to us in our studies should be seen as happening. And what occurs there should be seen not in terms or pictures or representations of what 'that something' truly is, but in terms of the different possible relations it might have, the different roles it might play, in people living out the rest of their lives—a relational rather than a representational understanding.

> Shotter (1997, pp. 1–2)

Reconciliation arises from the reconstruction or transformation of relationships through discourse. Ceremony and ritual provide an enriched form of discourse that nevertheless is mediated through language—of the word and of the body, of song and of dance. This opens up and extends the relationality among us. As Shotter (1997) says, 'In short, the 'things' supposedly in our 'inner' lives are not to be found within us as individuals, but 'in' the momentary relational spaces occurring between ourselves and an other or otherness in our surroundings' (p. 3).

What I am suggesting is that we have to learn to trust the dialogue more than we do at present. Perhaps like John Bunyan described in the allegorical *Pilgrim's Progress* (1964), we must rely more on faith in action, on our belief in the capacity of the human spirit to overcome trauma and pain and to create something beautiful in its place. After all, we have so many examples around us. Many great works of art were produced in the midst of incredible human suffering. Perhaps our job is to recognize that when all voices are heard equally, movement occurs toward satisfactory resolution without our having overly to guide it. We can learn to trust the dialogical process. Our work, then, is to render all voices intelligible to all listeners. For this process to unfold, translational skills may be required. Men may need to talk in ways that women can understand. Women may need to talk in ways that men can understand. The languages of immigrants may need to be translated into the dominant cultural language and vice versa. Ethnic minorities may need help in understanding members of the dominant culture. This translation is the role of the facilitator of the dialogue.

Perhaps our language can evolve beyond the concepts of perpetrator and victim toward a relational understanding of differential ways of responding to adversity. Perhaps we will use that understanding to forgive some wrongdoings, but not others. Some actions are so egregious that we cannot fail to separate the person from the remainder of humanity. But most wrongdoings fall within gray areas and are not clear-cut, more demanding of compassion than punishment.

Reconciliation depends upon the creation of common ground between people. Common ground is created through dialogue that requires a context of tradition. Common ground is easier to create between people from the same culture who can hear the same traditional stories (my Story 3). It is harder to create common ground between people from different cultures who have different traditional stories (my Story 2). In Story 3, the Elder forged an 'emotional truth that resonated between the parties.' He created a common ground of tradition and story. Within that context, reconciliation could happen because it was implicit in the stories he was telling. The local knowledge for how to reconcile was contained in his stories. My Stories 1 and 2 did not have a common ground of local knowledge for how to reconcile, so it did not happen. In Story 1, tension and conflict existed in the local interpretation of the Roman Catholic faith from the parish priest to family members and other friends. A shared story was not apparent. Nor did Alfred and Trina from Story 2 have a common ground. They came from different cultures and were not embedded in one or the other culture (or even a third, alternative culture) because of their isolation, so a common story could not arise.

Reconciliation arises from this common ground of story-telling, not from moral explanations or psychological defense mechanisms (which are not really defense mechanisms at all, but habits of memory). Defense mechanisms cannot be found in the brain. Rather, we have an amygdala, which mediates fight, flight, freezing, eating, and mating. When faced with a fearful situation, the amygdala signals the hippocampus to scan through memory and find something similar with which to compare this new, potential threat. The hippocampus does the best it can. Unfortunately, if the only memory is of trauma, hurt, and betrayal, these are the stories the hippocampus will send back to the amygdala. Only through learning and incorporating new stories and experiences (involving the frontal cortex) can new memory (which can be metaphor and doesn't have to have actually happened) be delivered to the amygdala to change our response tendencies. Reconciliation requires less of a threat response and more curiosity. In other words, we need to feel safe to reconcile. And traditional stories and teachings bring about that safety.

Law and order isn't all it's cracked up to be

My stories have taught me to disagree with Colleen Murphy (Chapter 4, this volume) about the importance of the rule of law. What we need more than law is relationship. Laws become unnecessary when we are accountable to each other in relationship (see Trial at Fortitude Bay). Law cannot compel behavior except through fear. Fear breeds the neurochemical context that is associated with fight, flight, freezing, not loving, and not eating. So instead of law, perhaps we need communion over food. We need to feast together and participate in ceremony and ritual. These actions change our neurophysiology toward desired goals of respect and appreciation.

A final criticism of European-American reliance on law comes from Foucault (1980). My interpretation of Foucault is that he makes the radical claim that even justice is nothing more than a tool manufactured to assist individuals/groups seeking differing, and often antagonistic, ends across time. Political and economic struggles, he asserted, should not invoke justice as legitimation. Instead, he says, we must understand its, and our, context and become aware of our underlying desire to alter political, and therefore power, structures. Hence, reconciliation requires equalization of power imbalances or it will not work.

Engagement, community, and political action

Carlos Maldonaldo (2005) has argued, and I agree, that healing occurs through political action (to change the conditions that bring about trauma and oppression, not necessarily to create more trauma and oppression through taking revenge upon the oppressors) and through telling one's story and feeling heard—through the engagement in a fellowship of community.

Deborah Spitz (Chapter 6, this volume) also points to this idea—that healing requires more than a therapist. It requires a community of others who can hear and be heard from. The repetitive retelling of tales of trauma to the same individual goes nowhere. Telling the story once and for all, in a context of communion and fellowship, while being engaged in a socio-political process to change the future for others so that the trauma can never happen again— this is healing. Judith Herman (1992) tells a beautiful story of how healing through political action happened to Freud's patient, Anna O., whose real name was Bernice Pappenheimer. Contrary to Freud's theory, Bernice really was sexually abused by her father and his friends. It wasn't fantasy. When Freud threw her out of treatment for being resistant and recalcitrant (i.e., not agreeing with him), she went briefly psychotic, was admitted to hospital, pulled herself together, and proceeded to go on a lifelong mission to create safe houses all over German-speaking Europe for young women who were being abused within their families, taking every opportunity to spread the news of sexual abuse, which is now well-known. The famous theologian and philosopher, Paul Tillich, delivered the eulogy at her funeral. Her story provides another example of relational healing. She did not heal her relationship with her father or with Freud, but she did heal, through being heard and through becoming politically engaged.

12.7 Engagement through story-telling leaves open the possibility of reconciliation

Reconciliation is not an external process that can be forced upon people who are not in community with each other. They must first be engaged. Then they can reconcile. A good story produces that engagement. It absorbs people's interest in listening. That's why we have to start with story. Reconciliation or restorative justice between individuals and in communities arises through dialogue and must remain consistent with local knowledge and practices. The error is to think that reconciliation comes from outside and that it must be forced upon people or that people must be taught how to reconcile. The same is true about forgiveness. Forgiveness must be produced. It cannot be applied like a principle. It either emerges or it does not. Kindness and love are similar. They cannot be insisted upon, demanded, or commanded.

Genuine relational healing practiced within a context of social justice will put Sharon Lamb's concerns to rest (cf. Chapter 10, this volume). A participatory, community model of reconciliation and restorative justice produces outcomes that arise as the emergent properties of dialogue. They cannot be forced on to people by authorities or experts. Outcomes, whatever the resolution, emerge from communicate actions that exist and are legitimate only in the domains of the perceivers' realities (Andersen, 1991). Legitimate outcomes are always consensual—all the shareholders agree. Enforced outcomes result from the application of a dominant paradigm upon minority shareholders. This is Lamb's concern—that women should not be coerced into kindness and forgiveness. In Chapter 9 of this volume, Pier Verhagen discusses the importance of forgiveness, so I will not elaborate on this subject, except to say that community must pre-exist acts of forgiving.

People need to be brought into dialogue, which may lead to punishment or to reconciliation. What I am suggesting is that we focus more on dialogue and resolution within the context of empowerment of local communities (subject to accountability requirements to other communities). The larger, dominant culture must relax what Hilde Lindemann Nelson (2001) calls its master narrative of retribution, punishment, evil people, criminals, and law. Local communities can be assisted to find their own way through the resolution process with more flexibility than current national policies allow. Punishment is not always the best approach. Only on the local level, and only through the relational action of talking and listening, can people decide what is appropriate. Lamb (Chapter 10, this volume) argues that many women in therapy are being coerced into forgiveness and kindness as if the truth does not matter. Similarly, when considering domestic violence, few want to hear the stories of the mostly men who commit these violent acts. It has become politically incorrect to see violence as a behavior maintained by social conditions and relationships within families and communities. We have attempted to pathologize violence instead of seeing it as a form of communication. Violence can communicate powerlessness, rage, frustration, and more. Its meaning varies with each communication. Yet, it has something to convey in the situations in which it is encountered.

Resolution requires listening and talking. We must listen to the stories of the violent as well as the stories of the abused. We need not pre-judge or demand a particular response to the violent or the abused but, instead, let that response arise from dialogue, supporting each shareholder in the discussion to contribute his or her own local knowledge about the foreground situation (the violent act) and the background situation (the context in which violence occurs).

The thoughts of all interested parties about what should happen to resolve a situation must be respected and valued, given precedence over theoretical principles that potentially are others' constructions, especially those of mainstream or dominant cultures (McNamee and Gergen, 1999). The voices of the stakeholders in the situation become the driving force of intent and direction.

Through the co-evolved process of talking about what happened for all participants (including the affected audience), new options and possibilities emerge (Swim *et al.*, 1998). Reconciliation may or may not emerge as a co-exploration, a co-participatory effort of social relations, from moment to moment, thought to thought, word to word.

Others will address the expansion of relational healing approaches into international relations. That is beyond the score of my work and experience. Nevertheless, I believe that dialogue and story-telling could prevent some kinds of international relationships from escalating into major disasters. For example, at a recent conference, a member of the audience questioned the wisdom of allowing Saddam Hussein's voice to be heard. I responded that the best outcome I could imagine for him was not sitting in a prison cell, but traveling across America, talking at every high school about the way in which he was financed by the US—in essence, created—to oppose Iran, and the ways that his story unfolded from that beginning to become what it was at the time of the US invasion. We need to understand the process by which Saddam Hussein was created and then destroyed, I said. We need to recognize that all of us are related to him, regardless of our country of origin. As real a man as he is, he is also symbol. He is us and we are him. He did what we imagined. He carried out American foreign policies, perhaps too well, and for this, he was eventually declared a criminal. Let him precipitate an international dialogue about how to prevent this from ever happening again. Let us dialogue about our responsibility to stop creating minor despots to oppose our current enemies, who change soon enough anyway.

12.8 Conclusions

My approach to families and communities in which relational violence has occurred requires an attitude of uncertainty about what should happen coupled with a curiosity about what involved parties believe should happen. I try to avoid bias accruing from training or my own beliefs (the stories that I live and that live through me). I attempt to facilitate a genuine interchange to learn from everyone how their participation in the traumatic event came about and what each person proposes to do to contribute to positive movement toward a better future. I ask each person to consider how they can reduce the burden of suffering for the others. Additionally, I try to move the conversation when appropriate to addressing the underlying sociopolitical disparities that prohibit effective solutions, encouraging people toward political activism to correct these disparities, knowing that even the action toward social justice can be healing, whether or not the larger culture responds. With the absence of socially constructed privileged information (from theory or from personal experience), I present myself as curious about each person's perspective. I want to understand their stories about how they became involved and remain involved and I want to respect their stories in their own right. In doing so, I become an advocate for everyone's concerns. Each person's painful life experiences must be heard and respected from all sides of a violent event. A conversational space is created for participants to have dialogical exchanges that have never before occurred, thereby catalyzing the emergence of new stories for healing of each person and for the community. Narratives of pain and trauma must be given credibility for all parties in order for change to occur within the dialogical space (Andrews and Clark, 1998).

Before the healing Elder engaged Robert and his family, Robert was seen as sick and imbalanced, a criminal, a drunk. A satisfactory reconciliation process enabled everyone to emerge as human and not intrinsically defective. All became equal relational participants in finding meaning and a shared future. When social labeling is eliminated, relational partners can search for meaning devoid of counterfeit constructions that lead dialogue into conventional interpretations and results (Swim et al., 2001). The search can be egalitarian where everyone can trust and believe in each other and simply talk about what is troubling or what change is desired.

Finally, a few comments on the importance of local community decision-making are in order. Outside the scope of my chapter are the limits that a nation-state or a province should place on local decision making. Communities may arrive at solutions that are outside the domain of what the remainder of the province or nation can tolerate. As a province, we would not, for example, tolerate the execution of the entire family of a murderer, though one could imagine that a local community might wish to exact this type of vengeance. The question becomes one of power balance between communities and federal agencies with a need for accountability. Communities must be accountable to each other in the same way that individuals are within communities.

Yet we are interested in empowering local communities to solve their own problems, including the problems of relational violence and using existent local knowledge and practices. We wish to deconstruct the idea that we know the proper response to trauma or that there is a proper response, for all of our responses are social constructions arising from our shared dialogue. We may conclude that punishment and imprisonment is inefficient, even unaesthetic. We may conclude that it does not reach our goals and that other means are needed. Or we may not. But dialogue is necessary for solutions to emerge. Mandatory sentences must be eliminated. Aboriginal communities must find their power to demand creative flexibility for healing social trauma.

References

Andersen T (1991). *The Reflecting Team: Dialogues and Dialogues About the Dialogues.* New York: WW Norton & Company.

Anderson H (1997). *Conversation, Language, and Possibilities: A Postmodern Approach to Therapy.* New York: Basic Books.

Anderson H and Swim S (1994). Supervision as collaborative conversations: connecting the voices of supervisor and supervisee. *Journal of Systemic Therapies,* **14**: 1–13.

Andrews J and Clark D (1998). Postmodern ideas and relational conversations in clinical practice. *The Family Journal: Counseling and Therapy for Couples and Families,* **6**(4): 316–22.

Bunyan J. (1964). *Pilgrim's Progress.* New York: New American Library.

Foucault M (1980). *Power/Knowledge. Selected Interviews and Other Writings, 1972–1977.* Toronto: Random House of Canada.

Gergen K and Kaye J (1992). Beyond narrative in the negotiation of therapeutic meaning. In: *Therapy as Social Construction* (eds S McNamee S and K Gergen). London: Sage Publications, pp. 162–85.

Herman J. (1992). *Trauma and Recovery.* New York: Basic Books.

Maldonaldo C (2005) The narrative practice of community psychiatry. *Journal of Narrative Therapy and Community Work,* **6**: 21–6.

McNamee S and Gergen K (1999). *Relational Responsibility.* London: Sage Publications.

Nelson HL (2001). *Damaged Identities, Narrative Repair.* Ithaca, NY: Cornell University Press.

Shotter J (1997). The social construction of our 'inner' lives. *Journal of Constructionist Psychology,* **10**: 7–24.

Swim S, Helms S, Plotkin S, and Bettye S (1998). Multiple voices: stories of rebirth, heroines, new opportunities, and identities. *Journal of Systemic Therapies,* **17**(4): 61–71.

Swim S, St George S, and Wulfe D (2001). Process ethics: a collaborative partnership. *The Journal of Systemic Therapies,* **20**(4): 14–24.

Index